www.brookscole.com

www.brookscole.com is the World Wide Web site for Brooks/Cole and is your direct source to dozens of online resources.

At *www.brookscole.com* you can find out about supplements, demonstration software, and student resources. You can also send email to many of our authors and preview new publications and exciting new technologies.

www.brookscole.com
Changing the way the world learns®

Counseling Diverse Clients

Bringing Context Into Therapy

Jeanne M. Slattery
Clarion University of Pennsylvania

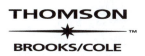

THOMSON

BROOKS/COLE

Australia • Canada • Mexico • Singapore • Spain
United Kingdom • United States

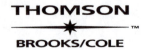

Executive Editor: Lisa Gebo
Acquisitions Editor: Marquita Flemming
Assistant Editor: Shelley Gesicki
Editorial Assistant: Amy Lam
Technology Project Manager: Barry Connolly
Marketing Manager: Caroline Concilla
Marketing Assistant: Mary Ho
Advertising Project Manager: Tami Strang
Project Manager, Editorial Production: Catherine Morris
Print/Media Buyer: Kristine Waller

Permissions Editor: Sarah Harkrader
Production Service: G&S Typesetters, Inc.
Art Editor: G&S Typesetters, Inc.
Copy Editor: Steven Baker
Illustrator: G&S Typesetters, Inc.
Cover Designer: Denise Davidson
Cover Image: The Studio Dog/Getty Images
Compositor: G&S Typesetters, Inc.
Text and Cover Printer: Webcom

Printed in Canada
1 2 3 4 5 6 7 07 06 05 04 03

For more information about our products, contact us at:
Thomson Learning Academic Resource Center
1-800-423-0563
For permission to use material from this text, contact us by:
Phone: 1-800-730-2214
Fax: 1-800-730-2215
Web: http://www.thomsonrights.com

Library of Congress Control Number: 2003107084

ISBN 0-534-56390-2

Brooks/Cole-Thomson Learning
10 Davis Drive
Belmont, CA 94002
USA

Asia
Thomson Learning
5 Shenton Way #01-01
UIC Building
Singapore 068808

Australia/New Zealand
Thomson Learning
102 Dodds Street
Southbank, Victoria 3006
Australia

Canada
Nelson
1120 Birchmount Road
Toronto, Ontario M1K 5G4
Canada

Europe/Middle East/Africa
Thomson Learning
High Holborn House
50/51 Bedford Row
London WC1R 4LR
United Kingdom

Latin America
Thomson Learning
Seneca, 53
Colonia Polanco
11560 Mexico D.F.
Mexico

Spain/Portugal
Paraninfo
Calle/Magallanes, 25
28015 Madrid, Spain

To my clients and students, my most important teachers.
To my friends and family, without whom I could not risk learning.

Contents in Brief

Contents

Chapter 3

Defining Culture and Context 32

Chapter 4

Oppression and Prejudice 60

Chapter 5

Values and Worldviews 84

Chapter 6

When Worldviews Clash   *110*

Chapter 7

Problems Resulting From Group Membership   *135*

Chapter 10

Egalitarian and Empowering Relationships *212*

Chapter 11

Making Meaning *235*

Chapter 12

Blame, Responsibility, and Control   261

Chapter 13

Finding Natural Supports: Outside and In   289

Chapter 14

Bringing It Into the Community: Group Identity and Group Transformation   313

Chapter 15

Rediscovering a Sense of Balance   338

Chapter 16

Highlighting Themes   360

List of Tables

List of Figures

Preface

Every book, like every person, has a context in which it developed and a worldview that characterizes it. Three points especially characterize this book:

Multiculturalism Is Relevant to Everyone. Most multicultural therapy books are written about culturally different clients and for culturally different therapists and students. While reminding us that not all clients are YAVIS; that is, Young, Attractive, Verbal, Intelligent and Successful, such books have left many wondering what a multicultural therapy book has to do with them, especially if they are not culturally different themselves.

This reaction is understandable. However, most Euro-American therapists *will* work with culturally different clients at some point in their careers. Although the number of Euro-Americans increased by 11.3% in the United States between 1980 and 1996, the number of African Americans increased by 26.4%, and the Latin American population almost doubled to 93.5% (J. W. Wright, 1998). Euro-Americans already are in the minority in California, Hawaii, and New Mexico—relative to other groups—which is a trend expected to extend into more states by 2025 (Campbell, 1996). Despite this, the majority of therapists who work with culturally different clients continue to be Euro-Americans. Therefore, learning about the roles of race and ethnicity is as important for Euro-Americans as it is for people of other racial backgrounds.

However, we must move beyond race and look at additional influences on our clients; these include culture, geography, gender, affectional orientation, class, family, religion, health, age, and ability. In 2001 approximately 24.5% of the population in the United States identified itself as Catholic, with 16.3% being Baptist, 1.3% Jewish, and .5% Muslim (Mayer, Kosmin, & Keysar, 2001). These percentages are likely to shift in the next few decades. The percentage of Jews in the United States has dropped in recent years, while people self-identifying as Buddhist or Muslim doubled between 1990 and 2001. In 1996, 3.5% of men and 2.1% of sexually active people in the United States reported having sex with someone of the same sex in the last twelve months (National Opinion Research Center, 1996, as cited in J. W. Wright, 1998), and nearly 18.7% of working-age people in the United States have a physical, psychological, or intellectual disability (Stoddard, Jans, Ripple, & Kraus, 1998). The percentage of the elderly population is expected to continue to increase over the next 25 years (Campbell, 1996). Our awareness of the influence of these multiple groups on our clients' values, goals, preferred communication style, and preferences for therapy can strengthen our assessments and our ability to work with our clients. Just as not all clients are White, not all people in any single group are the same.

Learning about the many contextual factors that make people who they are is not something that can be done overnight. It is part of a journey that can take a lifetime. As Kingsolver (2002) describes, this journey can sometimes be awkward, with frequent missteps taken even by the well-informed. Nonetheless, the journey is worth every step. Not only is it often enjoyable, it is necessary for learning to listen to people who are different. By necessity, this includes everyone.

Respect People and Their Differences.   I began writing *Counseling Diverse Clients* after years of hearing therapists talk about their clients in less respectful ways than they did about themselves when they were in the same situations. Even though they cut themselves slack when *they* had problems, they imposed high standards on the people around them, especially their clients. Furthermore, when they were "nice" to the people around them, they often engaged in caretaking behavior. In one conversation, an acquaintance of mine self-disclosed the personal biases and prejudices that were part of his decision to open the door for a veteran in a wheelchair. While he initially thought he was being "kind," he later realized that he had assumed that the man needed to be helped—despite the fact that the man was clearly capable of doing most things on his own, including traversing stairs.

I was concerned that many therapists didn't believe that their clients could make decisions for themselves or didn't have the resources to be successful and to function well. Therapists' expectations can become self-fulfilling prophecies when they expect less of their clients. People will behave down—or up—to expectations. This seems especially true when race, class, significant mental illness, or worldview come between therapist and client. When we believe in our clients, clients will believe in themselves and will believe they can do almost anything.

This book was as much influenced by my discussions with these therapists—people who were often well-intentioned and otherwise competent—as by my conversations with people whose beliefs were more similar to my own. I thank both groups for listening to me and for helping me clarify my thinking.

Listen for Worldview.   A major theme in this book is that therapists can and must listen in order to understand their clients' worldviews. Throughout the book I present broad differences among groups, while also emphasizing the often-large differences within the groups. Recognizing group differences provides a base from which we can work. Discovering ways to listen to our clients' individuality further develops our skills.

WHAT MAKES THIS BOOK UNIQUE?

Generally speaking, we are respectful of those we understand and like. Although most of us start out this way, by the time we have been in the field for several years, a lot of us seem less respectful. Why? Perhaps it's only that we do not understand our clients. This book, in exploring context, is intended to help new therapists—and their older brothers and sisters—become more understanding and empathic.

Understanding context can be difficult initially because it often requires us to look in different places than our clients may be used to looking. I outline and use several sets of guidelines throughout the book to help therapists see their clients' context, which can be too easily ignored sometimes. Although these sets are first described in chapter 2, they are further developed and used in different ways throughout subsequent chapters.

I believe that people learn more when ideas are presented in the form of stories. Consequently, I have included a number of stories and case examples. I have also been very much influenced by the patient protest literature, often written in the form of autobiographies. Many quotes from this literature inform this book and my ideas. I believe we can learn from our mistakes.

Helms and Richardson (1997) note that learning about context is often best done from within one's own cultural contexts. With this in mind, I have included a number of brief exercises throughout the book to help readers apply these ideas as readily as possible. Rather than skipping over these exercises, readers are encouraged to stop and think about the ways in which these ideas apply in their life or in those of the people around them. This balance of examples and theory can help readers learn and apply this material as rapidly as possible.

ACKNOWLEDGMENTS

Throughout *Counseling Diverse Clients* I have included a number of short and long case studies. Because of issues of privacy and confidentiality, most of the identifying characteristics of those who serve to inspire these descriptions have been changed so that the people involved might not even recognize themselves. Some cases are based on two or three different people with whom I have worked, and I draw on my understanding of their friends and family. A few are based on aspects of me. Sometimes, however, cases take on a life of their own. While descriptors have been changed, the underlying dynamics are true as I saw them. I want to thank the people who worked with me and inspired these descriptions. Learning occurs on both sides of the couch.

I also want to thank the people who talked with me about the ideas that are included in these chapters, as well as those who read and commented on earlier drafts, helped me with the research, and encouraged me or supported me during the book's gestation. Debi Jones Bean, Terry Bean, Crystal Park, and Randy Potter spent many hours talking with me about these ideas and challenging my thinking. My Wednesday lunch group—Carol Bolland, Kathy Fleissner, Kay King, and Jean Rumsey—was supportive throughout and challenged my thinking when it became sloppy. Sandy Ferringer, Pam Gust, Melanie Herzog, Crystal Park, Bea Slattery, John Slattery, and Linda Wilbur read drafts, talked with me about the ideas and gave me useful feedback about how to develop them. Sometimes my friends, colleagues, and family shared stories that helped clarify my thinking. Some of those stories are here, although the storytellers would likely be surprised by the changed context. Lisa Bria, Sandy Ferringer, Amber Kromer, Tracy Motter, Janina Jolley, and Whitney Smith looked for books, articles, and sources of obscure stories and quotes. Ten anonymous reviewers significantly influenced my thinking and helped me think about how to present my ideas, and I am very appreciative of their thoughtful comments. Finally, Julie Martinez and Sue Ewing were very supportive editors from the beginning and were very patient with my frequent questions. Michael Bass ushered the book through the production process, and Travis Tyre made numerous suggestions to make this book read more clearly and gracefully. I hope I am always lucky enough to work with people like them. While family, friends, colleagues, and reviewers caught a number of errors, any remaining problems are my responsibility alone.

I am also appreciative of my home, Clarion University, which gave me a sabbatical to work on the ideas in this book. My department and university supported me throughout this process, even when it occasionally inconvenienced the people around me. My family's support was also important. Although my children sometimes complained that I was working too hard, they were interested and encouraging (things that are just as important to a parent as to a child).

Finally, there were always people in the background who babysat or cleaned and gave me the hours and freedom to write. Thank you.

THE IMPACT OF CONTEXT

Last week Luisa fell asleep in the middle of her geography class. Mrs. Sanchez, her fifth-grade teacher, complained to Luisa's guidance counselor about Luisa's laziness and lack of motivation, "It's a shame, since she's so bright."

Luckily, Luisa's guidance counselor Julia talked to Luisa about what was happening. Luisa was very anxious, and she worried aloud about her brothers who were becoming involved with a local gang. Her mother had been beaten the night before and had whimpered in the next room throughout the night. Luisa's family had not had diapers for her younger sister (who had a bad case of diaper rash), and Luisa was trying to be mother to her siblings and her parents, without having all the skills. She was doing what she could, but she would often worry and have difficulty sleeping and concentrating on her schoolwork.

Quickly, Julia recognized that there was a problem, but it was not the problem Luisa's teacher identified. Instead of internal problems—being lazy and unmotivated—Julia saw that Luisa was worried about a series of events in her life that were largely outside her control. Shifting her teacher's view of the problem also shifted the way that everyone responded to her.

Generally, people recognize the external, unstable factors that contribute to their own behavior and attribute their problems to them (J. Greenberg, Pyszczynski, & Solomon, 1982; Jones, 1979; Zuckerman, 1979). Doing this allows them to save face and to see problems as out of the norm and changeable. Conversely, people tend to attribute their successes to internal and stable factors such as personality traits, abilities, and hard work and view their successes as a natural part of themselves.

Members of individualistic cultures like the United States tend to attribute problems in other people to laziness, incompetence, narcissism, poor insight, or other internal characteristics (Gilbert & Malone, 1995; Jones, 1979; Kenrick, Neuberg, & Caldini, 1999). Luisa's teacher ignored the contextual factors—her family problems—that might actually be affecting her performance and instead focused on the internal stable factors—laziness and poor motivation. Most people overestimate the effect of external factors on their own failures, while underestimating the impact of situations on others.

Spend a moment thinking about your own relationships with people you do and don't like. How does this match the predictions of attribution theory? When do you tend to be generous in your reactions toward others? When do you tend to be stingy?

These are generalizations with some important exceptions. First, the fundamental attribution error, as this phenomenon is called, is more common in individualistic cultures that extol individual responsibility and autonomy. Conversely, members of collectivist cultures like India and China tend to use situational explanations when describing strangers' behavior (Morris & Peng, 1994). Western cultures tend to ignore a person's context, while collectivist cultures tend to pay special attention to relationships *and* context. Euro-Americans tend to choose from polar opposites when identifying blame ("It's my fault" or "It's your fault"), while people from China and India are more likely to recognize that the fault may be both theirs and others' (Peng & Nisbett, 1999).

Second, although people tend to underestimate the impact of external factors, especially with people they don't like, they recognize these factors more easily in their friends (J. D. Brown, 1986; Martz et al., 1998; Sedikedes & Campbell, 1998). The fact that Julia liked Luisa made it easier for her to reframe the problem.

Third, people who are depressed tend to accept their failures as their "real self" and view their successes as aberrations (Abramson, Metalsky & Alloy, 1989). For example, a depressed student earning an A on an exam might say, "It was just an easy exam," or "She's an easy professor," or "I just happened to study the right stuff." Conversely, that same student may obsess about a C earned on a quiz and see it as an uncommonly clear reflection of her abilities and as a definitive indication that she will never make it into graduate school or be successful in her life and career.

Mrs. Sanchez was blinded by a semester of poor test performances, tardiness, and school absences. She didn't know that Luisa had performed well up until the third grade when her parents' marriage became increasingly violent. As a result, Mrs. Sanchez responded especially poorly to Luisa's problems in school and ignored both the explanations and the excuses. Luisa herself may accept Mrs. Sanchez's viewpoint, forgetting that things are different when she is not depressed.

LOOKING AT THE SOCIAL PSYCHOLOGY OF THERAPY

Although this book does not primarily grow out of a social psychological framework, social psychology is an important influence on it. In the United States, psychology has incorporated societal values of autonomy and self-reliance, and it tends to look at the individual at the expense of culture and context (Morris & Peng, 1994). These individualistic assumptions are consistent with and may even exacerbate the fundamental attribution error. This avoidance of context is especially notable when we as therapists work with culturally different peoples whose values and situational constraints are different from our own. Because we are less likely to be intimately aware of situational pressures on our clients' behavior, we are more likely to attribute their actions to dispositional or intrapsychic factors, and perhaps even unintentionally blame them for behavior that is beyond their control (Jones, 1979; Morris & Peng, 1994).

Unfortunately, Euro-Americans tend to be less willing to like, to listen to, and to give the benefit of the doubt to people whom they view as "different" (Morris & Peng, 1994; M. E. Rosenbaum, 1986). We may assume, for example, that Luisa's school absences are related to her lack of interest in schoolwork, until we take the time to listen to her story. Then, when we hear her fears about leaving her mother home alone in a dangerous neighborhood with a violent husband, we begin to see the ways that Luisa has been "parentified." In order to work successfully in the therapy process, we need to recognize and listen to other viewpoints, values, and strategies for solving problems and remain open to other solutions. We must question when our clients' approaches are either successful or problematic and when they automatically equate "different" with "problem."

The typical styles of social perception, including the fundamental attribution error, can cause concern and problems when we work with people outside the dominant culture. Because psychotherapy is an activity that often supports the status quo (D. W. Sue & Sue, 1999; Szasz, 1963), people entering therapy may act defensively and may prepare for actions that support the mainstream's values against their own best interests. We might assume that our clients' current behavior is their typical behavior, and we may forget about the situational influences, especially when a client is a member of a different cultural group (Jones, 1979; Morris & Peng, 1994). Therapists who have been trained in the assumptions of an individually oriented field may accept the ideals of autonomy and self-reliance without question. These concerns may become problems even when a therapist is raised outside the mainstream culture (Zhang, 2003c).

While this book focuses extensively on the importance of becoming aware of context and culture, it also highlights intervention strategies that go beyond simply becoming aware of context. Chief among these is an emphasis on learning to listen to and empower clients. In the process of meeting these goals, the book also spends considerable time looking at culture and arguing that culture is an essential factor to consider with all people, not just with racial and ethnic minorities. Every therapist must consider cultural issues, no matter what their clients' race or gender is and no matter how narrowly defined their clinical practice may be. Understanding cultural issues helps us assess our clients accurately, relate empathically with them, and identify barriers that may prevent clients from meeting goals.

This book defines culture even more broadly than do universal theorists (Fukuyama, 1990; Pope, 1995). Instead of looking only at issues of race, ethnicity, gender, affectional orientation, class, age, and ability, we will consider the effects of the broader context, including the nature of the system and temporal, historical, and situational factors. We will also pay attention to the observer's role in observations. In doing so, we will attempt to balance the extreme individualistic viewpoints that have been traditional in psychology with systemic and contextual views of human behavior.

Opening the lens this wide has the potential to dilute our understanding of any single group and decrease our ability to synthesize information from diverse sources to assess clients accurately (Helms, 1994; Locke, 1990). These are important concerns, but this book attempts to avoid the inherent problems of this approach by balancing nomothetic (group) and idiographic (individual) views of problems. Assessing cultural and contextual factors is an important part of this process. In the second half of this book, these ideas are extended to the therapeutic process. Throughout, this book examines cultural, contextual, and systemic factors that contribute to a greater understanding of these issues. This therapy process makes something meaningful out of what could otherwise be meaningless or destructive and translates insight into action in a way that leaves the client feeling stronger, more powerful, and more connected.

WHY IS CONTEXT IMPORTANT?

"When Mercedes, a woman in her 70s from South America, visited New York City for the first time, she looked around Manhattan in amazement. She turned to her daughter and whispered, See that man there? He sells newspapers, yet look how well dressed he is! The man, a Wall Street

TABLE 1.1	DIFFERENCES BETWEEN OBSERVATIONS AND INFERENCES	
Observations	**Inferences**
Observation: A fact; something that can be seen, heard, felt, or tasted.	Inference: Something concluded, often from observations; something often influenced by the observer's values.
Everyone can agree about the nature of an observation.	People may draw markedly different inferences about the same observations.
Additional observations may increase a person's confidence about the frequency of an event.	A range of observations increases the accuracy of a person's conclusions about the meaning of an event.

broker, was carrying *The New York Times*" (Montalvo & Gutierrez, 1990, pp. 51–52). Like Mercedes, we can miss or misunderstand context. When this involves clients in therapy, it can have serious consequences.

Recognizing Context and Thinking Critically

People often make an observation (e.g., "His face is red") and automatically draw an inference (e.g., "He's angry"). However, the red face may be due to a multitude of other factors such as a warm room, a sunburn, an allergic reaction, embarrassment, or even a red skin tone. Only in gathering additional information about the situation can we choose thoughtfully from among the options and make a full inference. People who are able to think critically and to identify multiple hypotheses for understanding a situation are better able to act more intentionally. Therapists must be able to hear their clients' viewpoints *and* recognize that other explanations are possible.

Thinking critically is important both for the therapist and for the client. Clients often are unable to see alternate ways of approaching the situations in which they find themselves. Broadening their picture can help them discover other ways of seeing both themselves and their culture and finding new ways of responding to problems (Watts, Abdul-Adil, & Pratt, 2002). By recognizing our conclusions as inferences rather than as facts, we take an important step toward becoming intentional experts rather than just being nice people or good listeners. By considering alternatives, we can also recognize paths through the situations in our clients' lives—paths that we might otherwise ignore when we align too strongly with their viewpoints.

Missing the Context in Therapy

What if something has a significant and negative impact on a group, or if it is perceived by the group members as having one, yet that impact is misunderstood or unrecognized by outside observers? A 1998 Princeton

Survey Research group conducted a poll of attitudes about homosexuality for *Newsweek* magazine (Peyser, 1998) that found marked differences between the opinions of gay and straight respondents. For example, a heterosexual population reported less discrimination against homosexuals and was less likely to believe that the country needed to work to protect gay rights. This population was also less concerned about issues of gay marriage and gay adoption rights.

Therapists, while generally being more liberal than the population as a whole, unfortunately are exposed to the overall population's viewpoints and prejudices (Bergin, 1991; E. W. Kelly, 1995). As a consequence, we may miss discrimination when it occurs or fail to acknowledge or challenge issues that are unique to a group. We may also under-recognize the impact of discrimination (Greene, 1985; Montalvo & Gutierrez, 1990; Steinpreis, Ritzke, & Anders, 1999). We can get stuck in our culture's beliefs about homosexuality and homosexuals—just as others do—and miss problems because "That's the way it is." Also like others, we can accept our culture's beliefs about African Americans, Asian Americans, Latins, and other minority groups. When we ignore or underestimate the impact of discrimination and oppression, however, we miss a therapeutic opportunity and reinforce the status quo.

Furthermore, we may make internal attributions about others by believing that other people's problems are their own fault and expecting clients to make fundamental changes in their personality or intrapsychic processes to change or to stop having the problems. Certainly, some portion of our problems—and our successes—are due to intrapsychic processes such as beliefs, ways of reducing anxiety, patterns in perceiving the world, and motivations, but other portions are just as likely to stem from the context in which we live. Common contextual factors include living in an unsafe neighborhood; being ridiculed for an accent, skin color, hair texture, or choice of partner; and having opportunities closed because of these factors. Still other problems may be viewed as the results of chance ("She was in the wrong place at the wrong time"). Part of our job as therapists is to recognize the relative influence of each of these factors and to help clients control the things they can recognize and to accept the things they cannot.

Nothing, however, is either one or the other. Context, intrapsychic factors, and chance collectively influence events. Luisa's poor performance in school may be due to being raised in a place where violence inside and outside the family compromises her every act and being in an environment where education doesn't accrue advantages for her (context), hopelessness is internalized (intrapsychic causes), and being unlucky enough to have a string of teachers who simply bided their time (chance). Positive changes in any one of these realms can buffer her from problems in the others.

Try to remember a time when something bad happened (something that was outside your sphere of control) like the death of someone close to you from a terminal disease. Imagine how you might feel and react if someone accused you of causing this tragedy. Imagine that you were not sure whether or not you were responsible for it—as perhaps how you felt as a child when your parents divorced. How is accepting responsibility for the tragedy advantageous? How is it disadvantageous?

Accepting Responsibility: Advantages and Disadvantages   There are some advantages, at least perceived ones, to accepting responsibility for life's problems. Samantha, like many children with a history of incest, accepted responsibility for being attacked ("It must have been something about me, how I was dressed, what I said, where I was . . ."). Her statements can be perversely helpful if they allow her to recognize a sense of control and responsibility in a situation that may feel totally uncontrollable (Ruggiero & Taylor, 1995; Shapiro, 1989, 1995). She may, as a result, be able to make some changes in her life that will keep her safe in the future such as avoiding eye contact, certain types of clothes, and places. She may even watch others vigilantly and travel with people she deems "safe." Depression often decreases as a sense of control increases (Shapiro, 1989, 1995).

Samantha's conclusion complements those made by many perpetrators of abuse ("I couldn't help myself; she was so sexy" or "Did you see the way she looked at me?"). In each case, responsibility for an action is easily shifted to the victim. It is easy to listen to a perpetrator's language and recognize how inappropriate it is. In one perpetrator's group, whenever a group member talked like this, the other group members would challenge the statement immediately, even when they had difficulty recognizing the same thoughts in themselves.

People's own beliefs seem to match those of victims and perpetrators. Park and Cohen (1992, in Park & Folkman, 1997) reported that college students who had a friend who died in the previous year tended to blame the friend for his or her own death. Park and Cohen attributed this to attempts to maintain a sense of control and personal invulnerability. For example, one participant's friend had gone out "walking when he shouldn't have," was hit by a drunk driver who jumped the curb, and was killed on the sidewalk. Adams and Betz (1993) noted that therapists were less blaming than the general population, but they also reported that male therapists tended to blame incest victims considerably more often than did female therapists, and they tended to define incest more narrowly, thus excusing some behaviors.

Although a child should be encouraged to find ways to feel powerful and safe, ultimately the responsibility to prevent abuse lies with the adult, not the child. Therapists need to help children who have a history of abuse recognize a sense of control without falling into the trap of self-blame (Shapiro, 1989, 1995). While there *are* things that the child can do to keep herself safe, she needs to learn that she is blameless and that the abuse was not about her, but rather about the person who hurt her.

Blaming Clients While Ignoring Context   Recognizing the distortions in an abused child's self-talk is easy. However, when therapists look at intrapsychic processes alone and do not recognize the role of context, they allow or encourage clients to blame themselves for things outside their sphere of responsibility. What is the impact of blaming Luisa for her failure to pay attention in class then treating the problem with a stimulant and not acknowledging the domestic violence that makes it so difficult for her to pay attention? Medicating her anxiety, having her monitor and challenge her self-statements, and teaching her relaxation techniques treats the symptoms alone and may even encourage her to think there's something wrong with her. These actions may motivate her to take control of her life, but they do so in ways that can be blaming and even iatrogenic.

When James, an African American businessman, attempted to control his environment rather than challenge the occasional "sucker punches" that he received at work and in his "tolerant" community ("We've got enough Blacks on this committee . . . "), he acted like Samantha. What did it cost him to accept and dismiss racism? Although it gave him some measure of apparent control, it came at the tremendous cost of internalized racism, depression, and self-blame. The freedom and complacency that the majority culture enjoyed came at his expense.

Sometimes, it's simply easier and useful to label a context as insane. As long as Samantha believed that her classmates' stepfathers were prostituting them and that her classmates were coping well nonetheless, she felt isolated, "broken," and "less than normal." Labeling her family and life history as "They're crazy, not me!" can be freeing. Sometimes, clients' psychiatric symptoms are normal—although perhaps not adaptive—responses to living in an insane world (Laing, 1967).

As long as therapists ignore the context of Luisa's, James', and Samantha's problems, we are likely to blame. However, when we can see the *whole* picture of our clients' world, we are able to intervene empathically and respectfully.

RESPECTING INDIVIDUAL FOCUS *AND* CONTEXT

Individual focus and context are like two sides of a circle, each completing the other (May, 1967). Looking at people without also seeing their context can be misleading. Likewise, paying attention to the context and ignoring individual contributions can rob a person of individual responsibility and control. The two must go hand in hand. By shifting between an individual focus—helping Samantha recognize that she has elements of responsibility and control—and a contextual focus—acknowledging the roles of time, place, and situation—Samantha becomes enabled in her efforts to recognize and cope with an insane world.

Seeing Parts Versus Seeing the Whole

Believing that only a piece of the picture explains everything about the whole is an easy thing to do. This fallacy can be seen in the classic story of the three blind people who ran into an elephant and tried to determine what it was. One felt its tail and decided that they'd run into a rope. A second put her arms around its legs and decided that they'd actually found a large tree. The third grabbed onto the elephant's ear and decided that, if it was a tree, it must be a palm tree with large leaves.

Obviously, by focusing on a single part, anyone can miss the whole, just as we miss the whole when we ignore context. In most situations, failing to identify an elephant by its parts causes no lasting problems. But, a client whose therapist misses the role of race, ethnicity, culture, family, affectional orientation, or history of abuse may feel self-blame and may not find effective coping strategies. Instead of being freed from old and useless constraints upon mind and behavior, the client may be further oppressed.

The goal of this book is to help therapists identify the old ties that bind their clients (and themselves) and find ways to challenge these ties. The next chapters are designed to help therapists discover and nurture unrecognized strengths and develop strategies that empower our clients. While this book examines context and the ways it affects people, it also looks at ways to make all therapies more effective and less iatrogenic.

ASSESSING CONTEXT

In an apocryphal story, a journalist from the United States was said to have written about gender roles in Kuwait. As the story goes, she observed that before the Gulf War women generally walked about 10 feet behind their husbands. After the war, she returned to discover that men now walked several yards behind their wives. She was puzzled by this turn of events and approached one of the women for an explanation of what had caused this change in gender roles. The Kuwaiti woman was said to have replied "Land mines." (See Mikkelson & Mikkelson, 2001, for their commentary on this story.)

Context is often ignored and generally obscured by our focus on the "problem." With a truly ambiguous figure (see figure 2.1), we often see only one of its guises until someone asks if we see the other. Even then, we often

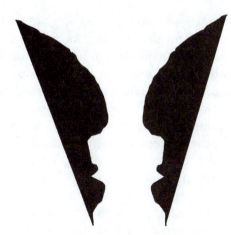

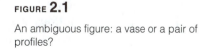

FIGURE **2.1**

An ambiguous figure: a vase or a pair of profiles?

have difficulty shifting our view from the faces to the vase (or vice versa). Our awareness of the initial figure often blinds us to other possibilities.

Our tendency to perceive a single figure may help us organize sensory data more rapidly, but it often can limit our ability to consider other possibilities. We have difficulty generating the real range of possible explanations for a phenomenon and often will have even more difficulty accepting alternate explanations as an adequate reframing of our observation. No matter how many times Dominique, a Euro-American social worker, was told that Mr. Washington, an African American construction worker, loved his children deeply, she saw only his gruff criticism of his sons and his sudden decision to send them to live with relatives as "proof" that he was a neglectful and abusive parent. Dominique had a difficult time understanding that Mr. Washington might criticize his sons so they could survive in an often mean and heartless world. Was it possible that he sent them off to live with people he hoped would be better parents to his sons? Could he do this because he loved them, rather than because he did not care?

Is this a Pollyannaish reframe? From the first moment Mr. Washington walked into the clinic, he had his arm around his oldest son and held his younger son's hand. During a session break, the three sat amiably on the front stoop of the clinic sharing a soft drink. During a very difficult session, Mr. Washington calmed down and became less critical when the full range of his feelings about his sons was reflected, to which I replied: "You've been very concerned about your sons, but I'm struck by how protective of them you are. You must love them very much." Which set of data is more important: the observations that led to seeing him as critical and rejecting or those that showed him to be loving and protective?

I had sent my daughters off with friends for several weeks that summer, and no one questioned my love for them (they even went to the ocean!).

Because my interactions with my daughters had generally been good, others may have judged my decision in a more benign light than they might have of Mr. Washington's decision to have his sons live with his relatives. Context forms the figure, which in this case was race, class, and gender influences that affected the perception of Mr. Washington's behavior. However, the conclusions drawn did not challenge the validity of the decisions. Could I have wanted a break from my kids? Might Mr. Washington have been looking for the best opportunities available for his sons?

Seeing context takes a special effort. We tend to become stuck in a single view of a complex and ambiguous "figure" without generating other options. Frequently, culture is an important piece of this context. Unless we are willing to broaden our perspective, we may, like the journalist visiting Kuwait, attempt to force a situation into our own cultural context. Unless we pay attention to context, we may—as in the case of Mr. Washington— ignore factors and draw different conclusions.

CHOOSING PLACES TO LOOK

Theory guides where we look for the "problem" and how we intervene. When we believe someone is depressed because of changes in dopamine levels in the brain, we prescribe medications to balance neurotransmitter levels. If, however, we believe that depression is a consequence of learned helplessness (Seligman, 1975), we provide settings to challenge helplessness beliefs and build self-efficacy. When we conclude that contextual issues shape the problem, however, we need to throw a large amount of data—everything outside the individual—into the pot. This huge amount of information could leave therapist and client overwhelmed by "trees" without identifying a path through the "forest."

Although it may be true that everything influences everything else, some things have a major impact and others have less impact. Research is the key to identifying the factors with major influences. Factors identified include, among others:

- Culture and group factors (Hofstede, 1980; Knight & McCallum, 1998; Steinpreis et al., 1999; D. W. Sue, & Sue, 1999)
- Number of major stressors experienced (Holmes & Rahe, 1967)
- History of success or failure both with that problem and with others (Bandura, 1997; Haaga & Stewart, 1992; Seligman, 1975)
- Nature of the work environment (Aquino, Russell, Cutrona, & Altmaier, 1996)
- Nature and quality of social supports (Aquino et al., 1996; T. Elliott, Herrick, Witty, Godshall, & Spruell, 1992; Latané & Darley, 1968)

- Attributions about events (Affleck, Tennen, Croog, & Levine, 1987; Beck, 1991; Curry, Snyder, Cook, Ruby, & Rehm, 1997; Frankl, 1959; Janoff-Bulman, 1992; Reed, Taylor, & Kemeny, 1993)

Often, we as therapists have to look where their clients do not (R. M. Epstein, Quill, & McWhinney, 1999). We must look at cultural factors when clients suspect only psychological ones, at psychological issues when they focus only on social and cultural ones, and at biological issues when they made either psychological or social concerns the sole focus. The guidelines in table 2.1 cast a wide net over biological, intrapsychic, systemic, and cultural contributions to current problems. In particular, this set of guidelines highlights three overlooked areas: (1) the nature of the symptoms and their individual and familial meanings, (2) the individual and systemic context for symptoms, and (3) the individual and systemic resources and barriers to treatment.

These guidelines describe issues for which there are identified and preferred treatments (cf. APA Task Force on Promotion and Dissemination of Psychological Procedures, 1995). In addition, they identify client-specific and relationship factors that help therapists tailor therapies and avoid the tendency to force everyone into "one size fits all" treatments (Meichenbaum, 2000a; Norcross, 2000).

Two Examples: Rosa and Abbey

Imagine two women walking into your office on the same day. Both have symptoms of moderate depression and suicidal ideation. If they have different contexts for their symptoms, different prognoses can be expected, as well as a need to intervene in different ways with each one.

Rosa grew up in a rich and supportive cultural framework and had many friends and relatives who believed in her ability to do anything she wanted to do. She was physically healthy and felt that she lived a charmed life. She fell in love with the social work field after having volunteered in the school system, and she decided to work in academe to train future generations of social workers. After having lived in upper middle-class Cuban American communities her entire life, she moved to a small town in the Midwest that had few other Latinas. She had at first been excited about the move, but after a short while she started to cry every day and have difficulty sleeping and eating. She thought about suicide almost constantly. Having previously been able to talk to friends and family about her concerns on a regular basis, she now could only do so by phone—and her family used the phone only to communicate information, not to talk about feelings. Her new "friends" did not know the long history that she shared with her old friends. She rarely felt heard and understood. When her

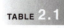

TABLE 2.1   QUESTIONS TO ASSESS DURING THE ASSESSMENT PHASE AND
THROUGHOUT THERAPY

Problem

Current symptoms
What symptoms does the person report? How severe are they? How chronic are they? When
did they begin? How much are they interfering with functioning? Are they specific to certain
situations or do they occur across situations?

Because clients often have difficulty reporting "bad" symptoms, therapists must be careful to
assess major concerns (especially about suicide) rather than expecting clients to disclose
them freely. Ask "What else?"

Beliefs about symptoms
What are the client's beliefs about what is wrong? What does the client believe about the appropriate treatment for his or her symptoms? Does he or she expect to get better?

Personal history of psychological disorders
Has the person experienced symptoms similar to or different from current symptoms at some
time in the past? What was helpful then?

If he or she received formal treatment in the past, how might this affect current treatments?
Were previous therapists respectful? Hopeful? Effective? Empowering? Is current therapy an
extension of previous work or, from his or her viewpoint, is it focused on the same old issues?

Family history of psychological disorders
Does the person's family have a history of psychological disorders or symptoms? How have
family members handled these problems? Specifically, has suicide been used to cope with
psychological problems?

Current Context

Recent events
What negative or positive events have occurred recently at home, work, school, and in important relationships? What ongoing stressors are present in the client's life? Are reactions pro-
portional or disproportional to the stressor?

Physical condition
Can any medical conditions account for the symptoms being reported? Have these been
ruled out?

Drug and alcohol use
Is the person taking any medicinal or recreational drugs that could be causing symptoms? Is
he or she taking any street drugs that could be interacting with other medications prescribed
to treat symptoms?

Intellectual and cognitive functioning
What are the client's intellectual strengths and deficits? Could symptoms be caused by cognitive deficits?

Coping style
Is the person applying generally adaptive or maladaptive coping strategies? When is he or
she most successful in coping with the problem? What works? Are coping strategies generally short-term or long-term solutions?

Self-concept
What are the client's beliefs about himself or herself (e.g., "I'm helpless with regard to the
winds of fate")? What beliefs about himself or herself or about past problems are particularly
helpful? Does he or she have a generally strong or weak sense of self-efficacy?

Sociocultural background
In what culture was this person raised? If the person is an immigrant, how long has he or she
been in this country? Why did he or she come to this country? What are the client's connections
to his or her homeland? What is the level of acculturation? What other group identifications such
as race, affectional orientation, gender, age, physical abilities, and the like are most important?

(continued)

TABLE 2.1 *(continued)*

How does the person's culture or group influence reactions to symptoms? How does cultural background influence the therapist's assessment of symptoms? Could the behavior be "normal" in the client's culture and not in the therapist's (or vice versa)? Could differences in group identification influence the nature and quality of the client/therapist relationship?

Religion and spirituality
What, if any, religious affiliation does he or she report? Is this important to the person? How do religious beliefs influence current functioning? Does a supportive network exist?

Resources and Barriers

Individual resources
What does the person do particularly well? What does he or she feel good about? How can persistence, loyalty, optimism, and intelligence become resources for treatment? How might these attributes undermine treatment?

Social resources, such as friends, family, school, and work
How positive and supportive are the client's family, friends, and relationships with coworkers? Are these relationships sufficient in both quantity and quality to meet the client's needs? Do any relationships increase or decrease the client's stress levels? Do these relationships empower the client or undermine him or her?

Community resources
What agencies, if any, are involved? How supportive are they? How well do they work together? Do they undermine each other's recommendations or are they open and collaborative in sharing information ?

Community contributions
How does your client contribute to the community? Does this feel useful and meaningful to him or her? Are your client's contributions acknowledged by important people in his or her support system? If so, how?

Mentors and models
What real, historical, or metaphorical figures serve as pillars of support or spiritual guides? How have these figures handled similar problems? Note: Some models may be primarily negative in tone. What are the positive aspects of these "negative" models?

Obstacles and opportunities to change process
What things might serve as potential obstacles or aids to the change process? These can be financial, educational, social, intellectual, and the like. What does he or she believe will (or might) happen if change occurs? Does he or she imagine events such as marriage dissolving, family working together more effectively, or losing financial support?

Therapeutic relationship
What sort of relationship do the therapist and client have? Can the client be honest about symptoms, actions, side effects, and concerns? Can he or she honestly disclose the level of compliance with the therapist's recommendations? Does he or she feel comfortable contradicting the therapist or correcting any misconceptions made?

department chair began verbally attacking her in a smarmy and vague way, her colleagues distanced themselves and let the attacks continue. Her depression deepened.

In the second example, Abbey, a Euro-American grandmother who had been dysthymic most of her life, became more depressed after a hysterectomy in her mid-30s. She had little energy, was constantly fatigued, and had difficulty sleeping and eating. She reported having frequent headaches and stated that her mother, aunts, and older sister endured similar symptoms after menopause. She also said that no one had been able to help them.

She described her childhood as "okay," but reported a variety of behaviors that suggested severe neglect, including having had several broken bones ignored by adults around her. Abbey and her family lived in severe poverty—earning about $6000 a year—and did not receive any federal living support. As if this were not enough, a number of significant stressors occurred; most notably, her youngest child was diagnosed with cancer.

Rosa has a strong probability of being able to recover rapidly. She had handled stressors well in the past and had developed good coping mechanisms. Her current problems come in the midst of a series of acute stressors—the move, a separation from her support system, and the personal attacks. These were not preceded by either family or individual histories of depression. Additionally, she has considerable resources to bring to bear on this problem. She has a good familial and cultural support system—both she and her family are well-respected in her home community—and she is in the process of developing a strong support system in her new community. In fact, she reports that her new support system is better than she expected it to be. She is active and productive and, although her department chair was not supportive, colleagues in other departments have helped her test her perception of this situation and brainstorm responses. She has good coping mechanisms and, although distressed about her current problems, she does not really believe that she will continue this way forever.

Abbey's prognosis was poorer because, unlike Rosa, she did not see herself as able to be helped. She has a significant number of female relatives who attribute their depression to hormonal factors beyond their immediate control, and she believes these attributions. She also has a history of overlooking her considerable chronic and acute stressors. She failed to recognize her history of neglect and abuse, for example, even when it was identified. If she can ever acknowledge the context of her depression and challenge her self-concept that stems from this context, her mood will probably lighten. Abbey's one advantage is her poor level of functioning, which will likely allow her to perceive even relatively small improvements in functioning as significant and meaningful.

> Given what you know about these two women, how would you intervene? Would you do something different for one than for the other? If so, why?

ASSESSING CONTEXT IN THERAPY

Because stepping outside of a cultural frame is difficult, three tools can highlight aspects of context—family relationships and functioning, community connections, and the cultural and historical contexts—that often get ignored. These tools are:

- Family genogram (McGoldrick, Gerson, & Shellenberger, 1999)
- Psychosocial history or community genogram (Ivey, Ivey, & Simek-Morgan, 1997)
- Timelines

Each tool looks at the presence (or absence) of clusters of events to identify factors that played a special role in the presenting problems. The interview process should assess contextual issues that serve either as facilitating factors or as obstacles to change. The following discussion presents an approach to using these tools. In subsequent chapters, specific case histories are examined and implications for their use are discussed at greater length.

Family Genogram

The family genogram is a visual means of identifying and organizing hypotheses about familial factors that may contribute to the problem. Simple genograms may include genealogical material, but they can also show relationships, patterns of mental health diagnoses and substance abuse, and some of the major events in the family history. Most genograms include basic information such as the number of marriages, number of children from each marriage, birth order, and deaths. Other genograms include information on disorders running in the family—such as alcoholism and depression—alliances, and living situations. Their form is only limited by the imagination.

Generally, males are identified with a square and females with a circle. An X through an individual's marker indicates a death. The index person or identified patient's marker is usually identified with double lines. Spouses are connected by horizontal lines. Separations and divorces are indicated by, respectively, single and double slash lines through the marriage lines. Children are connected to their parents' marital lines by vertical lines, with the line getting hatched to signify adopted children. Miscarriages are indicated by a small, solid circle instead of a figure identifying its gender. Birth, marriage, divorce, and death dates may be indicated by initials, such as *b* for birth and *d* for death, followed by the year (e.g., b. 89). Numbers in the markers identify ages. Circles made from hatched lines around several family members indicate family living arrangements that would otherwise be unclear. A filled-in space at the bottom part of a person's marker generally indicates substance abuse, and a filled-in space on the left indicates physical or psychiatric problems, depending on the genogram's use.

Knowledge about the nature of relationships among family members is important for the therapist to acquire. Are family members close to each other or distant? Do they have frequent and intimate relationships or rare

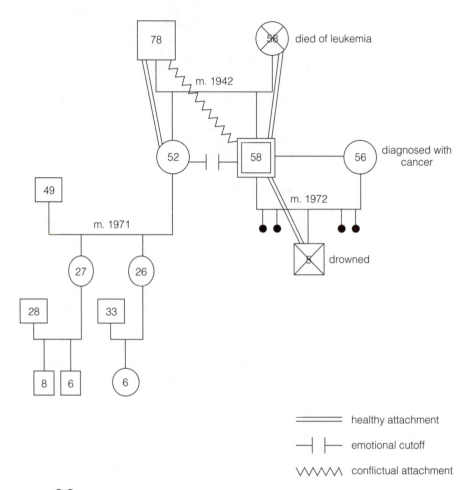

FIGURE **2.2**

A family genogram for Mervyn, a 58-year-old Euro-American male.

and difficult contact? Cutoffs, alliances, enmeshments, and stressful relationships are indicated by the nature of lines that connect the individuals (see figure 2.2).

An Example: Mervyn Mervyn, a 58-year-old Euro-American male, requested therapy when his physician asked for a psychological consult after concluding that a series of minor infections and other illnesses had no physical basis (see figure 2.2 for Mervyn's family genogram). Although Mervyn initially had a very limited view of the "problem," this perception was enlarged when he considered the impact of the deaths of his mother and son; his wife's miscarriages; and his conflictual and emotionally distant relationships with his father, sister, and wife. All of these factors, including his elderly father's illness, affected his sense of community. Deaths and losses in his family almost selectively affected the people he loved the most. As he is the same age as his mother was at her death and his nieces and nephew are about his son's age, anniversary issues may also play a role in his current functioning.

He noted how his symptoms increased in severity after a visit with his great-nieces and great-nephews. He really enjoyed his time with the children, but he experienced a confusing set of feelings after the visit, perhaps in part because the kids were the approximate age of his son at his death. This genogram helped Mervyn view his symptoms as stress and depression rather than as a series of difficult-to-manage infections.

Because family genograms are a standard part of family therapy and have been well-described elsewhere (McGoldrick et al., 1999), this book does not cover them in great detail. Nonetheless, they are an important source of hypotheses—as opposed to facts—about an individual's and family's behavior and symptoms.

Psychosocial History and the Community Genogram

In addition to understanding the ways families function, understanding the ways clients relate to their greater community can be extremely helpful in therapy. In the course of a psychosocial history, questions like those in table 2.1 begin to expand our understanding of the client and the "problem." Perhaps most importantly, we can assess the nature of connections with self, others in the community, and the culture. In the course of this assessment, we can help the client recognize obstacles to change, find areas to be strengthened, and use available resources. We can then identify areas of strength and weakness and determine where the person is currently "out of balance."

Psychosocial histories are frequently presented in written form, but the nature of connections—an important part of a person's context—can be easily drawn to describe the connections in the person's life. Such descriptions are especially useful in therapy sessions, where therapists may want to highlight a few points about the nature of connections, rather than summarize the vast amount of information that can be gathered in the course of an interview.

Illustrating the nature of these connections in a community genogram (Ivey et al., 1997) can be done with many of the same identifiers used in family genograms. The easiest way is to identify the client (or family) by drawing a circle or other symbol in the center of the page and connecting the client to the various resources or stressors that play a role in his or her life. Positive and supportive relationships are generally indicated, as in family genograms, with a double line. More tenuous relationships are indicated by a single line, and enmeshed relationships are suggested by a triple line. Conflictual relationships are identified by a lightning bolt and emotional cutoffs by a single, interrupted line.

The most obvious relationships to include on a community genogram are those involving spouses, children, and families of origin. However, others relationships may have a major impact, albeit less obvious, and these will also be important to assess. They can include a child's school, a child protection agency, a church, or the workplace, as well as friends, babysitters, and neighbors. Each of these can be either a significant support or stressor.

Community genograms can be drawn in the course of a therapy session. But unless they are drawn with a theory guiding them, they can become unsystematic and can lead to the therapist overlooking important areas. For that reason, forms such as that shown in table 2.1 can be useful in guiding assessment. In tabular form, the community genogram can store large amounts of complex information that would otherwise be overwhelming. Because these guidelines assess areas that are important to most people, a written psychosocial history often is much more complete, and thus more useful, than a drawn community genogram.

An Example Most notable about someone who values connections as much as Mervyn said he did was how few supportive relationships he had (see table 2.2 and figure 2.3). Although a professional in his community could be expected to have a number of significant and positive relationships at his stage of life such as a wife, children, grandchildren, friends, and contacts with business associates and community members, Mervyn had very few. In fact, he had conflictual and superficial relationships with family members, a pleasant but shallow relationship with his next-door neighbor, and demanding and conflict-ridden relationships at work. He reported having no close friends, no hobbies, and no spiritual or community involvement. His coping mechanisms were poor, and they tended to isolate him even further from the people in his life. Rather than helping him solve problems, his natural coping mechanisms tended to create additional ones. Life's circumstances had contributed to his being in a very different life situation than others of his age, who were generally stable in their jobs and looking forward to retirement. Also, they had become involved grandparents and were expecting a dozen or more years of good health. Mervyn, however, was a man out of balance without any positive connections as potential supports. Instead of being firmly grounded on both feet, he wobbled on a single toe.

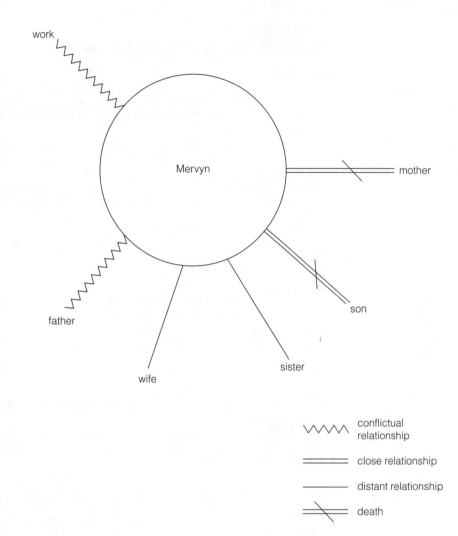

FIGURE **2.3**

Mervyn's community genogram.

However, Mervyn did report significant strengths that could become assets in therapy. He was a hard worker who believed in his ability to solve problems in an action-oriented manner. Rather than being angry with his physician for referring him to a psychologist, he was relieved that there was something he might be able to do to resolve his symptoms. Although he could not immediately identify a course of action to follow in this situation, he expected that an "expert" would be able to. This was facilitated by the strong, positive relationship that he and his therapist developed almost immediately.

TABLE  2.2   MERVYN'S PSYCHOSOCIAL HISTORY

Problem

Current symptoms
Reports a history of infections and other relatively minor, but extremely bothersome illnesses during the last two years. These have led to his taking one brief medical leave.

Beliefs about symptoms
Saw symptoms as primarily medical in nature, although willing to consider his physician's suggestion that symptoms are psychosomatic in origin.

Personal history of psychological disorders
No history of psychological symptoms reported, although the therapist can infer some degree of depression following his son's death (based on reported history). Client has never seen a therapist.

Family history of psychological disorders
None reported. His family (the father, in particular) has strongly negative feelings about expressing negative emotions and problems.

Current Context

Recent events
Wife has been diagnosed with breast cancer. She has quit her job and is unable or unwilling to perform many chores around the home.

Physical condition
His symptoms have baffled his physician, and medical syndromes have been ruled out.

Drug and alcohol use
Only moderate social drinking has been reported. He denies drug use.

Intellectual and cognitive functioning
Average intelligence. He is persistent, with strong problem-solving skills.

Coping style
He describes "swallowing things" and working harder when under stress. He does not talk to family or friends because he believes he will "overwhelm" them, although he is willing to talk to and listen to his neighbor.

Self-concept
He sees himself as a good person, but buffeted by fate. He tends to see his past as a series of failures and bad luck. He is pessimistic about the future and about his ability to make any effective change in life.

Sociocultural background
He is a middle-class male in a rural Euro-American community. He reports being fair-minded and is concerned about issues of justice.

Religion and spirituality
Although he had been active in the Catholic Church until his son's death, he now describes himself as an agnostic.

Resources and Barriers

Individual resources
Describes himself as responsible, dedicated and determined. He considers himself able to identify a problem and attack it successfully. He reports having enjoyed gardening and camping in his early adulthood, but reports that they "wouldn't work now."

Social resources, such as friends and family
He has a superficial friendship with a neighbor. He reports being afraid that he would "overwhelm" his friend if he shared his stressors or tried to do anything that would make the relationship more genuine.

(continued)

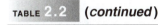 **TABLE 2.2** *(continued)*

Family relationships are distant and often conflictual at the present time, although he reports having had close relationships with his wife, mother, son, and sister in the past. His mother died from leukemia, and his son drowned.

Work
He describes himself as a "workaholic," although he does not enjoy the number of hours he works. He does not feel appreciated; in fact, he feels taken advantage of. But he is concerned that he could lose his job if he suggests changes.

Community resources
He has yearly physicals with his doctor and makes visits to handle "infections" most months. No other agencies are involved.

Community contributions
None exist currently. He had been a Boy Scout leader and an usher in his church until his son's death.

Mentors and models
He sees himself as being like Job; that is, being showered with problems but surviving them. He also sees himself like JFK (i.e., courageous, with strong convictions). He remembers his mother during times of stress and wishes he were more like her. He admires his employer whom he describes as decisive, efficient, and capable.

Obstacles and opportunities to change process
Afraid that setting limits with his wife, family of origin, or work would have negative consequences—that they would, respectively, be overwhelmed, be rejecting, or be anxious to fire him. Nonetheless, he is "tired of living like this" and is "willing to do anything" to avoid feeling this way.

Therapeutic relationship
He is open and honest about symptoms because "That's what you're here for." He is not concerned about the possibility that the therapist might be overwhelmed. He feels listened to and understood. He accepts minimal direction and extends work in therapy tenfold.

Timelines

People exist in a family and systemic context that can be assessed readily by family and community genograms. They also exist in a temporal context. A timeline is a useful device to identify clients' temporal and historical contexts.

A timeline is just what it sounds like—a line from birth to the present. It describes all major events that affect clients and their immediate family. It is both a handy organizing system for information and an organizing device to mark the temporal contiguity of events. A timeline generally starts with the kind of information that is gathered in the course of doing a family genogram. Components include dates of births, deaths, marriages, divorces, and the like that involve the immediate family. In addition, it records both the mundane events, such as a voluntary job change, and unusual events, such as being charged with statutory rape.

Consider looking at a timeline as a kind of informal version of the Social Readjustment Rating Scale, or SRRS (Holmes & Rahe, 1967). Instead of simply listing stressors in the last year, as the SRRS does, this approach

TABLE 2.3	TIMELINE FOR MERVYN
March 1948	Mervyn's parents marry.
December 1948	Mervyn's sister Martha is born.
April 1952	Mervyn is born. Mervyn describes his early childhood as relatively uneventful, but denies having close relationships with any of his family members.
1971	Mervyn meets Johanna. They begin dating.
1972	Mervyn and Johanna marry. Money is tight. They live with his parents and decide to delay having children for a few years. This living arrangement is conflictual.
1975	Mervyn and Johanna move into their own home and begin trying to have children. Their relationship with his parents improves. Conceiving turns out to be more difficult than they had expected.
1977	Mervyn's mother is diagnosed with leukemia. Johanna miscarries.
1978	Johanna miscarries again.
November 1979	Johanna is pregnant again.
February 1980	Mervyn's mother dies unexpectedly from complications related to leukemia. His father says, "You're not going to embarrass me by crying are you?" He never cries.
April 1980	Johanna delivers their son David prematurely. He spends one month in neonatal intensive care. Johanna spends much of this period at the hospital, crying. Mervyn spends more time at work.
1981	David thrives. Mervyn describes himself as a "devoted and happy father." Work goes well. Johanna miscarries again.
1983	Johanna miscarries twice more.
September 1986	David joins the Boy Scouts, and Mervyn becomes a troop leader. He remembers enjoying this job and being good at it.
November 1986	David drowns while playing on a frozen creek near their house. Johanna is depressed for months and doesn't leave the house. Mervyn doesn't cry, but he works long hours. Although he had been an usher in his church previously, he stops attending altogether. He now describes himself as an agnostic. His friends complain that they don't see him anymore.
1987	Against Johanna's wishes, Mervyn gets a vasectomy.
1990	As his company downsizes and leaves the area, Mervyn loses his job. Because he is two years short of being vested, he loses his employer's contributions to his retirement.
1991	Mervyn looks for a job, but does not find one for eight months. He takes a one-third cut in pay. Mervyn is diagnosed with an ulcer.
1992	The business goes under, and Mervyn loses his job. This time, he finds a job within four months, but it is another low-paying job with no retirement program. He begins to work long hours to earn overtime and is diagnosed with hypertension.
1993	Johanna, a receptionist for 15 years, gets a first warning at work about her excessive absences. Mervyn's ulcer flares up.
1994	Johanna is diagnosed with breast cancer and has a mastectomy.

(continued)

TABLE 2.3	(continued)
1997	Johanna finds another lump and has a second mastectomy. She takes extended sick leave from work. Mervyn's father becomes more infirm and begins to require significant care. His sister refuses to get involved because she lives farther away. Most visits with his father end in a fight. Mervyn visits his doctor 10 times this year because of apparent infections.
1998	Johanna is asked to quit her job because she has not worked since March of 1997. Mervyn's employer has begun expecting him to work 70 hours each week. Although he doesn't want to work these hours, Mervyn is afraid to refuse. He is referred to a series of specialists for the infections.
1999	Johanna is again diagnosed with cancer. Mervyn's specialists say that they have ruled out all possible physical causes. They recommend a consultation for psychological causes. He is skeptical, but agrees.

looks at stressors and major events from the client's *idiosyncratic* point of view throughout the lifespan. For example, flying may not be a stressor for most people, but being told to fly across the country as a requirement for one's job could become a major stressor for anyone who may already be phobic about flying. Additionally, the timeline provides an opportunity to look at clusters of stressors and the client's reactions to them. Losing a job is almost always a stressor even when there are no other major issues, but the impact can be worse when it happens at a time when one's child has been diagnosed with cancer or the mortgage has been foreclosed on or the marriage is rocky. Also, the person who experiences four major stressors in a relatively quiet period can be expected to perceive these stressors differently than the person who has had major stressors throughout life.

Often, this assessment process picks up reactions to these stressors, which may include depression, suicide attempts, ulcers, and increased drinking. How does the person respond to stressors? Do relatively trivial stressors overwhelm the client or can clusters of stressors be handled well? Has this pattern of reactions changed through time? Is the person seeming to become more easily overwhelmed or hardier and more resistant to stress? What sorts of job-related, interpersonal, or familial stressors seem to overwhelm the client? Do these stressors have a theme, such as personal threat, loss of control, or perceived abandonment?

An Example   As Mervyn's timeline makes apparent, he had fairly average levels of support during his early adult years. However, these became scattered and less supportive over time. His mother and son died, he lost a good job because of a downsizing, his wife became ill, and he grew afraid of overwhelming her (see table 2.3). He noted that he withdrew from the people who had been important to him because he believed that his showing emotion, sharing problems, or asking for help were signs of weakness, as they had been in his family of origin. This is a common pattern for males of Northern European extraction (McGoldrick, Giordano, & Pearce, 1996). He also admitted being afraid that someone else would die.

Apparently, support and connections were useful to him. He reports being happier during periods when he had stronger family connections and was more involved with his community. These components have important implications. If he had not been happier during these periods, therapy would not encourage him to strengthen these sorts of connections; rather, it would focus on other predictors of healthy functioning.

BRINGING THESE ASSESSMENTS TOGETHER

These assessments make clear that Mervyn experienced significant family and life stressors, had few personal and interpersonal supports, and had limited adaptive coping mechanisms—except perhaps his tendency to avoid problems by working harder. Although he suggested that the lack of interpersonal and familial supports was relatively unimportant, we might question this when looking at his timeline. Each of these problems suggests possible places to intervene.

The strengths that become visible in these assessments are equally important. Mervyn is an active, hardworking man with a history of being productive in his community and being well-connected to his family. He is a person who believes he has been given a raw deal in life, yet he also tends to believe in the ability of experts to "solve" them. He seems to be very persistent in seeing problems through. Even his family's taboos about focusing on and speaking about problems, while generally problematic for him, reveal a hidden strength. Once his concerns have been acknowledged, he may prefer to address them rather than continue to obsess about them.

These assessment tools are useful, but they are only a source of hypotheses. They are best evaluated by comparing them to developmental and cultural norms. What are typical paths for his age and cultural group? No one would have been surprised that Mervyn had no children when he was 23, but they might think it was very unusual for a 58-year-old. If Mervyn had been a Latino rather than Euro-American, having only two children would have seemed unusual. However, simply being unusual does not mean that a discrepancy is problematic. Following up on these concerns with an assessment of the meaning of these areas is an important step.

See table 2.4 for examples of questions that might have been raised in response to Mervyn's psychosocial history.

What does it mean to have lost your only child or not to have grandchildren later in your life when your peers are beginning to dote on theirs? What does it mean not to be involved with a church at this point in life—despite it having been very important earlier? Note that Mervyn uses a biblical reference to describe himself even now.

Spend some time doing your own family genogram, psychosocial history, and timeline. What patterns do you see in your own life? How has your life been similar to the norms for your age cohort and cultural group? How has it been different? How have these differences affected you? How might the accidents in your life and your decisions influence how you see your clients' problems?

It is also important to consider whether contextual issues affect the client in clinically significant ways. For example, the presence of marital conflict can be a significant clinical issue when working with an externalizing child, but the effects of marital conflict on children in general seem to create problems through their impact on parenting (Fauber & Long, 1991). In other words, when expectations and structure remain clear, when discipline is consistent, and when parents continue to be warm and involved, marital conflict has little impact. Separations and divorces do not necessarily cause a child to have problems.

What this means, of course, is that family genograms, psychosocial histories, and timelines are, like other assessment tools, only sources of hypotheses to help guide treatment. In the course of collecting more information—during the assessment process and during therapy—some hypotheses can be ruled out.

INTERVIEWING FOR CONTEXT

Because the assessments have been described separately, one might conclude that they should also be assessed separately. This can be useful at times, especially when a therapist suspects an unusual confluence of events and wants to highlight these with the client, but in many cases, psychosocial histories, family genograms, community genograms, and timelines are assessed simultaneously, as this brief segment shows.

EM: *Wow . . . As you've been talking, I've been listening to the number of stressors you've described for the last several years. Let's spend a couple of minutes looking at them. (Self-disclosure, open probe)*

MERVYN: *Sure. It's been rough lately, but when I was a kid it wasn't so bad. I lived in the country, in an area where everyone knew everyone else. Everyone watched over us kids. It was kind of nice then.*

EM: *Then? (Encourager)*

MERVYN: *It all seemed to change when my mom died. We'd been living with my folks for several years, but then I got a job in another town, and we got our own place.*

EM: *When was that? (Closed question)*

MERVYN: *1975. We'd decided to try to have kids, but it took about five years. David was born in 1980, two months after my mom died. (Silence, tears up)*

EM: *That sounds like a hard time. (Reflection of feeling)*

MERVYN: *It was. I was always much closer to my mom than my dad, and I wanted her to see our son David. She died just before he was*

TABLE  **2.4   HYPOTHESES RAISED BY MERVYN'S PSYCHOSOCIAL HISTORY**

Problem

Beliefs about symptoms
Medical issues have been addressed and ruled out. Will he accept the referral to therapy and the suggestion that problems are psychosomatic in nature?

Personal history of psychological disorders
Why now? Will he be open to receiving treatment at this time?

Family history of psychological disorders
Family taboos, such as expressing negative emotions and disclosing problems, may serve as a barrier to effective therapy.

Current Context

Recent events
The drop in income, an increase in household chores, and his wife's illness factor into his increased stress.

Physical condition
His symptoms have baffled physicians, and medical syndromes have been ruled out. Symptoms are probably psychological in nature, but the doctors continue to explore other explanations.

Drug and alcohol use
This is unlikely to interfere with treatment.

Intellectual and cognitive functioning
Intellectual and cognitive skills may facilitate treatment.

Coping style
His tendency to "swallow things" may interfere with treatment. His tendency to work longer during times of stress may help, but only if he is able to think divergently and try new solutions.

Self-concept
He has external loci of control and responsibility, yet he is hardworking and persistent. Is he ambivalent about his ability to control his world? Perhaps the therapist can see the positive end of this ambivalence and expand his ability to exercise some control. He sees himself as a good person and thus undeserving of the bad things that have happened in his life.

Sociocultural background
Do his cultural background and gender interfere with his ability to handle his feelings adaptively? Does he have a support system in which he can share these feelings? While issues of autonomy are probably addressed satisfactorily, are intimacy needs satisfied?

Religion and spirituality
Is his church truly unimportant or has it become a place where he feels cut off and isolated from a spiritual community. (See his response in the "Mentors and Models" section.)

Resources and Barriers

Individual resources
He is high in self-efficacy, which should facilitate therapy. He has few hobbies that might otherwise help him relax.

Social resources, such as friends and family
Does he enjoy little support from friends and family because he has to be the "strong one" or because the relationships are conflictual?

How does he feel about not having children and grandchildren at this point in his life? Does this leave him feeling "different" and isolated from "normal" society?

(*continued*)

TABLE 2.4 *(continued)*

Work
While he feels competent at his job, he does not feel appreciated. Is this another source of stress?

Community resources
He has not used community supports other than his physician. Are there sufficient supports to help him handle stress well?

Community contributions
He does very little away from work other than take care of the family. Does he internalize these activities to support his sense of self as a competent contributor to society?

Mentors and models
He sees himself as a person showered with problems, but a survivor nonetheless. He admires decisiveness, efficiency, and competence, but also warmth and emotional connection.

Obstacles and opportunities to change process
Who would do the things that need to be done if he didn't do them? Will he be a good person if he doesn't do them? Can he harness his self-efficacy in other areas for therapy?

Therapeutic relationship
Will he use therapy effectively since he does not transfer concerns about disclosure to the therapy situation? Will his ability to accept this form of support and his ability to extend homework assist therapy?

born, prematurely. And it wasn't just that. When Mom died, Dad told me, ordered me, not to embarrass him or anything by crying. (Pause) That's one of the things that I keep remembering. (Pause) I didn't cry when Mom died, when Jo miscarried, when David died. I just couldn't. (Pause) And it continues. I've been working 70-hour weeks lately, worrying about Jo—she has cancer again. One or the other of us seems to be sick all the time.

EM: *Wow! That's a lot. (Feedback)*

MERVYN: *Yeah, it was . . . .*

This dialogue focuses primarily on developing a timeline for a short and especially problematic period of Mervyn's life. Whereas Mervyn initially described the problems in his life, Em was able to change his focus from the problems to the things that worked well. Because Em started with Mervyn's concerns and then validated them ("That's a lot . . . "), he was able to accept the implicit reframe: "You're not a weakling; you're a fighter."

At the same time that Em was assessing a timeline, she was also beginning to sketch out a family genogram with a few initial hypotheses about the nature and quality of Mervyn's support systems. At this point, he talked primarily about the support that he didn't have or had lost. Along with this pessimistic view of his resources, he tended to focus on how he had *not* coped, rather than how he *had*.

Introducing Grays

Context includes the events and people that may influence current problems. Rather than accepting clients' stories about their problems at face value, therapists often want to challenge descriptions drawn with large brushes in black and white. Mervyn described his father as cold and emotionless and his mother as warm. When Johanna was ill, she provided little help or support. He talked as if he had few resources—a perception that may significantly contribute to his feelings of stress.

Were there any bright spots in Mervyn's life? A stronger therapeutic interview, rather than being simply a source of initial hypotheses, would recognize and enlarge some of these grays, as Em shows next:

MERVYN: *I didn't cry when Mom died, when Jo miscarried, or when David died. I just couldn't . . . .*

EM: *Everyone grieves in different ways. How did you handle it? (Normalization, open question)*

MERVYN: *I was the caretaker. Somehow, I made all the arrangements for the funeral and got the reception together afterwards. Jo had fallen apart, and I kept moving the whole time, thinking that my mom was there beside me. Since then, I've been working 70-hour weeks and worrying about Jo—she has cancer again. One or the other of us seems to be sick all the time.*

EM: *Wow! That's a lot. What have you done to make it through this? (Feedback, open question)*

MERVYN: *Make it through? I don't usually think about it that way, but I suppose I have, haven't I? (Pause) Hmm . . . Well, I complain about work, but it's also a haven. I don't have to think there, and I feel like I've accomplished something. And, before Jo got so sick and before I lost my job, we used to travel all over, staying at little bed-and-breakfasts and visiting antique shops. (Pause) I used to paint, too. Those things helped. (Pause) Well, I suppose I also think about myself as a modern-day Job and that if he could handle things, so can I, although (Laughs) maybe my shoulders aren't as broad as his.*

EM: *(Laughs) It sounds like they're pretty broad! (Feedback)*

With little additional work in the second dialogue, Em was able to get Mervyn to reframe the problem, to recognize his strengths, and to acknowledge his resources. He was not cold and unfeeling, but grieving in one of many ways. Rather than only being "sick all the time," he also found resources in the present and past that helped him cope. When Em asked, "What have you done to make it through this?" she encouraged Mervyn to pay attention to his resources. When he accepted and developed her ideas, he agreed that he was competent, with resources to bring to bear on this and other problems. In beginning to identify and highlight these resources, which is a therapeutic strategy, the therapist continued to assess his psychosocial history and the nature of his community resources.

CONCLUSIONS

Ignoring context and thus committing the fundamental attribution error is easy. When context is ignored, people tend to ascribe negative and stable attributions to others and ascribe more positive and unstable attributions to themselves (J. Greenberg et al., 1982; Jones, 1979; Zuckerman, 1979). This shift in attributions seems to be dependent both upon one's attitudes toward another person's group, and the amount of knowledge known about the person.

This chapter examines a number of techniques to assess a person's personal, temporal, community, and familial contexts and their meanings. These techniques include (1) the family genogram, (2) a psychosocial history or community genogram, and (3) timelines. These are tools to help therapists gather and present a fair amount of information rapidly, as seen in the first section of dialogue between Em and Mervyn. They also help introduce greater complexity into both the therapist's and the client's views of the problem, as seen in the second section. In the latter, both client and therapist invest more time, but they get a more sophisticated result. Subsequent chapters explore a number of other ways these assessments can supplement and enrich the therapy process.

Assessment is not something to be performed merely in the initial sessions and then dropped. Rather, it should be synthetic to the therapeutic process. Initial assessments identify the general direction, treatment goals, and interventions of therapy, but assessments *during* therapy help refine these initial goals and increase understanding of the client's worldview. Furthermore, strong assessments require sensitive listening and a clear understanding of a client's verbal and nonverbal language, which of course depend on empathy and empathic responses. Clues for enriching understanding and empathy are found throughout this book.

Defining Culture and Context

Up close, it's only random splotches of paint. But a few feet away the blue, red, green, and yellow dots in Seurat's famous impressionist painting *A Sunday Afternoon on the Island of La Grande Jatte* begin to resolve into people, umbrellas, and a sprawling park. What had at first appeared to be haphazard has begun to look methodical.

Some people are organized. Others are disorganized. Some are polite and considerate; others are awkward and rude. In a way, people seem to be best characterized by their differences.

When Americans, for example, venture abroad and see other peoples and cultures, the differences can become strikingly clear. In the former

Soviet Union, the average person has less private space, yet many seem content with what would feel like constant boundary violations to people from the United States—who can complain about a house with only 500 square feet per person! Not only is this way of life simpler, but the people actually seem happy with fewer possessions. Russian stores and museums, in contrast, are so much larger and more imposing than many in America. Moscow, in particular, can make a foreigner feel lost and uncomfortable. In Minsk and St. Petersburg, however, public spaces feel more intimate and less formal and overwhelming—at least until one views the Hermitage.

Russians seem to place a great deal of value in their country's appearance. The subways are lined with spotless works of art (compare this to urban graffiti in New York and Chicago). The streets are rarely littered, and debris is picked up rapidly by the babushkas who tend the streets. On any day, rubbish can swirl along the sidewalks, and people will walk right on by without noticing.

UNIVERSAL AND FOCUSED APPROACHES TO THERAPY

Under normal circumstances people look at others' behavior without seeing the patterns or they attribute the patterns to traits rather than to contextual issues, such as culture or situations. Once outside one's own culture, patterns get a little easier to see, although these patterns are still difficult to interpret, particularly when not imposing one's own worldview and values. Noticing the patterns is important, but how they are interpreted makes a significant difference. Should a teacher view the behavior of a student from mainland China as being due to social anxiety or to cultural dictates to avoid self-disclosure and to be respectful toward authority figures? Should a grandmother's frequent discussions of her friends' deaths be seen as a morbid preoccupation with death and dying or as an awareness and acceptance of death common in her age cohort? Interpreting these behaviors works best when the cultural frameworks and context are taken into account.

Unfortunately, people often think of culture as a complication to their understanding of others (Hall, 1997; Hays, 1995; S. Sue, 1999), rather than as a useful factor in the assessment process and a helpful resource in identifying intervention strategies. As a result, psychology and the other social sciences have tended to look first at general patterns and have ignored the effects of race, ethnicity, class, and other aspects of culture. This is a dangerous assumption considering that one-third of the U.S. population is currently made up of racial and ethnic minorities—nearly 45% of all students in the public school system and about 75% of all people entering the workforce (D. W. Sue, Bingham, Porché-Burke, & Vasquez, 1999).

This chapter introduces the concept of culture and defines it broadly (Fukuyama, 1990; Pope, 1995; D. W. Sue et al., 1999). It also further explains context and the role of context in people's interactions with others. Additional coverage includes how context can be useful in helping therapists better understand their clients.

The broad definition of culture, or universal approach to the issue, involves the following factors:

- Race
- Ethnicity
- Class
- Gender
- Age
- Religion
- Affectional orientation
- Ability

With such a range of cultures, most people will belong to more than one cultural group, with some being more salient at some points than others. Culture significantly influences clients' worldview, yet it is easy to overlook when people often inappropriately attribute its effects to personality—as the example of the Chinese student and grandmother implies. An important goal is to search for a balance between finding commonalities among individuals and recognizing unique cultural differences.

In contrast, some authors (e.g., Helms, 1994; Helms & Richardson, 1997; Locke, 1990; D. W. Sue et al., 1999) have decried a universal approach, arguing that it has the potential to become inefficient and may even dilute efforts to increase the effectiveness of therapy, especially among disfranchised groups. For example, Locke was asked to present on African Americans to a class in which students had been allowed to choose an article on any cultural group different than their own. Locke was appalled to discover that the students had not chosen to read about African Americans or any other racial or ethnic groups that they were most likely to work with in the future. As a consequence, they were no more prepared to work with these populations than before, even though they may have believed they had become more culturally competent and aware. He argued that courses in multicultural counseling should focus specifically on those "overlooked" groups: African Americans, Asian Americans, Hispanics, and Native Americans.

Toward a Universal Approach

With the problems that Helms (1994; Helms & Cook, 1999) and Locke (1990) describe, why should therapists take the kind of broad view of culture and context proposed by them? Without a breadth of understanding, therapists can too easily overlook the range of factors that influence their clients. By acknowledging the range, however, their understanding will become significantly more complex . . . and realistic. Without a broad view, people can become divided, and they can ignore issues faced by groups outside of the traditional racial and ethnic minorities (D. W. Sue et al., 1999). Here, Lorde (1984a) describes this problem:

> Somewhere, on the edge of consciousness, there is what I call a *mythical norm*, which each one of us within our hearts knows "that is not me." In america, this norm is usually defined as white, thin, male, young, heterosexual, Christian, and financially secure. It is with this mythical norm that the trappings of power reside within this society. Those of us who stand outside that power often identify one way in which we are different, and we assume *that* to be the primary cause of all oppression, forgetting other distortions around difference, some of which we ourselves may be practicing. (p. 116)

The goal of this chapter is to combine breadth and depth and to provide an overarching approach to recognizing and working with cultural differences and the clients who reflect them. Its specific focus is on three aspects of culture. First, the aim is to be inclusive in the definitions of culture and difference and to move beyond race and ethnicity to include issues of class, gender, age, affectional orientation, religion, and ability. Some of these concerns are common to a number of culturally different groups. Second, while there are some issues that characterize many groups—particularly oppressed groups—other issues such as cultural worldview and culture-specific or context-specific issues are unrelated to oppression per se and are peculiar to individual groups. These issues must also be considered in the course of effective therapy.

Finally, not all members of a particular group will have problems with every issue, even if it is a common concern among members of the group. These three layers of difference: (1) cross-cultural patterns of oppression, (2) group-specific issues, and (3) individual differences should be considered when working with all clients. Too many groups exist to introduce within a single book all the cultural issues involved, so it must be said that learning about cultural differences is a journey, not a destination.

THE EFFECTS OF CULTURE

Culture directly contributes to people's habits, communication patterns, family structure, values, norms, and expectations, even in places they do not expect. People of different cultures may eat different foods, spend their time in different ways, and celebrate different holidays. They may perceive coming of age, sex, sexuality, and their bodies differently. Euro-American women, for example, tend to perceive beauty as something that results from being thin and young, while African American women value thinness less and see beauty as something that comes from individual flair. They also expect to become more beautiful as they grow older (D. Sue, Sue, & Sue, 2000). In addition, different members of a culture experience different patterns of privilege and oppression in their daily interactions with other members of their group and with other groups. Understanding one's own culture and those of clients will help therapists understand their clients' needs and will show them effective ways to intervene.

Without being directly taught, people learn about how they should speak and how closely they should stand. They learn to make eye contact at some points and to look away at others. People learn how to dress for particular occasions and when and how they should appear for them. These patterns are often subtle and rarely directly communicated, yet they often define a culture so well that a foreigner can be identified without even opening his mouth.

A culture's values about time, independence, intimacy, autonomy, achievement, and the like influence behaviors and how others perceive them. Some actions such as deciding to have more than two children, keeping a three-year-old in diapers, or sharing a bed with a five-year-old may be typical in one culture, but be seen as unusual and problematic by another. Both the "problem" behavior and the observer's judgments are, however, grounded in valuing decisions. Should a child be encouraged to individuate or to stay close to parents? The answer one gives to this and to similar questions will determine his or her actions and the way he or she is viewed by others.

A Bahamian student commented on the habit of U.S. students of gathering their books and possessions before the end of a class period (P. Rigby, personal communication, April 19, 2002). The girl noted that when she first came to the States she considered this behavior to be very rude ("You should listen to elders until they are finished talking"). After living in the States for a while, she recognized that this behavior not only reflected differences in respectful interactions with elders, but was also grounded in the time orientation common to most North Americans—a group that never wants to be late to the next class. Perhaps this is a different, equally valid, indicator of respect.

Finally, group membership within a society, has meaning. Belonging to a group, as discussed further in chapter 4, may either afford a person privileges or deny them. Group membership may also afford privileges in one setting and deny them in another. An example is when an African American male is welcomed in some social settings, but Euro-Americans cross to the other side of the street or grab their purses when they spot him. Group members often signal their membership when it may be otherwise un-clear—and even when it is clear—to "outsiders." They do this with cloth-ing, jewelry, hairstyles, and names that signify their membership and com-municate their attitudes about being connected to the group.

Relative Roles of Individual and Cultural Differences

Sometimes, people overlook cultural issues, misunderstand others' inten-tions, and inappropriately attribute their observations to traits. However, at other times they search for cultural issues to help them understand others. L. M. Fygetakis (1997) describes this process for one woman:

> It used to drive me crazy when I was little and we would visit the relatives in Greece. They would always ask me, "Which are you? Are you Greek or are you an American?" Of course, if you didn't want to get lectured on the supreme importance of Greek civilization and our proud heritage in de-mocracy, philosophy, theater, the Olympics, etc., you knew what you had better answer . . . except I always said, "Both!" (p. 158)

This woman's relatives presumably wanted to know her cultural iden-tity for two reasons: (1) whether she valued Greece's contributions to West-ern culture and, more importantly, (2) whether she identified with the United States or Greece—with all that it entailed. The latter question as-sumes an essentialist position, where all Greeks, U.S. citizens, women, les-bians, and others are believed to share common characteristics. This as-sumption can lead to an overreliance upon stereotypes. The validity of this essentialist assumption is examined next.

Using a statistical analogy, two cultures can be thought of as being like two distributions with different means; their standard deviations can also differ. Two cultures may be only slightly different on a particular dimen-sion, as in figure 3.1a, or very different, as in figure 3.1b. Despite these smaller or larger between-group differences, there may be significant within-group differences that can be greater than the difference between the groups (S. Sue, Zane, & Young, 1994). This variability may be so great that it makes using only a single criterion to identify the members of each group very difficult. For example, while men and women are statistically different in their mathematical abilities on standardized tests, the ability to identify the gender of the test taker based on math scores alone is quite poor until the very high end of the distribution (Hyde, Fennema, & Lamon, 1990). However, people tend to "sharpen" these differences, so that differ-ences between the two groups appear larger than they really are (Eagly, 2000; Kenrick et al., 1999). Even with numerous predictor variables such as race, ethnicity, gender, age, and the like, the ability to predict accurately rarely reaches 100% because of very tall and physically aggressive women and short and nonaggressive men.

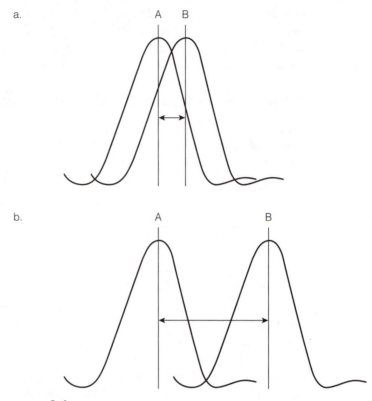

FIGURE **3.1**

The relative importance of between and within group differences in cultures where there are (a) small between-group differences or (b) large ones. In the second set of distributions it would be much easier to identify the individual's "culture" accurately.

These issues are significantly complicated by the fact that most racial and cultural groups, as they are commonly discussed in the literature, are extremely diverse (Hardy, 1990; S. Sue et al., 1994), including many groups that consider themselves to be very different from one another and who may not even get along amiably. The term *Asian American* generally refers to people who trace their lineage to non-Soviet Asia and to the surrounding islands, including China, Japan, North and South Korea, the Pacific Islands, the Philippines, and Vietnam. Native Americans trace their culture to one of between 547 and 1000 native peoples (Helms & Cook, 1999). Latins may trace themselves to the Caribbean and Central or South America. Blacks may be African American, Afro-Caribbean, or African. Whites living in different parts of the United States, while superficially similar, may have dramatically different values, goals, and concerns (cf. D. Cohen, 1998; D. Cohen, Nisbett, Bowdle, & Schwarz, 1996).

Make a list of your friends and relatives or other people you know well. Try to rank them according to the following variables as fairly as you can: height, verbal skills, mathematical skills, empathy, emotional expressiveness, and aggressiveness. If necessary, separate your groups into High, Medium, and Low amounts of each attribute. Pay attention to the attributes you use to rank the members on your list. Do you use the same kinds of behaviors for each person? If not, why not? Complete your rankings before going on to the next paragraph.

Now, go back and look at the patterns in your lists. Highlight all of the members of one sex. Do your rankings follow gender stereotypes? Does any one person match all of his or her gender stereotypes? Would gender be sufficient to separate the males and females on your list? Why or why not? If you were to use different behaviors to define each behavior, would this change your rankings? If so, how? If you feel that your rankings were distorted by the kinds of people you used for your "sample," go back and add other people who are extreme on one or another of your dimensions. How does this change your findings?

Research with one group is often generalized to other superficially similar groups, and this complicates understanding. Members of the larger group may be studied without distinctions being made among peoples of different origins. An example is Asian Americans from different countries of origin (S. Sue et al., 1994). Cultural and historical factors of these disparate, but superficially similar groups are sometimes ignored at great risk. For example, although Mexican Americans have a history of oppression and relative powerlessness, Brazilians coming to this country often have had a very different experience, having been members of the majority group throughout their lives and not having experienced a history of oppression (DeSouza, 2000).

Limitations of Using Culture as a Predictor

Culture is an important predictive variable, but as the exercise shows, all members of a group clearly are not alike. Helms (1994; Helms & Cook, 1999) argues that this is partially due to the tendency to use demographic variables such as Latina, female, or lesbian as though they are necessary indicators of cultural or socioracial background. For example, biracial children or those adopted outside their race may identify by their minority status, while some may incorporate the customs, traditions, and values of one group and share the social and political experiences of others.

Susie was a college student who had been adopted from Korea as a toddler and raised by Euro-American parents. She was baffled when strangers discriminated against her as an Asian American and voiceless when her classmates asked her to comment on her experiences as an Asian American. While she recognized her obvious ethnic background, she identified as White. Her experiences, values, and sense of identity were very different from either those of an exchange student from Korea or of a first generation Korean American with whom she is physically more similar—and more similar to her Euro-American adoptive parents with whom she identified. On the other hand, she experienced many of the same stereotyping, prejudices, and discrimination that other Korean Americans did.

These examples begin to separate racial identity, which is the understanding of one another as racial beings and the manner in which one appears to others as racial beings (C. E. Thompson & Jenal, 1994). People who appear White may identify as a member of another racial group and vice versa (cf. McBride, 1996; Sandler, 1993). Even within the same family, people of the same racial background may self-identify differently (Karrer, 1990).

> I, as a woman of Asian racial background, may declare myself a woman of color because I see myself as belonging to a group of ethnic/racial minorities. However, my (biological) sister could insist that she is not a woman of color because she does not feel an affiliation with our group

TABLE  **VARIABLES TO ASSESS WITH NEW CLIENTS, DEPENDING UPON THEIR ETHNICITY, SEXUAL ORIENTATION, CLASS, RELIGION, HISTORY OF SEXUAL ASSAULT, AND MARITAL STATUS OF PARENTS**

Ethnic Immigrants and Their Descendants
- Place of birth
- Number of generations in the United States
- Nature of family roles and structure
- Nature of gender roles
- Language spoken in the home
- English fluency
- Educational status
- Economic status
- Degree and kind of acculturation into the majority culture
- Cultural traditions practiced
- Religion
- Community and friendship patterns with other ethnic immigrants and the majority group
- Nature of experiences bringing them or their ancestors to this country

Note: From Diller, 1999; Erickson & Al-Timimi, 2001; Ponterotto, 1987; Yi, 1995.

Gays, Lesbians, and Bisexuals, and Transgendered People
- Relationship status
- Levels of self-acceptance and acceptance from family, friends, and coworkers
- History of discrimination and physical and/or sexual assault
- Relative size and level of political activism in the local GLBT community
- HIV status of self and partner
- Number of AIDS-related deaths within social circle
- Suicidality, particularly among adolescents
- History of substance abuse, particularly among lesbians

Note: From Cochran, 2001; Goldfried, 2001; Greene, 1997.

Socioeconomic Class
- Expectations of economic culture such as strength, athletic prowess, particular form of beauty, interpersonal relationships, and aesthetics
- Degree of awareness and acceptance of dominant culture's values
- Mechanisms for meeting expectations
- Mechanisms for resolving potential conflicts between economic culture and dominant culture around the above
- Styles of expressing anger and frustration

Note: From Liu, 2002.

Religion and Spirituality
- Relevance and importance of religion to life
- Current level of commitment to religion relative to desired level
- Motives for religious involvement (intrinsic or extrinsic)
- Religious attributions for past mistakes and current problems, as well as beliefs about the possibility of redemption
- Tendency to dichotomize people, including therapists, into good/bad, like me/not like me
- Perceived conflict between life and salient religious or spiritual doctrines
- Degree of perceived support within church or spiritual community
- Number of religious adherents relative to community as a whole
- Perception of religious adherents in greater community (and vice versa)

Note: From Bergin, 1991; Worthington, 1988.

(continued)

TABLE **3.1** *(continued)*

History of Sexual Assault
- Age when assaulted
- Education
- Marital status when victimized
- Duration of abuse
- Frequency and severity of abuse
- Presence of other types of abuse
- Nature of the relationship between client and perpetrator such as relative, friend, or stranger (positive, negative, or neutral)
- Nature of the relationship between client and perpetrator (positive, negative, or neutral)
- Nature of the relationship between client and significant others
- Reactions of significant others to disclosure of the abuse
- Coping mechanisms

Note: From Courtois, 1988; Follette, Alexander, & Follette, 1991; Hindman, 1989; Rind, Tromovitch, & Bauserman, 1998.

Children of Divorced Parents
- Appraisal of level of control
- Attributions about divorce
- Style and effectiveness of coping strategies
- Level and nature of parental conflict
- Psychological health of parents
- Quality of parenting strategies and nature of relationship with parents
- Quality of support network including family, school, and community

Note: From Pedro-Carroll, 2001.

goals, even though she is a person of Chinese ancestry. Does her nonaffiliation take her out of the group of people of color? Or does she remain in it regardless of her own self-identification because of her obvious physical characteristics? Generally, in the context of identities based upon racial and physical characteristics, ascribed identities will, rightly or wrongly, continue to be attributed to individuals by others. It is left up to individuals themselves to assert their identities and demonstrate to others that they are *not* what they might appear to be upon first notice. (Chan, 1997, pp. 240–241)

Assessing only race and ethnicity would cause some to rely on stereotypes and to make inaccurate predictions. Assessments must also be made of place of birth, number of generations one's family has lived in the United States, family roles and structure, the language spoken in the home, English fluency, educational and economic status, degree of acculturation, cultural traditions practiced, religion, and community and friendship patterns (Diller, 1999; Saba & Rodgers, 1990; Yi, 1995). See table 3.1 for variables to assess when dealing with new clients.

A recent immigrant from Nicaragua working as a dishwasher and living in substandard housing will face different issues than will the well-educated son of Mexican immigrants who works as a stockbroker. While both are Latinos and may be the same age, the concerns they bring to therapy will

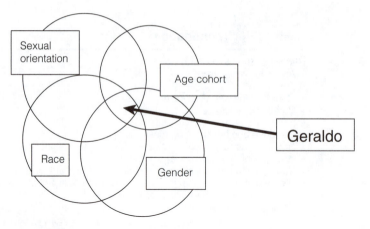

FIGURE 3.2

Geraldo is influenced by multiple, overlapping contexts (i.e., race, sexual orientation, age, gender, etc.), no one of which can fully explain him.

probably be very different. The Nicaraguan immigrant may be struggling more with issues of poverty, a language barrier, and cultural misunderstandings, and may worry about his family remaining in his native village. The Mexican American stockbroker's concerns may involve his parents' unhappiness with his degree of acculturation and abandonment of traditional values, the shifting roles and structures within his family, and his attempts to achieve professional success without denying his ethnicity and traditions. Seeing culture without the moderating variables of class, education, and degree of acculturation severely limits the therapist's ability to understand these two very different men.

The variables that Diller (1999) and Yi (1995) identified can be important when working with Latinos, but other variables will be useful as well. These may include the gay population, women, or people with a history of sexual assault (see table 3.1). In effect, race and ethnicity may be the first—but only the first—branch on a decision tree that enables therapists to make finer predictions about the nature of the issues that a client may face. Nevertheless, the predictions made by following this decision tree should be, at best, a first approximation. Many clients identify with and are influenced by multiple cultural groups (see figure 3.2); in fact, it may be more than a thousand cultures and roles at any one point in time (Pederson, 1990, cited in Ridley, Mendoza, Kanitz, Angermeier, & Zenk, 1994).

Geraldo is a gay Latino from Cuba, but he is also elderly and well-educated. These multiple influences can be recognized when Geraldo becomes Geraldine, an elderly and well-educated lesbian from Cuba. The sex change alters predictions about the issues that may be influencing him.

Geraldine, in identifying herself as a lesbian, both violates the cultural mandates for indirectness and face-saving that also control Geraldo's behavior, but it also acknowledges her sexuality and sexual behavior despite gender-specific cultural prohibitions about discussing them (Greene, 1997; Vontress, Johnson, & Epp, 1999). These prohibitions are important to Cuban Americans, but they are incomprehensible to Brazilians, who often do not differentiate between heterosexuals, homosexuals, and bisexuals in the way North Americans do. Their argument is "There's no sin south of the equator" (DeSouza, 2000).

Although Geraldo is an elderly, male, gay, and well-educated Cuban immigrant to the United States, not all of these groups influence him equally. He can be expected to identify with some groups more than others and be influenced by other group identifications (Ridley et al., 1994). Elliot (1999), for example, quotes one Afghan tribesman whose ideas strongly state this idea:

> Firstly we are Pushtuns . . . and secondly we are Moslems. Lastly we are either (this with a dismissive wave) "Afghans or Pakistanis." (p. 52)

This sense of group membership may fluctuate depending on the circumstance—such as being the only Cuban American in the room, as opposed to being one of many—and it should be assessed early in treatment.

Furthermore, Geraldo's cultures only partially convey who he is. His experience contextualizes him. How and when did he come to the United States? How has his income changed since going there? Has he been able to be open about his sexuality? What have been the consequences? Has he felt dismissed, marginalized, tolerated, or perhaps accepted?

Similarly, Tolman (1991) discusses the socialization process that creates ambivalences about sex and sexuality among young women and causes some to deny their feelings. While most women receive messages about inhibiting their sexuality, this socialization is complicated by other cultural factors. For women with a history of sexual abuse, dissociating from their body is consistent with messages about gender roles, but it may also be a way of protecting themselves during the abuse or from memories. A lesbian's ability to become aware of her sexuality may be complicated by messages that she should not be aware of her sexual feelings and, especially, her attraction to other women.

Culture Influences Rather Than Determines

Instead of determining who a person is and what her or his issues are, context provides a rich set of hypotheses about the unspoken issues that a new client confronts (Vontress et al., 1999). Upon meeting Patience, a 24-year-

Spend a few minutes thinking about the cultural groups that define your identity. What is your race and ethnicity? What is your gender, affectional orientation, religion, physical ability, and age cohort? Which of these seem most important to you? Are other group memberships important? If possible, rank these in terms of how much each influences who you are. Would you have ranked these differently at other points in your life? If so, why?

old Euro-American woman with a history of sexual assault, her therapist began assessing these predictor variables. Who assaulted her? Was she able to disclose the assault? How did her family and friends respond to the disclosure (refer to table 3.1). As the therapist was discovering facts about her: (1) molested by a favorite uncle from age 8 until she was 12, (2) refusal by single-parent mother to believe her when she disclosed the abuse, and (3) that her most recent and most serious boyfriend dropped her like a hot potato upon learning that she had been raped, the therapist began to make some guesses about important issues affecting her.

She began to wonder about Patience's beliefs about the relationship between love and pain. Does Patience believe that love must occur in the midst of pain, chaos, and crisis, as she experienced with her uncle? Does she have difficulty seeing a calm and continuously supportive relationship as loving? Does she believe that she has the right to share her feelings and to be assertive about them? If she shares her thoughts and feelings, will she be believed and accepted? Will her thoughts and feelings be taken seriously and acted upon or will they be dismissed and belittled? Although these are reasonable hypotheses, they cannot be accepted as givens and must be investigated in the course of therapy.

THE IMPORTANCE OF GROUP MEMBERSHIP

Some of these cultural groups will seem to be "normal" or to have no effect if the group is a majority group ("It's just the way people are"). In fact, many White clients will not report that their race and ethnic background are important to them. Many, however, will report that religion is a very important influence. The fact that race and ethnicity do not *seem* to have a significant influence may lead some dominant group members to complain that, relative to other groups, "I don't feel I have any culture of my own" (Diller, 1999, p. 23). Therefore, some may become envious of ethnic groups that have a strong cultural history that is distinct from mainstream U.S. culture.

Take a few minutes to describe a friend. What do you include in your description? Why?

Minority group membership, on the other hand, can have a disproportionate impact and influence upon who a person is. When this is true, it does not mean that dominant group culture has had no influence, but that minority group membership explains a larger proportion of the variability in the differences from mainstream expectations and norms. Similarly, chimpanzee and human DNA are 99% alike (King & Wilson, 1975). Although this 99% is important in determining those things that are similar such as number and relative placement of arms, legs, eyes, and ears, the relatively small *differences* are incredibly important in differentiating between the two species.

Relative Importance of Different Group Memberships

Chances are that the descriptions given to the last question were of the unusual attributes of a person such as being 6' 4", freckled, red-haired, and always smiling, rather than of the many common characteristics in one's culture or community, such as having two eyes and two legs. Descriptions probably also depended on who might be receiving the information and why. When one wants to uniquely identify another, common responses include aspects that are different from the norm. Hair color would be useful in a family that included every possible color of hair. Hair color, however, would not be useful if everyone was a redhead. On the other hand, if a person was or should be a member of a group, aspects that were *similar* to other members of the group would be used. When introducing a friend to the basketball team and explaining that she would like to join, descriptions of her would include her height, her work ethic, her long hours spent in practice, and her skills as a team player.

By extension, two cultural groups may be very similar to one another, but the differences between them may be perceived to be especially important and frequently reported both anecdotally and within the research literature. Differences within a group may be de-emphasized in order to maintain group cohesiveness. For example, while the average size of reported sex differences is smaller than that generally reported in the psychological literature (Hyde & Plant, 1995), these differences distinguish two groups that are important both biologically and culturally. The importance of gender in any culture is clear when one thinks about their reactions to discovering that a friend or acquaintance has recently had a baby. Most people would ask, "Is it a boy or a girl?" perhaps even before inquiring about the health of the mother or child. As a result, the differences in the mathematical ability of men and women have been emphasized, even though they are small relative to the variability in mathematical ability between them.

Minority group membership may seem to have a disproportional influence on an individual's identity because of the importance of these differences in defining who he or she is in terms of cultural norms. Furthermore, minority group members must remain aware of the dominant group both to protect themselves and to discover ways to adapt to, or succeed within, the dominant society (Fiske, 1993; Lorde, 1984a; Wood & Mallinckrodt, 1990).

Being a member of a dominant cultural group may *seem* to have little effect on members, but it influences their values, behaviors, and customs. Without an awareness of the relativity of these, everyone might accept others' outlook and values, even when they are not true. What appears to be givens—that Whites are the majority of the world's population and that virtually everyone has a computer—are not. One's cultural worldview may blind them to differences, especially as to how others see the world.

THE EFFECTS OF EURO-AMERICAN CULTURE ON THERAPY

Katz (1985) describes how Euro-American culture can be deceptively "plain vanilla," yet have real and unexamined implications for the therapy process and its choice of goals (see table 3.2). The culture's individualistic and autonomous assumptions might cause therapists and clients to conclude that the clients' problems are intrapsychic rather than cultural or systemic and to believe that clients should take charge of their own problems. Middle- and upper-class individuals with this cultural background often believe that problems are best resolved by thinking and talking about them (Helms & Cook, 1999). Thus therapies are often highly dependent upon verbal skills, insight, and a thinking style that is open to the scientific process. On the other hand, the autonomous orientation of Euro-American culture can lead both therapists and clients to believe that they must *do* something to make things different. Clients, especially males, often enter therapy feeling weak because they have been unable to solve their problems on their own.

Furthermore, while some psychiatric syndromes are identified as problems in almost every culture as well as by the vast majority of individuals within these cultures, some syndromes are culture-specific (Al-Issa, 1982). Pathology is often identified by the degree of divergence from dominant cultural norms (Fontaine & Hammond, 1994; Katz, 1985). In this case, the greater the difference between the values and behaviors of Euro-American culture and the client's behavior, the more likely it is that the person will see the differences as a problem. This is always a greater concern when context has been removed and when a rationale for the behavior cannot be seen. For example, people are more likely to think that someone who is muttering and hitting her ear has a problem, but not if they are told that she has a bug in her ear.

This individualistic and autonomous orientation may cause therapists to derogate clients. Janet has an external locus of control and blames society for closing off options ("Employers are afraid to hire lesbians"). Nanci is accused of being "dependent" for thinking of her elderly mother's needs before her own. The rational, scientific, and materialistic basis of Euro-American culture can cause therapists to misunderstand Hiroshi, who is seen as superstitious because he checks the almanac every day to determine his fortune, which he hopes will answer the problems he faces.

In sum, Euro-American therapists who want to move beyond the monocultural assumptions of the dominant culture will need to become at least

TABLE 3.2   WHITE MIDDLE-CLASS CULTURAL COMPONENTS AND HOW THEY INFLUENCE A THERAPIST'S ACTIONS AND PERCEPTIONS DURING THERAPY

Component	Description	Implications for therapy
Rugged individualism	The individual is the focus and is valued for being independent, autonomous, and able to master his or her environment.	Problems are (1) intrapsychic in nature rather than systemic, (2) best solved by oneself, and (3) resolved by knowing oneself and taking charge. People may believe they are weak if they need help in doing this.
Action orientation	People must do something to solve their problems.	Controlling their lives and environments is useful. Problems are caused by being passive. Clients must replace inaction with control and mastery of their environment.
Status and power	External credentials, material possessions, and prestige determine one's social status and power.	Therapists are experts who earn their expertness from paper credentials. They know the cause and appropriate treatment better than their clients.
Communication rules	A person must use standard English to discuss problems and should do so directly and assertively.	Clients should discuss their issues in fluent English. Therapists should reflect feelings and concerns raised by clients. Clients who do not discuss concerns directly are "passive," "not insightful," "dependent," or "unassertive."
Time	Time is a valuable commodity that can be quantified.	Therapy appointments are scheduled for a fixed amount of time, starting and ending on time.
Aesthetics	The "best" people exhibit European physical and cultural attributes.	Clients who do best in traditional therapy are young, attractive, verbal, intelligent, successful (YAVIS), and white.
History	Anything worth knowing or being has its basis in Europe or in White America.	Clients are seen as pathological to the degree that they vary from Western values and individualistic frameworks.
Family structure	The male-dominant nuclear family, with the female doing the majority of the caretaking is the normative and ideal socialization unit.	Clients and families differing from these ideal, gender-based family roles and structures are "abnormal."
Rational empiricism	Everything of importance can be quantified. That which is rational, objective, linear, and parsimonious is best.	Traditional Western theories and measures are preferred, and they describe a client's experience better than the client can. Psychological experience is preferred over physiological experience.

Note: Modified from Katz, 1985.

moderately bicultural and knowledgeable about the issues, values, and unique behavioral and interactional patterns of their clients' cultures. This occurs in a context of knowing oneself and recognizing common patterns of thinking, feeling, and behaving, while also appreciating the uniqueness of a person's culture and patterns of social oppression (Croteau & Hedstrom, 1993; Fontaine & Hammond, 1994). Neither this self-knowledge nor the understanding of widely differing cultures can occur overnight, but it is part of a lifelong journey that is enriched through reading and by learning about other groups.

Normality: Perceiving the World Through Culture's Filter

One's perception of events occurs in a cultural and valuing context that influences what they view as normal (G. S. Howard, 1992; Katz, 1985; E.W. Kelly, 1995). While suggesting that others respect cultural and subcultural differences, Fontaine and Hammond (1994) also emphasize the importance of cross-cultural *similarities* and suggest that therapists use standards from their own life as benchmarks to assess their clients' behavior. This clearly is valuable during the course of therapy ("How would I feel if my partner said that?" or "This child is much more active than other 8-year-olds I've seen"). Although using one's own experience can lead to parochial assessment and decision making, Fontaine and Hammond remind therapists to continually examine their objectivity and point of view by discussing their clinical hypotheses with others sharing more commonalities with the client.

Consultations around cultural issues may require that therapists question the culturally limited meanings of their perceptions. For example, Minuchin and Nichols (1993) oppose the status quo of Euro-American culture, arguing that words and phrases such as being alone, giving in, dependency, and initiative "carry an aura that comes from the value our culture places on the rugged individual" (p. 58). When confronted, most people can think about ways to compromise without feeling like they are lost. They may even be able to create a win-win solution. Many clients, however, have a difficult time turning to others for help, seeing this dependency as a sign of "weakness." Moving beyond the values with which anyone has been raised can be difficult. However, helping a client to reframe a problem and to challenge accepted values is an asset both to the culturally different and to those of the dominant culture. "We can be dependent without being weak."

To some degree, being able to move beyond a valuing stance requires exposure to other values and being challenged to change this point of view. As discussed in chapter 6, this change is more likely to occur when people have recognized the costs of their beliefs or the benefits of others'. Attitude change is also more likely to happen when the other person or group is more attractive, powerful, or personally important. As a result, it is possible for the members of the dominant group to change their beliefs and values, but there are greater impediments for them than may exist for other members of the minority group.

Because most people identify normality based upon what is typical in their experience, being a member of the dominant group creates the background against which these differences are compared. If most people in a culture maintain good eye contact when talking, they are more likely to see this as the way things should be and may then ascribe positive intentions to eye contact and negative intentions to its absence. For example, Euro-Americans generally see maintaining eye contact during a conversation as showing interest in the other person's ideas and as being respectful. In contrast, they view limited eye contact as exhibiting social anxiety, being ashamed, or lying. Nonetheless, eye contact is not universally accepted as a measure of respect and interest (Ivey & Ivey, 2003). In fact, African American, Asian American, and Native American cultures hold this behavior in low regard. Members of these groups often perceive eye contact with someone of greater power or authority as rude and unbecoming. Note that each culture ascribes negative intentions to behaviors that are atypical within their own group.

The fact is that people tend to compare their observations to expectations derived from their cultural background. Zhang (2003a) describes an African American colleague's misperceptions of a Native American audience's reactions to his talk. Zhang's colleague concluded that his talk was "a complete failure . . ., they are not interested," because the audience was silent (p. 94). Zhang, using the same data, argued from a different sense of "normal" and asserted that the talk had been well-received. While an African American audience is more likely to demonstrate its interest by being active, asking questions, expressing emotions, and even talking directly to the speaker, Native American audiences tend to be silent even when interested. Zhang notes that Native Americans, as well as many Asian Americans, consider asking questions of a speaker to be immodest and disrespectful. Furthermore, both groups may fear that if the question is seen as ridiculous, the questioner could lose face. These groups use the same nonverbal and verbal responses, but exhibit them and interpret them differently.

The tendency to see one's own experiences as normal can put blinders on therapists, as was the case with Samantha in chapter 1. She had been raised in a household where her stepfather prostituted her to his friends. When she entered middle school, she believed this was a "normal" experience that her friends avoided talking about. This perception colored her expectations about dating relationships and made her adolescence difficult. The contradictory messages she received made things even more difficult. On the one hand, prostitution was normal, yet it was never discussed outside the home or in the media.

If therapists are going to work with clients outside of their own race, class, gender, and the like—and most do on a daily basis—they must learn to challenge what they see as normal. As Samantha discovered, just because something happens frequently does not mean that it is a normal or adaptive behavior. Clients will present with problems that therapists may have never seen before, and this will require stepping outside of personal history to determine whether these are indeed problems. Therapists must learn to help their clients think divergently about their experiences and recognize multiple ways to solve a problem, and therapy must involve examining the costs and benefits of each solution ("Does it work?"). Pragmatic therapists who recognize that a current solution is successful can often leave the "problem" alone.

For example, a common assumption is that children should be allowed to be children and not be forced prematurely into a parenting role. Larry, whose mother had operable brain cancer and was bedridden for several years while she recovered, took exception to a classroom discussion of the disadvantages of parentifying children. He argued that in the best of all possible worlds, he would like to have both of his parents healthy. However, he needed to be able to do something useful during his mother's recovery in order to cope with what otherwise would have been overwhelming anxiety and grief. He felt that cooking dinners, watching his younger siblings, helping them with their homework, and mowing the grass gave him ways of coping successfully with an otherwise extremely difficult situation. In fact, he was given more responsibility and was allowed to enjoy a few age-appropriate privileges, including joining the Boy Scouts, playing basketball, and visiting friends.

Family therapists tend to negatively view children in parentified roles, but many adults report having successfully handled being parentified. In fact, many therapists and others in the "helping" professions have this component in their background. High functioning teenagers with strong verbal skills and effective coping mechanisms often thrive as parentified children, especially when they are simultaneously encouraged to be kids (Minuchin, 1974; Boyd-Franklin, 1990). Unfortunately, some family therapists see the parentified children who attempt to compensate for weak or mentally ill parents and do not have the verbal skills and coping mechanisms to do the job well. Instead of jumping to conclusions, it may be better to wonder what actually works. Minuchin (1974) would challenge the rigidity of a system that has a parentified child, whereas Berg (1994) and O'Hanlon and Weiner-Davis (1989) might examine this solution and wonder when and how this role works and when it doesn't.

Stop and think about yourself. Are there times when you have trouble controlling your temper and times when you don't? What's different about these times?

THE EFFECTS OF CONTEXT

Sartre (1946/1965) describes people as being influenced by and understood best in their own context. If one person wants to know another, he or she "must inquire first into the situation surrounding [them]" (p. 60). Context, like culture, influences what people do. It colors why people do things and when and where behaviors will be accepted and negative responses drawn.

The effects of context can readily be seen with assertiveness. Assertiveness is a set of behaviors involving the way one expresses thoughts and emotions in a direct fashion. It includes recognizing one's legitimate rights and acting in one's own best interest without hurting others in the process (Halonen & Santrock, 1997). This is difficult for ethnic minorities in some settings (Wood & Mallinckrodt, 1990). Table 3.3 shows how Asian Americans may be comfortable being assertive in relatively less formal situations and with people of lower status, but be very uncomfortable doing so in more formal settings such as at work or in therapy. Native Americans, particularly those from agrarian groups, generally favor indirect ways of expressing themselves and may hint or tease as ways of expressing their opinions. However, who can be teased and who cannot is generally culturally proscribed. Traditional Latinas may receive significant support for being assertive at school or at work, but they will need to find ways of expressing their thoughts and feelings at home that are accepted within the cultural framework. Even Euro-Americans, who generally value assertiveness, often find that assertiveness is more difficult, particularly (though not always) with authority figures than with friends. Furthermore, Euro-American females often report having more difficulties being assertive than their male counterparts, perhaps because of gender messages that require them to be nice and considerate of others' feelings (Gilligan & Brown, 1992).

These contextual issues may compromise therapeutic work in the here and now whenever it fails to take into consideration that observations made in one situation may be different than in another. Beverly recognizes this variability in the following example:

BEVERLY: *Clare, you've had a very difficult time expressing your feelings here today, and I only discovered that I misunderstood you by accident. I wonder if it's this difficult for you to say how you feel when you're at home or with your friends. (Feedback, implied question)*
CLARE: *Often . . . but it seems worst when I'm stressed. Sometimes, I feel like I can't be clear about anything here. I just can't talk about everything that's happening at work. It's so overwhelming . . . .*

Context also affects the way people perceive events. Like culture, being aware of context or ignoring it can cause people to draw very different interpretations of their observations. Jackson, a 15-year-old African American, began drinking and using drugs heavily around the age of 10. He began skipping school and hanging out at all hours of the day and night with his friends. When he went home, he stayed in his room, rarely came out, and often slept 14 or more hours a day. Although he had previously been

TABLE 3.3   SOME COMMON CULTURAL PATTERNS TO ASSERTIVENESS

Assertiveness-related Values and Context	Effects of Cultural Values
African Americans Behavior and attitude are more likely to be perceived as more aggressive than those exhibited by Euro-Americans. Expressing true feelings is seen as "dangerous" in many contexts.	Often inhibit expression of true feelings "in public."
Arab Americans Family and group needs seen as more important than individual needs.	May have difficulty identifying individual needs and may feel guilty when they do, especially when individual needs come at the expense of the group.
Men generally act as head of the family, although women exert their influence in many ways.	Women are more likely to influence decisions indirectly or nonverbally, rather than directly.
Asian Americans Assertiveness seen as impolite. Emotional expression in public is not valued, and people will attempt to ensure that both parties "save face."	Assertiveness does not bring success. In informal situations, such as with friends or members of their own race, expression is easier than in more formal situations (with authorities, in counseling, in the classroom, or even with strangers). Assertiveness is associated with higher anxiety and guilt.
Respect and deference is valued and is given to authority figures such as elders and men.	Greater deference given to those seen as having more authority.
Contradictory viewpoints are not perceived as incompatible and can coexist. Synthesis or choosing between poles is unnecessary.	Tend to seek win-win, or conciliatory, solutions to challenges.
Subordination of individual to group needs is expected.	Expression of individual needs inhibited.
Modesty is expected.	Giving and acknowledging compliments seen as "immodest."
Subtlety is seen as respectful and an indication of manners, education, and refinement.	Direct confrontations seen as rude, immature, unmannered, and insensitive.
Harmony and balance are valued.	Assertive responses may be avoided to maintain harmony. Increasing confidence in the ability to be assertive especially appropriate.
Euro-Americans Assertiveness valued.	Assertive responses often encouraged by peers and family members.
Individual needs generally valued over group needs.	Group needs not highlighted during decision making.
Tend to use arguments and counter-arguments to examine the validity of a proposition and choose the "right" answer.	Individual needs chosen at the expense of group needs. Compromises chosen less frequently.

(*continued*)

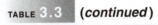

TABLE 3.3 *(continued)*

Assertiveness-related Values and Context	Effects of Cultural Values
Being assertive often seen as aggressive grab for power, especially when a power differential exists.	Assertiveness generally easier to express with friends, where there is little power differential. Assertive expressions easiest with strangers.
Women and girls are expected to be "nice" and to take care of others.	Assertiveness often easier for men to express than for women, especially when it might hurt others.
Latin Americans Respect, obedience, and deference to elders and family valued.	Socialization, especially for girls, is for teaching respectful and conforming behavior.
Assertiveness viewed as undermining of authority and disrespectful.	Assertiveness more difficult with men and authority figures. Formal situations are less threatening than with family, especially with parents and grandparents. Assertiveness is generally easier for men than women.
Native Americans Nonaggression, cooperation, and deference, especially toward elders, are valued.	Indirect expressions of feelings and attitudes are acceptable; direct expressions are proscribed.
Focus is on group needs over individual needs.	Purpose of communication is to maintain group harmony, not to assert individual needs.
Anger seen as the cause of negative energies that "pollute" others. Eventually, anger can cause physical illnesses.	Anger often repressed and may be related to alcoholism or other "problems in harmony."

Note: From Duncan, 1976; Erickson & Al-Timmi, 2001; Gilligan & Brown, 1992; Gonzalez-Ramos, Zayas, & Cohen, 1998; Tafoya, 1990; Peng & Nisbett, 1999; Wood & Mallinckrodt, 1990; Wang, 1999; Zane, Sue, Hu, & Kwon, 1991; Zayas & Solari, 1994; Zhang, 2003.

very close to his grandmother, he began to avoid her as well as other members of his extended family.

Jackson's mother and aunt, who were raising him, attributed these changes to his being bad ("He's just like his father"). He internalized this description—he liked the connection to his father—but he talked readily in therapy about being scared, especially about having the people who were close to him leave. The father he had been close to had walked out on the family four years earlier and was now believed to be drinking and using drugs. Four of his closest friends had died in the last three years, each under unusual and traumatic circumstances. His great-grandmother, one of his closest confidants and mentor, had died of a brain tumor the year before.

Knowing his history of losses can easily change the way to perceive his behavior. As seen in his community genogram (see figure 3.3), Jackson had

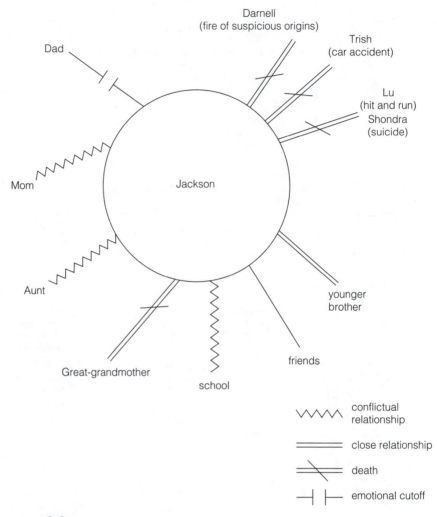

FIGURE 3.3

A community genogram for Jackson at age 15.

a number of significant losses. Although he had had a chaotic home life during his early childhood, these losses came rapidly over a short period of time and were correlated with the onset of his symptoms (see table 3.4). Unfortunately, his family seemed to perceive his connections with others like those drawn in figure 3.4, and they significantly underestimated the impact of these losses. From their point of view—without context—death or absence seemed to remove these significant individuals from his genogram. They also focused on their conflicts with Jackson at the expense of the connection. They underestimated the impact of his relationship with his

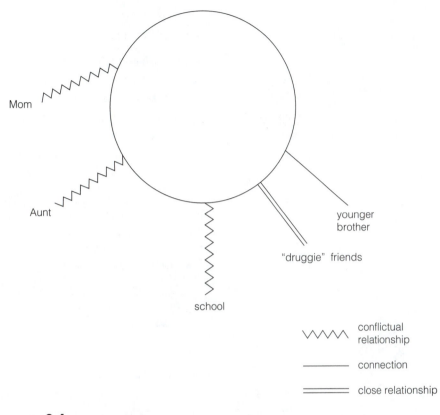

conflictual relationship

connection

close relationship

FIGURE 3.4

Jackson's family's apparent perceptions of his community genogram.

brother and exaggerated the strength of his relationships with what they called his "druggie friends."

Rather than being "bad," Jackson seemed to be depressed and afraid about who was going to leave next. His "devil-may-care" attitude and excessive sleeping could be seen as evidence of depression (Paniagua, 1998). His drug and alcohol use easily could be attempts to self-medicate. Rather than hating his family, which was something they believed he did, his history of being close to them motivated his willingness to continue valuing their opinions. However, he was afraid they would leave him, and he was even more worried that they would discover what a "terrible" kid he was. His social withdrawal (another possible symptom of depression) seemed to be an attempt to distance himself from people he was afraid would leave him or who would judge him in the same light as he judged himself.

Context changes everything. Knowing the context for Jackson's behavior allowed a reframe that turned out to be amazingly effective. He was seen eight times over a period of four months. He became less depressed

TABLE 3.4   **JACKSON'S TIMELINE**

July 1983	Jackson's parents get married.
June 1984	Jackson is born.
August 1985	Jackson's brother Jake is born.
September 1985	Jackson's father begins to work for the post office.
May 1987	Jackson's father is warned about drinking on the job.
March 1988	Jackson's father receives a second warning about drinking on the job.
June 1989	Jackson's parents fight while he is drinking. His mother receives a black eye.
1990	Jackson's father receives two tickets for DUI. His parents fight frequently. His mother ends up in the hospital on one occasion.
January 1991	His parents separate for a period of two months. His father continues to deny having a drinking problem.
September 1991	Jackson's great-grandmother is placed in a nursing home after breaking a hip.
1992	Jackson's father loses his driver's license and his job. He begins to work for Wal-Mart. His parents' fights become more frequent.
1993	His parents separate for one month. The fighting continues.
June 1994	His parents buy a house.
August 1994	His parents separate, this time permanently. They move in with Jackson's grandmother.
September 1994	Jackson's father disappears for three months.
December 1994	Jackson's mother begins to date David.
June 1995	Jackson's parents divorce.
September 1995	Jackson's mother marries David.
1995–99	Jackson sees his father once and receives no Christmas or birthday presents. He begins to fight with his mother and stepfather ("You're not my real dad").
January 1996	Darrell dies in a fire of suspicious origins.
1996	Jackson begins using drugs and becomes sexually active.
October 1996	Trish dies in a car accident.
June 1997	Jackson's great-grandmother is diagnosed with a brain tumor.
December 1997	Lu is killed in a hit-and-run accident.
February 1998	Jackson's great-grandmother dies.
October 1998	Jackson's baby sister Tylina is born.
December 1998	Jackson's friend Shondra commits suicide. Jackson had not believed she would take her own life.

and interacted more positively with his family. Accepting his family's definition of the problem—the drug abuse—and overlooking his strong connection with family members—and his significant history of losses—had the
potential of creating a self-fulfilling prophecy that would put him at even
greater risk. Sometimes, refusing to accept a reductionistic explanation of
a problem, backing away, and looking at alternative causes such as the
significant losses can be much more useful than intervening primarily with
the more proximal drug use (Emery, Fincham, & Cummings, 1992).

Seeing context differently can change how an event is viewed, and
it can be difficult to see, as with the ambiguous figure (figure 2.1, p. 11).
Madanes (1999), for example, describes a "relatively simple" case heavily
influenced by context. Her student was seeing a man whose father had died
two months earlier. The man's grief, not surprisingly, failed to respond to
antidepressants so his physician hospitalized him. At that point, he became
so depressed that he could not work, and he soon learned that his job was
in jeopardy. Madanes suggested that her student normalize her client's grief
response, saying that it would heal within a year. She told him to leave the
hospital and return to his family and job. He did and felt better immediately—although Madanes' student was fired "for disregarding the hospital
hierarchy" (p. 47). Paying attention to context rather than just biological or
intrapsychic factors can be as difficult as swimming against the current and
can be viewed, as Madanes says, as a "subversive" act.

Dangers of Perceiving Context

Seeing people in context can be de-pathologizing. Nonetheless, they need
to be held accountable for their behavior (Davison & Higgins, 1993). This
problem can be seen in an excerpt from Mr. Stevick, a teacher of Benjamin
Smith, who went on a racially motivated shooting spree in 1999.

> My hope in [our ability to identify and help troubled students] has not
> been completely shattered, but my naive belief that such bigoted or dan-
> gerous people would stand out clearly or have transparent beliefs has been
> shattered. As you read and hear more about this case, be cautious about
> attempts to demonize this student and others like him: I saw Ben laugh
> and smile, and this is perhaps part of what makes this horror so troubling.
> It is the banality of evil. These are not people in places besides our own,
> people who exude hatred at all times. Rather, they are people in our midst,
> people you may not notice, people with whom you may have a cordial ac-
> quaintance. Many who can be quite disturbed in one context may not ap-
> pear that way in our interactions with them. (D. Stevick, personal com-
> munication, July 7, 1999, reprinted with permission)

Stevick's letter identifies one of the "dangers" of ignoring context:
When people see how others behave in one situation or context, they may

conclude that this is how people behave in all settings. On the other hand, when people see context, they may excuse behavior or see it with overly rosy glasses ("He was under so much stress!). The point is not to *excuse* people or to overlook problems (see chapter 12), but rather to be aware that there may be times when there aren't problems. This can be a solution in the making, and there will also be times when there are problems. A good assessment will look at all of the contexts for a person's behavior without ignoring it in order to maintain the relationship or by focusing on the problem and neglecting the relationship (Clark, 1998).

CONCLUSIONS

When behavior's antecedents or context are not known, perceiving people and their behaviors pejoratively becomes easy. For example:

> DAD: *Ceci, go to your room! You are not to hit your brother!*
> DECI: *But Dad! I was just sitting here, and Joey hit me!*

Or,

> AUNT MIMI: *Matt? Stop crying!*
> MATT: *(Sniffing) But I just dropped the last glass of milk on my foot, and the glass broke, and I think my foot is broken, too!*

Knowing about Joey's behavior and Matt's spilt milk will probably change the interventions of both Ceci's father's and Aunt Mimi. Although Ceci's father may not say "Go ahead and hit your brother," he is less likely to intervene in a negative manner, at least toward Ceci. Sharing a full community genogram (see figure 3.3) shifted Jackson's mom's and his aunt's views of his behavior and reframed his behavior in a way that Jackson could accept. What had been senseless and "bad," now had considerable meaning—meaning that each could accept in a positive way.

An awareness of context allows therapists to reframe behavior, but it also enables them to identify clear solutions to a problem (Berg, 1994; de Shazer, 1988; O'Hanlon & Weiner-Davis, 1989). "When does the problem not happen, even a little?" is a good question that is very useful therapeutically. Knowing that Ceci is more likely to have a tantrum when she is tired, and less likely to when she gets to bed by 8:30 p.m., her father can locate and identify effective solutions. More importantly, this solution is based on a less pathological view of the problem—Ceci is tired rather than bad—a reframe that mends relationships instead of becoming barriers to them. Notice that reframing Jackson's behavior also served to heal his relationships.

This contextualized picture of human experience works best when the broad patterns in human experience and the uniqueness of individuals are recognized. The former abstraction helps therapists recognize patterns associated with race, class, age, gender, and the like, even though the associated danger of falling into stereotyping exists. Remaining aware of moderating variables such as degree of acculturation, fluency, degree of community support, and individual differences can reduce this danger.

OPPRESSION AND PREJUDICE

My oldest daughter's class was put into reading groups in first grade. I remember wondering whether she was in the "good" reading group and being thrilled to discover that she was, in fact, a Bluebird. I looked around at the other group members and saw that she was one of The Few. She was a Reader. I remember looking at some of the other children, those who were not privileged to be a member of my daughter's reading group, and I felt sorry for them because they could not read as well.

The reading group divisions disappeared at the beginning of second grade, and I no longer knew who read well and who did not. I discovered what I could have told you anyway, that these children each had their unique strengths and weaknesses. They were athletic, empathic, creative, good problem solvers, and well-behaved. I began to look at them in ways that went beyond the simplistic definition of reading level and saw them as people.

Obviously, I knew that there were many other attributes to consider and value, but at the beginning of first grade I was worried about how my daughter was going to do in school. She had just had a cataract removed and was largely blind in one eye. Focusing on the reading groups gave me one way of controlling my anxiety about her vision, her health, and having her in school. It also gave me a benchmark to help me identify whether she was going to be okay. I became less judgmental as I grew more comfortable with her vision and her school—and as artificial group divisions disappeared.

THE DEVELOPMENT OF GROUP DIVISIONS

Have you ever been on a team for a sport, a sorority, or a fraternity? How did you view the opposing teams you played against (or the other sororities or fraternities)? If competition and prejudice developed, what factors contributed? What was different when your team did *not* react negatively to other teams or groups?

Group divisions characterize the world: the United States versus Russia, Blacks versus Whites, women versus men, or a school, a department, even a grade against another. The dynamics of these divisions were readily demonstrated in Sherif's classic "Robber's Cave" study (Sherif, Harvey, White, Hood, & Sherif, 1961/1988). In it, two groups of bright, apparently well-adjusted White boys were set up in Robber's Cave State Park. Each group was initially unaware of the other and spent the first several days performing activities that were considered normal parts of any camping trip. The groups readily acquired their own identities, leaders, and names (e.g., the Rattlers and the Eagles).

At this point, the study researchers (Sherif et al., 1961/1988) initiated a four-day tournament that consisted of tug-of-war, baseball, a treasure hunt, tent pitching, and other games and competitions. The winning team members received trophies, medals, and camp knives, while the losing members got nothing. From the outset, the competition was hot. Fights broke out, a team's flag was burned, names were called, and a raid was conducted on the other team's cabin. When the Eagles won the tournament, the Rattlers stole the Eagles' trophy knives. The resulting confrontation was so heated that the two groups had to be physically separated and restrained to prevent a full-scale battle. As might be expected, at the end of a two-day period of cooling off, the boys continued to describe the opposing group as "sneaky," "smart-alecky," and "stinkers," even while they generally described members of their own group as "brave," "friendly," and "tough."

These descriptions were given despite the researchers' efforts to match the groups beforehand.

How did these changes come about? At least one way to think about this is as a type of self-fulfilling prophecy (Kenrick et al., 1999). The members of each group probably *were* brave, friendly, and tough, at least when working together with their own group members. However, when competing with the other team for limited resources, they saw the other team as a threat and they acted competitively and aggressively—as sneaky, smart-alecky stinkers! This, of course, confirmed the other team's expectations and increased that team's probability of also acting in a competitive and hostile fashion (Eagly, 2000).

As seen in this study (Sherif et al., 1961/1988), two or more groups brought together will generally (1) compete against one another, (2) see the members of the other group stereotypically (the out-group), and (3) put down the out-group's members. While they do this, they will hold the members of their own group (the in-group) in higher esteem. Prejudice and discrimination are most likely to occur when

- *Only a single winner can be had or limited resources are available* (Sherif et al., 1961/1988).
- *When the out-group is less powerful* (Fiske, 1993).
- *When situational cues suggest prejudice is acceptable* (Dovidio & Gaertner, 1999; Fiske, 1993; Noel, Wann, & Branscombe, 1995; Pryor, LaVite, & Stoller, 1993).
- *When people belong to a group that they view as "beneath them."* In this case, they often need to find other ways to support their sense of self-esteem (Crocker, Thompson, McGraw, & Ingerman, 1987).

Competition among groups and resultant prejudice and strife are not inevitable, and simple contact is not enough to reduce it (Sherif et al., 1961/1988). Several interventions, however, have been shown to reduce prejudice. These include having groups work cooperatively at a single task or against a common enemy (Sherif et al., 1961/1988); priming self-concepts, values, and norms that are inconsistent with prejudice and discrimination (Fiske, 1993); and creating a task that no single individual can complete on his or her own (Cook, 1985). See table 4.1 for an example.

Blaming the Victim and the Just World Hypothesis

Kenrick and his colleagues (1999) argue that prejudice against out-groups and attempts to support one's in-group is one consequence of the Just World hypothesis. They note that "Successful individuals . . . want to believe that they are entitled to their economic successes—that they have earned

TABLE 4.1	FACTORS THAT INCREASE AND DECREASE NEGATIVE AND PREJUDICIAL RESPONSES TOWARD OUT-GROUPS

Increased Competition
- Task is competitive.
- Task can be completed independently.
- Only a single winner, or group of winners, is possible. Example: Only the top 5% of the class can earn As.
- There are limited resources. Example: "What *you* get reduces what *I* can get."
- The other group is seen as less powerful.
- Membership in the in-group is not secure, especially when attempting to impress members of the in-group.
- Cues indicate that being prejudiced is acceptable. Example: Telling off-color jokes.
- Person is not reminded that fairness and responsibility are valued.
- Self-esteem is poor.
- Members of other group are anonymous and faceless.
- Differences among groups are highlighted.

Decreased Competition
- Task is cooperative in nature.
- Task *must* be completed with others' help.
- Multiple winners are possible.
- Unlimited resources are available.
- The other group is of equal or greater status.
- Membership in the in-group is secure.
- Situational cues indicate being prejudiced is not accepted. Example: A Human Resources office promotes and expects fairness toward protected groups.
- Person is reminded that fairness and responsibility are valued.
- Self-esteem is good.
- Other group's members are seen as individuals.
- Similarities among groups are highlighted. Example: Groups are seen as American citizens in opposition to terrorists.

Note: From Crocker et al., 1987; Dovidio & Gaertner, 1999; Fiske, 1993; Noel et al., 1995; Pryor et al., 1993; Sherif et al., 1961/1988.

their positions in life 'fair and square'" (p. 402). To believe that our successes are fairly won, we have to believe that others' failures are also fair.

Although hard work and perseverance account for a few of the differences between individuals, situational and cultural factors, as well as pure chance, certainly play roles in how well we do. These factors influence our successes and failures and encourage us to continue or cause us to give up. Being unaware of these contextual factors can generate a sense of hopelessness among out-group members that may perpetuate problems, which can be another kind of self-fulfilling prophecy ("What can I do? It won't get me anywhere").

When we are unaware of context, it's easy to engage in victim blaming and not focus on the perpetrator's actions and potential political, social, and contextual factors ("Why was she walking there?" or "What did he do to provoke them?"). Victim blaming has "positive" consequences for the rest of us. As long as we believe that rape, domestic violence, assault, and discrimination are problems caused by the victim instead of being symptoms of greater societal issues, the rest of us can safely step back and absolve ourselves of responsibility for both the problem and its solution. When we do so, our beliefs parallel the perpetrator's ("It's not my fault" or "She was so sexy" or "He provoked me"). To the degree that we accept the status quo without acknowledging the roles of context and by ignoring the sociopolitical uses of power and control, victims are twice injured (Raine, 1998). The personal *is* political.

Many individuals and groups are able to recognize this re-victimization. For example, as an adult, Horace was very angry at his mother who was also the object of serious domestic violence by her husband. She had done nothing to stop the terrible verbal and physical abuse that Horace and his sisters received at their stepfather's hand. His mother admitted to being appalled by the abuse, but thought of herself as an "innocent party" and failed to understand his anger toward her. Horace believed that his mother had colluded with the abuse by refusing to leave her husband and by failing to protect her children. He needed to have her move beyond her self-absorption and empathize with her children's viewpoints and needs. Horace wanted his mother to accept responsibility for her failure to act and to admit that her husband's actions had very real consequences—then and now. So, Horace asked her to affirm that the children had not been "bad" and that they had not deserved the abuse.

Neither the oppressor nor the oppressed is truly free. Horace's responses to his mother failed to acknowledge the real limitations on her behavior—financial, emotional, physical, and cultural—that made leaving her husband difficult. Horace's anger stemmed from an idealization of his mother and belief in her ability to respond freely—in a way that few parents truly are. Mothers are supposed to see all and know all, as is generally evidenced by their amazing and often prescient abilities (Hindman, 1989): "If she could tell I ate a chocolate bar, how could she not know about the abuse?" Mothers are often depicted as the serene and all-loving madonnas of Renaissance art ("How could she fail to protect me?").

SEEING STEREOTYPES, PREJUDICE, AND DISCRIMINATION

Sherif and his colleagues (1961/1988) describe competition as a "normal" or typical part of recognizing group differences. Group divisions have significant consequences that can include competition, stereotypes, prejudice, and discrimination. Stereotypes are positive and negative beliefs, prejudice is negative attitudes and feelings, and discrimination refers to behaviors that block opportunities based on group membership. The boys in

Imagine being introduced to someone who is gay, Muslim, or Latino. What are your initial reactions toward people in these groups? Will you make attempts to get to know them better or will you likely try to avoid them?

What do you think about people from these groups? Do you believe they are likely to be smart, funny, and hardworking? How about moral, immoral, or amoral? What do you think will be their strengths and weaknesses?

the "Robber's Cave" study initially had negative beliefs (stereotypes) about one another and tended to see the other group as sneaky, smart-alecky, stinkers. They also had negative feelings toward the other group (prejudice) and would naturally avoid them (discrimination) when given the opportunity. Stereotypes, prejudice, and discrimination become oppressive when they prevent a group from realizing its own potential.

Although prejudice, stereotypes, and discrimination often occur together, they are not necessary correlates. One group can have a negative attitude toward another group without acting on it. Reasons for the restraint may be that they know it would be wrong or because they are unable to act. On the other hand, one might not even be aware of negative attitudes, and certainly not report these—except in contexts where these attitudes are elicited and accepted (Banaji, Hardin, & Rothman, 1993; Dasgupta & Greenwald, 2001; Greenwald, McGhee, & Schwartz, 1998). Furthermore, whereas a person might not act in a prejudiced manner because group norms may prevent it, he or she may act in a discriminatory manner when other factors justify discrimination, as when the criteria for a position are ambiguous (Dovidio & Gaertner, 1999). Yet, these implicit biases may better predict nonverbal behavior than self-reports of racial attitudes (McConnell & Leibold, 2001).

In addition, most people hold negative *and* positive attitudes toward discriminated groups (Eagly, 2000): "Women are such wonderful, nurturing beings, but they just aren't as smart or assertive." These positive stereotypes can prevent a group from entering certain spheres when doing so is seen as inconsistent with certain roles and expectations ("Because they are so nurturing, women could never make it in management"). This prejudice and resulting discrimination are generally only seen when the affected group is agitating for greater rights or resources. Finally, discrimination can happen without negative feelings or attitudes, especially if it occurs unknowingly or in the context of "That's the way it's always been done," as in "I think women are great! We've just never hired any women for that position before."

Stereotypes are not necessarily bad, and they may even be adaptive in the sense that they are just a kind of concept. They can be a way of organizing the huge amounts of data that people experience each day into simpler ways of looking at the world. They can even be useful in therapy, as when Ghisela, a woman with a history of sexual abuse, first enters therapy and her therapist wonders about her ability to trust and to believe that her therapist will be a stable and predictable person in her life. However, when stereotypes are overly simplistic ("Nobody with a history of sexual abuse can ever trust") or are rigid and unmodifiable in the face of contradictory evidence, they can be problematic. Stereotypes are most useful when they are used to generate working hypotheses instead of seen as inevitable and unchanging descriptive laws ("Many people with a history of sexual abuse have difficulty trusting, but not all are incapable of it. Ghisela, in fact, is often quite gullible").

Our difficulties in predicting behavior from a simple knowledge of predictor variables come, at least in part, from the fact that it is the *meaning* we give to events that influences how people react, not the events themselves. The person's history, context, and belief system influence the meaning we give events.

SEEING SOCIAL INEQUITIES AND SOCIAL CONTROL

Buddhist teachings describe three types of pride that divide people:

- I believe that I am better than you.
- I believe that I am less good than you.
- I believe I am just as good as you.

Each of these principles involves some sort of objectification of self or other and fosters artificial distinctions among people. Buber (1970) recommends that we identify and challenge this tendency. As we identify and attack sources of oppression, privilege, and other kinds of objectification, we also encourage more real and authentic relationships.

Oppression

Hays (1995) defines oppression as the political and social inequities that marginalize or exclude groups of people. Oppression is often difficult to recognize because people may see oppressive acts as a norm or even as the way things *should* be (Steinpreis et al., 1999). Should women be paid as much as men for the same job or should men be paid more because, as some argue, they have a family to support? Should health care be available to all families, regardless of their income, class, and parents' sexual orientation or should it be available just for certain types of families? Is having different expectations and privileges fair and reality-based, or is it discriminatory and oppressive? Seeing oppression requires an ability to step outside of the common habits of perceiving the world in order to identify other possibilities.

People on both sides of the divide have difficulty seeing oppression. G. Greenberg (1997), however, notes that it is "[therapists'] expertise in understanding and giving voice to people's suffering [that] allows us to focus on its social origins" (p. 266). To be effective therapists we need to see the major traumas (e.g., rape, war, and murder) and learn to recognize the impact of more subtle sufferings. Most of us would recognize a lynching as a racist act; however, most oppression is much more difficult to see. It flavors the nature of daily interactions imperceptibly, as seen in this children's rhyme, "If you're light, you're right. If you're brown, stick around. If you're black, stay back" (M. Wright, 1998, p. 43). Similarly, Bartky (1975, in Pinel, 1999, p. 114) describes oppressive comments as including "innocent chatter, the currency of ordinary social life, or a compliment ('You don't think like a woman'), the well-intentioned advice of psychologists, the news item, the joke, the cosmetics advertisement. . . . Each reveals itself, depending on the circumstances in which it appears, as a threat, an insult, an affront, as a reminder, however subtle, that I belong to an inferior caste."

Because much of the oppression that exists is an integral part of daily life—in our nursery rhymes; vocational choices; and preferences for skin color, eye shape, hair color, and hair texture—it often goes unidentified. Oppression is like walking around with two-pound ankle weights—impediments that are overlooked until removed. Prejudice, discrimination, and oppression occur from outside and within the out-group, as when a parent uses color to reprimand: "Child, you get your black butt over here right now!" (Liu, 2002; M. Wright, 1998). Also, these statements are part of a ubiquitous system of social control. When Fahard's classmates call the top-achievers "Einsteins," it directly communicates that being too smart—like not being smart enough—is socially unacceptable.

Oppression is often associated with economic deprivations and loss of political power. Job barriers, glass ceilings, and political and social roadblocks are an everyday, "normal" part of life, yet often invisible. Kennedy (1976), for example, described the invisibility of political forces in this manner:

> Unless you are political or intellectual, events like the Depression are seen as personal events. We thought of the Depression as something that made the pipes freeze; we thought it hit us because Daddy didn't move his taxi stand and because he broke his hip. It was only later I found out it was a national phenomenon. (p. 31)

Ogbu (1986) reported that some minority group members, especially those that see these barriers as permanent instead of temporary, develop a collective institutional discrimination perspective, a belief that discrimination's effects will make it difficult for them to advance into the social and economic mainstream through their individual efforts alone. Working hard in school or on the job will not be "worth it" if hard work is not generally followed by the typical middle-class rewards of access to jobs, promotions, and increased pay. Instead, many African Americans reject middle-class Euro-American goals and believe that advancement can only occur through struggles to change the system or by bypassing typical routes that lead to middle-class goals.

TABLE 4.2   AREAS OF HETEROSEXUAL PRIVILEGE

- If I choose to be with other heterosexuals most of the time, I can be.
- My behavior and achievements are not seen as a reflection of my sexuality. I can do poorly and have it be *my* fault. I can do well without being "a credit to gays everywhere." I don't enter a situation and have to *prove* that I'm okay, smart, and a good friend.
- I can sit in a class or group without having to explain or defend my sexuality. No one will ask me, "Tell me about . . .," as though I know everything about everybody who is "like me."
- I can criticize my government and express my concerns about how much I fear its policies without having my opinions dismissed as those of an out-group member.
- When I am pulled over by a police officer or when my taxes are audited, I can be confident that the actions were not based upon my sexuality.
- I can expect that the police officer and auditor will be "like me" and, if they treat me unfairly, I do not have to worry about whether or not the treatment was because of my sexuality.
- I can go to my local mall and easily find posters, greeting cards, books, and children's magazines that depict other heterosexuals.
- I can go home from many meetings of organizations feeling that I do or can belong, as opposed to feeling isolated, out of place, outnumbered, unheard, unwanted, feared, or kept at a distance.
- I can go to a restaurant, get a hotel room, walk into a store, and take a class without wondering whether or not I will be allowed in or be mistreated because of my sexuality. I don't need to travel miles out of my way just because I have been mistreated at some establishment in the past.
- When I need legal or medical help, I don't need to worry about whether my sexuality will work against me.
- When I have "one of those days," I don't need to ask myself whether negative situations had prejudicial overtones.
- I can walk down the street holding my partner's hand, and I can kiss in public and disclose my sexual orientation to people without them saying or thinking, "Ooh, yuk!"
- I can marry a person to whom I am sexually attracted.
- We can file our tax return as "married."
- I can qualify for my partner's medical insurance and retirement benefits.
- I can visit my partner in the intensive care unit at the hospital and make end-of-life decisions for him without the hospital staff looking for a "real" relative.
- My partner and I can adopt without having people wonder about how our sexuality will affect our children.
- Our children can go to their friends' houses without having their friends' parents criticize our sexuality or attempt to prevent them from seeing one another.
- My partner can go to the school and make decisions for our children without the school demanding to talk to their "real" parent.
- Our children can endure problems, and our relationship can have problems without people relating them to our sexuality.
- I can rent a movie with major characters who are "like me" without having the characters' sexuality be trivialized or used as an easy source of humor.
- I can turn on the TV or open a newspaper and see others "like me" widely represented, often in positive ways.
- I can open our children's textbooks and find others "like me." When issues of national heritage are described, I can expect to discover that heterosexuals made them what they are.
- I can tell my family and friends about my sexuality without worrying that they will never talk to me again or that they will disinherit me.
- I can bring my partner home to meet my family and wonder only about whether or not they will like him, not whether they hope it's "just a phase."
- I can disclose my sexuality to my friends without having them assume that I'm attracted to them.
- I can expect people to feel comfortable while talking to me about my partner and sexuality, and I can expect that they will acknowledge the fact that there are other aspects of me.
- If I move into a new house or apartment, I can be reasonably sure that my neighbors will not respond negatively if I choose to disclose my sexuality.

(continued)

TABLE 4.2   *(continued)*

- When my neighbors meet my partner, I can expect that they will respond pleasantly, or at least neutrally.
- Furthermore, I can expect my new neighbors not to attempt to keep their children from us.
- I can worship in my faith without the rabbi, priest, or minister referring to us and our lifestyle as "abominations."
- I can be religious without people thinking this is a contradiction in terms.
- I can talk about my partner at work without my sexuality becoming a focus of gossip.
- I can lose my job or miss out on promotions on my own merits, and I do not have to worry that the decision was related to my sexuality.
- I can be aggressive, passive, or feminine and be interested in weight lifting, decorating, and cooking without people attributing it to my sexuality, although they may relate my interests to my gender.

Note: Adapted from McIntosh, 1989.

Finally, many people internalize oppression and make it their own, in effect, becoming part of the problem that perpetuates oppression. Watts and his colleagues (Watts et al., 2002) complain about the violent, antisocial, irresponsible, and misogynist lyrics that are often part of rap music. They note that young African American men adapt to societal oppression "by creating the character armor they need to protect themselves. They exude 'cool' and 'hard' exteriors that are a challenge to penetrate" (p. 48). Nonetheless, there are multiple images of any group. Watts and his colleagues use positive images from rap music in their psycho-educational support group to challenge the young men with whom they work to think critically about the negative images.

Privilege

Sometimes, oppression can be recognized only when its polar opposite, privilege, is seen. Because of factors such as class, gender, race, and ethnicity, some have privileges that others do not (Helms, 1999; McIntosh, 1989). See table 4.2 for a discussion of heterosexual privilege. Privilege that accrues from class, age, race, gender, and affectional orientation makes life easier and simpler for the privileged group, and it often does so in ways that are readily overlooked, as in "That's just the way it's supposed to be" (Helms & Cook, 1999; McIntosh, 1989; D. W. Sue et al., 1999; Yi, 1998). A Euro-American priest named J. Carroll (1996) described the difficulty he had with seeing oppression and privilege before he became actively involved in the Civil Rights movement:

> I accepted the assessment that Freedom Riders who courted arrest and the "direct action" demonstrators who defied redneck sheriffs did so for the sake of the now ubiquitous television cameras. Dr. King . . . wanted too much too soon. Freedom now! . . . I hated Bull Connor, but I also

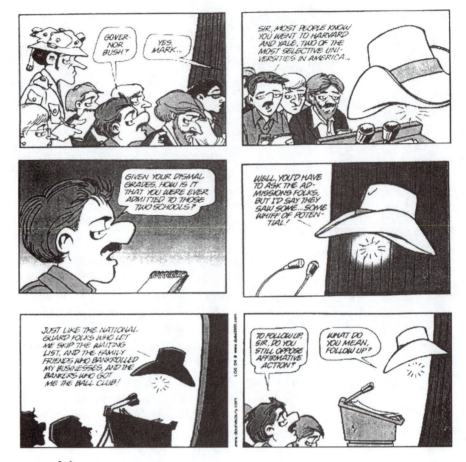

FIGURE 4.1

We may be blind to the role of privilege in our lives. (*Doonesbury* © 2000 G. B. Trudeau. All rights reserved). Reprinted with permission of Universal Press Syndicate.

thought the demonstrators he seemed to take such pleasure in clubbing brought it on themselves. And when . . . Medgar Evers was assassinated in Mississippi, I was appalled by the deed but critical of Evers also. . . . To me, Evers had been a misguided man who'd made the plight of his people worse, not better. (p. 133)

Doonesbury lampooned the ability of then-Governor George W. Bush to recognize the effects of privilege in his life (see figure 4.1). While Governor Bush may have been an easy target for ridicule on these grounds, everyone is vulnerable to the same criticism. Recognizing privilege requires that people step outside of their context and acknowledge the pieces that were fairly earned as well as the ones that came too easily.

Sometimes, it can be difficult to identify the source of privilege. I was in a drugstore in my small college town recently and watched the difficulties that two African American students were having in trying to return a hair dryer without a sales slip, a problem I've never had. Were their difficulties because they were African American? Was my experience with making a return easy because I'm not? Were their problems caused because they were students? Were the difficulties a result of the clerk's not recognizing them? How would these students explain the clerk's actions? Would they, like me, assume that they were being accused of shoplifting? Any comparison of one's own experiences with the plight of these students might highlight the degree to which one's own life is privileged and the students' is not. Note that areas of privilege often overlap: Some people's freedom from such hassles probably stems from sources such as their race, class, age, and interpersonal skills, and perhaps the history of such interactions in a small town.

Becoming aware of privilege is often difficult because it requires that we give up the Just World hypothesis (Kenrick et al., 1999; McIntosh, 1989; Razack, 1998; cf. Richie et al., 1997). We want to believe that life is what we make of it, that life is fair, that our society is just, and that life's rewards are commensurate with the work we put into it. Becoming aware of privilege means that we must also recognize that rewards sometimes come about through no virtue of our own and that others' misfortunes are sometimes unrelated to their actions. Becoming aware of privilege may also mean becoming aware of ongoing covert and overt discrimination (Hall, 1997). These are important things to remember in the therapy room:

> KOJI: *You've been talking about the problems you've had since losing your job and your confusion about why you lost it. It sounds like this is especially confusing because you thought you were doing everything right—you were there earlier, stayed later, had high productivity, and had even received recognition for your designs. Given what you've said about how you've been treated as a sex object at work, I wonder whether you see this action as gender-biased, too. (Summarization, interpretation in the form of a closed question)*

The privilege that is granted to heterosexuals (see table 4.2) should be applied across the board rather than being offered only to select groups (Hall, 1997; McIntosh, 1989). Everyone deserves to belong, to be seen as "normal" and "okay," to be expected to do well, to be evaluated on the basis of their work, to be given the benefit of the doubt in questionable situations, and to have their sexual orientation—as well as their gender, race, and class—made irrelevant when it comes to decisions about personal or professional competence. Privilege benefits the in-group, but it is oppressive to those groups that have not been endowed with it:

In proportion as my racial group was being made confident, comfortable, and oblivious, other groups were likely being made unconfident, uncomfortable, and alienated. Whiteness protected me from many kinds of hostility, distress, and violence, which I was being subtly trained to visit in turn upon people of color. (McIntosh, 1989, p. 11)

SEEING THE CONSEQUENCES OF OPPRESSION

School Performance

Pay attention to how others' expectations influence the way you perform. Does your boss think that you can do the work? Is your work viewed with an expectation that you will fail or succeed? How did your parents view you as a child? How did your teachers see you? Where have you performed best? Where was your worst performance? Do you work better when people acknowledge that you are competent or incapable? When are they supportive or unsupportive?

Successful performance of a task requires some degree of acceptance of, and internalization of, a domain's values and work ethic. However, in the process of becoming socialized to that realm—or perhaps just living in a society full of stereotypes and discrimination—we also learn negative stereotypes about our group (Banaji et al., 1993; Greenwald et al., 1998). Women aren't "supposed" to be good at mathematics. Men aren't "supposed" to talk about intimate and personal issues with other men. African Americans aren't "supposed" to perform well in school.

As we discussed in chapter 3, there are people who are like the stereotype and people who are not. However, some people who are not like the stereotype, such as men who enjoy intimate and personal friendships, may believe these messages about limits on their behavior and attempt to conform to them. This is an oppressive outcome of stereotypes (Steele, 1997).

One of my very bright friends explained her ambivalence about high school in this way, "My mom said girls shouldn't do well in school if they're going to get guys." Although she did well, she did not do as well as might have been predicted based on her later performance on the SATs.

Stereotypes are harmful, and they inhibit performance on a stereotype-relevant task when the category is salient (Steele, 1997, 1998). Activating stereotypes either directly or indirectly undermines students' task-related self-confidence and their predictions about their performance on a gender-related task (Stangor, Carr, & Kiang, 1998). When African Americans are asked to record their race before completing a difficult academic test, they perform less well than when race is not mentioned or when the test is described as race-neutral (Steele & Aronson, 1995). These performance deficits occur even when the students are interested in the task and see themselves as having significant strengths in that realm.

Steele (1997) suggests that negative stereotypes inhibit women's performance on mathematics-related tasks and African Americans' abilities on academic tasks in general and cause problems in predicting these groups' academic performance on SATs and GREs. Osborne (1997) notes that this sense of disfranchisement from school is true most often for African American boys and less true for other groups. Steele argues that stereotypes and the sense of inadequacy that they cause become an integral part of the personality, they intimidate group members into performing less well on stereotype-related tasks, and they lead to declines in self-efficacy and motivation. They create attitudes like, "What does it matter how I do on this test? I can't do well. I won't get anywhere with it."

This self-fulfilling prophecy is further reinforced by a real history of discrimination (Landrine & Klonoff, 1996; Steele, 1998; Whaley, 1998). Across cultures, stigmatized groups perform more poorly on intelligence tests and in school achievement—even when there are no racial differences between the groups (Ogbu, 1986). This performance deficit disappears when members of the stigmatized group immigrate to a country without prejudice against that group, as has been described for Japanese Bukaru who immigrated to the United States.

Stereotypes limit a person's perceived horizons (Steele, 1998). It is easier to act in ways that fit the stereotype than in ways that challenge it. Regardless of the course taken, the "stereotype constrains a person because it anchors the interaction, weighing it down, and holding it back" (Fiske, 1993, p. 623). It takes energy to attempt to disprove the stereotype. One's response to the stereotype will depend on how the following questions, among others, are answered:

- How much work is required to challenge the stereotype?
- How much risk will the work entail?
- Will I need to challenge these expectations continuously or only initially?
- Are there easier ways to resolve this dilemma?

Regardless of how we answer these questions, when we accept the dominant culture's values and attitudes, we can expect performance-related deficits, for the same reason that many of us have seen our own fluency or performance drop when we have been under stress. In contrast, others may maintain their self-esteem and self-identity by retreating from risky interests and values and investing in places where they can reasonably expect to be successful (Josephs, Larrick, Steele, & Nisbett, 1992; Stangor et al., 1998; cf. Hardy, 2001; G. H. Williams, 1995).

Hope, Self-Esteem, and Views of the Future

Stereotypes and discrimination may inhibit performance, but limited family resources, family stress, poor schools, disengaged teachers, uninterested peers, and distressed neighborhoods can undermine hope for the future and expectations of success. Failing to see a reasonable probability of success, rooted in real socioeconomic disadvantage, preempts any positive association with school even before it has a chance to form (Steele, 1998).

This is one way of interpreting the marginal success of Project Hope, a Milwaukee project started in the early 1990s to lift participants out of poverty. The program's proponents hoped it would remove the economic barriers that kept welfare recipients in poverty, but the income and employment gains made by participants who had been predicted to succeed were very modest at best and considerably below predictions. DeParle (1999) reported that, relative to members of a control group, the participants in this program worked 10% more hours per week. Fewer remained continuously unemployed over a two-year period than in a comparison group (6% versus 13%), and somewhat more worked their way out of poverty (27% versus 19%). However, there was no significant increase in program participants' incomes, at least without wage supports.

Lawrence Mead, who examined the high levels of depression that many of the Project Hope participants were in when they entered the program and that remained at follow-up, concluded that inner-city poverty is "rooted in an underlying culture of defeat," rather than only a lack of jobs (quoted in DeParle, 1999). Although the program challenged economic barriers, social and emotional barriers continued to prevent upward mobility.

Furthermore, the program's designers failed to recognize the impact of other values on work patterns. Some participants, for example, said they preferred to work less and spend more time with their families, even if doing so meant staying poor, which is certainly a stance adopted by some who are much better off.

Psychological and Physical Health

Despite our culture's emphasis on internal responsibility (Humphreys & Rapoport, 1993), societal factors have real consequences on mental health (Elligan & Utsey, 1999; Guyll, Matthews, & Bromberger, 2001; Harris & Kuba, 1997; Horne, 1999; Landrine & Klonoff, 1996). Elligan and Utsey conclude that racism and oppression should be implicated in the frequency of stress-related diseases such as gastrointestinal disorders, high blood pressure, cardiovascular disease, and stroke, as well as depression, suicide, substance abuse, antisocial behavior, low self-esteem, and decreased satisfaction with life among African American men. The roles of environmental and cultural factors in domestic violence and eating disorders are well accepted (Harris & Kuba, 1997; Horne, 1999). Internalized racism and psychosocial stressors are associated with abdominal obesity in an Afro-Caribbean population (Tull et al., 1999).

| TABLE 4.3 | **APPROACHES TO CULTURALLY AWARE ASSESSMENT AND TREATMENT OF EATING DISORDERS IN WOMEN OF COLOR** |

Additional Areas to Assess
- *Deviations from eating patterns typical of her family and culture.* Although simple deviations are not necessarily problematic, how might these patterns indicate differentiation from or rejection of the culture?
- *Concept of beauty.* Has it changed? If so, how and when? Is her sense of beauty consistent with her cultural background? Does it reflect internalized and oppressive images that she cannot achieve?
- *Racial identity.* What is her current level of racial identity? How does her racial identity interact with and change her body satisfaction, concept of beauty, and eating patterns?
- *Cultural self-hatred.* How might this be reflected in the use of food? For example, does she restrict food intake as a reflection of self-loathing?
- *Self-destructive eating patterns other than those described in the DSM-IV (1994).* Do patterns include compulsive eating and ritual dieting after binge-eating episodes? The DSM-IV diagnosis "Eating Disorder Not Otherwise Specified" should be considered for clients with atypical symptoms.

Unique Therapeutic Goals
- Incorporate knowledge of the meaning of food and cultural eating patterns into therapeutic interventions and relapse prevention plan.
- Normalize behavior as appropriate and identify treatment goals that are consistent with cultural eating patterns—such as religious fasting—while brainstorming alternative coping strategies.
- Develop a healthy spiritual base to help women feel grounded enough to explore the issues that underlie their eating disorders.
- Develop a supportive peer group, community, and family and identify healthy role models. These can provide a positive sense of self and culture as well as mediate against negative messages received from the dominant culture.
- Develop a healthy respect for her community, culture and, by extension, family. She will need a strong support system, but it must be defined broadly. She must develop a sense of systemic and cultural belonging while maintaining a positive self-identity.

Note: Modified from Harris & Kuba, 1997.

Culturally aware assessment and treatment means keeping the possibility of cultural and environmental factors in mind when working with clients of color. Table 4.3 is an example of ways in which cultural issues can be incorporated into our work with culturally different clients. Although these issues specifically address eating disorders, they should also be considered for other disorders and problematic behaviors.

COPING WITH OPPRESSION AND BEING OUTCAST

Members of an oppressed group can be defeated by their environment and can develop disorders related to oppression. They can also be mobilized into action, with good or ill intentions. Minuchin (Minuchin & Nichols, 1993) talks about this galvanizing experience in this description of his own upbringing:

I grew up Jewish in a town in which graffiti read: "Be patriotic; kill a Jew." But I got drunk on the Argentinean music, learned the local ghost stories, fought if another child stepped on a line I drew in the earth or if someone wet my ear, just like other rural Argentinean children. In issues of defiance we had no alternatives. I fought and was beaten "with honor" by children older and stronger than me. I grew up Argentinean, but without knowing it. My sense of pride and honor, the need to keep my good name even if it meant challenging windmills, had little to do with Russian Jewry—it was authentically Hispanic. Part of a despised minority, I learned to despise my Jewishness, to try to pass, and to hate myself for it. I grew up divided, internalizing the prejudices of the Argentinean majority and fighting the unfairness of prejudices both inside and outside myself. (p. 8)

Minuchin (Minuchin & Nichols, 1993) attributes this sense of division and feeling "outcasted" to the development of his personal strengths, resulting in his becoming a sensitive and empathic family therapist fighting for the underdog. However, the 1999 Columbine High School massacre has also been ascribed to group divisions. One student was quoted as saying, "The school was cliquish and extremely divided. . . . There was a lot of tension between the groups. It was almost continuous conflict between each one" (G. Wright & Millar, 1999, p. 5). In this case, the division was largely based on class and status at the school. The "jocks" and "preppies" were in power and "right at the bottom of the food chain, . . . the students who could not fit into any of the other groups, the quiet, brooding, intelligent ones." These students "were invariably shunned by the other tribes, and frequently bullied, verbally and physically," with unfortunate consequences (p. 8).

Why the extreme differences between these two outcomes? Perhaps they depended, in part, on the options the groups perceived as being available to them. Minuchin, who was raised in a relatively wealthy and influential family, likely saw options that the Trenchcoat Mafia of Columbine High didn't see—even though both Eric Harris and Dylan Klebold were very bright and their families were apparently very well off. Perhaps more importantly, Minuchin perceived the Jewish enclave in which he was raised as a very nurturing, extended family. This nourished him and his sense of justice. Harris and Klebold, in contrast, were part of the Trenchcoat Mafia, a group characterized by its sense of alienation. Unfortunately, this group was not large enough to provide the protection that immersion in a culture can allow (Greene, 1997). Harris and Klebold were allowed to objectify the "enemy," while Minuchin empathized with it; Minuchin's sense of justice thrived even after he was thrown in prison (Minuchin & Nichols, 1993).

Harris and Klebold hated their enemies and found a way to attack them; Minuchin empathized with his oppressors without identifying with them and searched for a way to foster justice in every country in which he lived. Painter (1996) describes yet another way of handling such conflict.

Sojourner Truth described her meeting with Abraham Lincoln in an open letter that was later published in her memoirs. In the letter, she describes her meeting with Lincoln as a grand, even playful discussion between two equals who recognized each other's greatness. For example, Lincoln, in a manner that was uncharacteristic of powerful white men of that era, reportedly stood up when she entered the room, greeted her warmly, and shook her hand. When she responded that she had never heard of him before he had become president, Lincoln "smilingly replied, 'I had heard of you many times before that'" (p. 206).

Truth's description, however, is contradicted by her omission from Lincoln's own journals, although he did describe the earlier meeting (Painter, 1996). Lucy Colman, who was also at this meeting, reported that Lincoln was three and a half hours late to the appointment and treated Truth condescendingly. Painter notes that Colman's report is consistent with other descriptions of Lincoln from this period, including the autobiographies of Frederick Douglass, who reported that Lincoln was gracious with "exceptional" Blacks and only under extraordinary situations, but otherwise maintained a Jim Crow White House with all of the inherent inequality that that implied.

Painter (1996) speculated about these discrepancies and attributed them to two factors. First, compared to other political leaders of the period, Lincoln had behaved graciously. He had, after all, allowed Truth and Colman to enter the White House and meet with him. More importantly, acknowledging Lincoln's slight would diminish not only Lincoln, but also Truth and admitting that she was not treated respectfully would give credence to the idea that she—and Blacks by extension—was not equal to Lincoln and did not deserve to be treated well.

Think about the dilemma Sojourner Truth faced. She could describe her meeting with the president accurately, and diminish Lincoln and herself in the process or she could distort it with the inherent distancing from reality that it would entail. What are the costs of admitting prejudice and discrimination? What are the costs of denying them? Her decision may have been an unconscious process, but perhaps it was a conscious one made to build support across racial and class boundaries, while she was fighting against other types of oppression. Perhaps she thought that his behavior was good enough given the times.

These stories describe different approaches to coping with oppression. Project Hope seems to be an example of how learned helplessness develops at the societal level—how it attacks whole neighborhoods that have given up in the face of obstacles and low expectations (DeParle, 1999). Steele (1997; Steele & Aronson, 1995), Stangor, and his colleagues (1998) described this phenomenon that occurs even among people with high self-confidence and a strong history of academic performance. Depression, hopelessness, and academic underachievement have been attributed to poverty, stress, and oppression as have a host of other psychological disorders (Elligan & Utsey, 1999; Landrine & Klonoff, 1996). Klebold and Harris fought against their oppressors by killing them. Truth openly denied (or accepted) the existence of some types of oppression in her work toward racial equality. Minuchin empathized with the underdog and fought against oppression within families and societies, becoming a noted family therapist in the process (Minuchin & Nichols, 1993).

THERAPEUTIC IMPLICATIONS OF IDENTIFYING OPPRESSION

When we work with people who have faced cultural barriers or any type of oppression, we should think about how they handle the problem. Do they attribute the problem to internal or external factors? We may help our clients recognize situational and cultural factors and in the process help them shift their locus of responsibility to one that is more external. While it may be healthy to have an external locus of *responsibility* in response to an oppressive environment, an internal locus of *control* is often useful (D. W. Sue & Sue, 1999; Shapiro, 1989, 1995; cf. Watts et al., 2002). This can be seen in chapter 5. Josh, for example, concluded that the poor schooling in his community was a racist issue (external locus of responsibility) and decided that he could do something about it (internal locus of control). At this point, he can choose either adaptive or maladaptive ways of making changes—something akin to Minuchin or to Harris and Klebold. Our goal is to help clients identify ways of addressing problems in healthy and growth-promoting ways, both in the short term and over the long haul (T. Robinson & Ward, 1991).

Certainly, it's important to identify environmental stressors, prejudice, and discrimination, but it's equally valuable to distinguish between benign environments and those that are more malignant and oppressive. Goffman (1986) is struggling with this dilemma in the following description:

> And I always feel this with . . . people—that whenever they're being nice to me, pleasant to me, all the time really, underneath they're only assessing me as a criminal and nothing else. It's too late for me to be any different now to what I am, but I still feel this keenly, that that's their only approach, and they're quite incapable of accepting me as anything else. (Pinel, 1999, p. 114)

Goffman's statement may be adaptive and self-protective to the extent that it allows him to recognize real prejudice and discrimination and externalize it appropriately. However, if he finds it difficult to differentiate between people who accept him and those who don't and then treats all people as though their kindness is mere artifice—or even engages in behaviors that confirm their stereotypes—we must challenge his own involvement in his revictimization and stigmatization (Pinel, 1999). This is also an important aspect of working with people who have a history of incest or sexual assault.

An Example

The ideas developed in the previous sections can be seen in this example: Rashelle, an African American teenager, had been depressed and at times actively suicidal for several years. Her grades had dropped, and she likely became depressed when she moved to a high school that was populated predominantly by Whites. Her mother and aunt, activists in the '70s, had "given up" and now seemed to be dysthymic. When Sherene, an African American school psychologist, talked to Rashelle about her attitudes toward being African American, it was clear that Rashelle had very ambivalent feelings. She was proud of her racial heritage, but she saw her appearance and kinky hair as coarse and ugly. She only wanted to date "white boys," and she foresaw few opportunities for success in her future.

Discussions with her revealed that Rashelle saw no place for African Americans at her school. She and her therapist brainstormed ways to address this problem and, along with several other interested students, the two began an informal support group. It used community members as mentors and others who worked to beef up the library's resources of ethnic and racial minority authors and developed an internship program with African American-owned businesses. Her depression—and her mother's!—decreased markedly. Sherene served as a positive model for Rashelle demonstrating that she could succeed *and* be true to her cultural heritage. Sherene took a nurturing and mentoring stance toward their relationship, a move that positively affected Rashelle's self-esteem and self-efficacy.

Rashelle's response to herself and others before and after therapy were very different (see table 4.4). Rashelle had viewed her body, self, and future negatively. She had claimed to see her race positively, although this was contradicted by her specific attitudes about herself and her community. While she initially had a few weak connections with others, these bonds were made significantly stronger and more meaningful by the end of therapy. As she began developing positive connections with herself, her race, and her community, her depression lifted.

CONSEQUENCES OF OPPRESSION ON THE OPPRESSORS

Although we have focused on the consequences of oppression on the oppressed, which included performance deficits, lost dreams, and a sense of hopelessness and alienation, oppression may also have significant

TABLE 4.4   RASHELLE'S FUNCTIONING BEFORE AND AFTER THERAPY

Problem	
Before Therapy	**After Therapy**
Current symptoms Reports moderate depression, overeating, and a lack of interest and motivation since starting at new school.	No symptoms reported.
Beliefs about symptoms Had not noticed that she was depressed and thought it was "normal" for her.	Decided that she had been depressed because she had felt isolated from her culture and devalued as an African American.
Personal history of psychological disorders Apparently dysthymic since moving to a new school.	Showed increased depression as she approached graduation.
Family history of psychological disorders Several family members had a history of mild depression (dysthymia).	
Current Context	
Recent events A move from a predominantly African American school to a predominantly Euro-American community and school predates her depression.	
Physical condition Health is unremarkable. Biological causes of her symptoms have been ruled out.	Recently broke her arm in a car accident.
Drug and alcohol use No current or past history reported.	None reported.
Intellectual and cognitive functioning Above average intelligence, especially on verbal tasks.	Good problem-solving ability.
Coping style Withdrawal, crying, daydreaming.Tends to go to best friend or mother to talk out problems.	Is action-oriented and creative in her approaches to problems.
Self-concept Saw self as ordinary at best. Did not expect to have anything to offer to others.	Recognizes her significant intellectual and leadership strengths. Is hopeful about herself and her future. Sees her actions as part of family tradition of activism.
Sociocultural background Preferred Euro-Americans as friends and dates. Preferred Euro-American ideals of beauty and culture. Disparaged her "kinky" hair and saw herself as "ugly."	Maintains a few Euro-American friends and dates, but also develops friendships and dating relationships with other African American students. Has begun to dress "African" and read African American literature.
Religion and spirituality Attended church regularly but at her mother's behest.	Attends church sporadically. Involvement frequently is self-initiated and more meaningful to her.
Resources and Barriers	
Individual resources Bright. A good student, reads voraciously.	Bright. A good student, strong leader. Active and involved in her community.

(continued)

TABLE 4.4 *(continued)*

Before Therapy	After Therapy
Problem	
Social resources, such as friends and family Few (and only peripheral) friends at new school.	Has developed several close friends in a larger multiracial group.
Passive and uninvolved with family, although fond of her younger cousins.	Has close relationships with several family members. Has begun to write her family history with her grandmother's help. Has begun to "mentor" her two younger cousins.
School B student. Feels isolated.	A and B student. Expects to go to college. Is acknowledged as a school leader and receives considerable support from teachers and peers.
Community resources No other agencies involved.	No other agencies involved.
Community contributions Saw self as impotent and unable to identify contributions to the community at large.	(1) Peer-critiqued friends' school papers, (2) began an informal support group for minority students, (3) developed a program on ethnic and minority authors for school, and (4) initiated an internship program with minority businesses for minority students. Family, school, and most peers have responded well to these contributions.
Mentors and models Few and only weak mentors. Saw no positive picture of what her future might be like.	Identified several African American models and mentors in her community, including her aunt and grandmother.
Obstacles and opportunities for change Significant hopelessness ("That's just the way it is. . . .") Internalized dominant culture's attitudes about African Americans.	Respects and listens to authority figures. Wants to believe things can be different.
Therapeutic relationship Positive, although adopted a one-down stance.	Positive and egalitarian.

consequences for the oppressive group. L. Brown (1998), for example, describes the ways that being bright, White, and middle-class constrains the girls she studied and leads them to become out of touch with their own thoughts and feelings. Cheryan and Bodenhausen (2000) describe several ways that being stereotyped in positive ways interferes with Asian American students' performance on mathematical tasks.

Lorde (1984c) also argues that ignoring or suppressing oppression damages everybody. However, indignant and focused anger can be liberating and empowering:

> If [my children's] full bellies make me fail to recognize my commonality with a woman of Color whose children do not eat because she cannot find work, or who has no children because her insides are rotted from home abortions and sterilization; if I fail to recognize the lesbian who chooses

not to have children, the woman who remains closeted because her homophobic community is her only life support, the woman who chooses silence instead of another death, the woman who is terrified lest my anger trigger the explosion of hers; if I fail to recognize them as other faces of myself, then I am contributing not only to each of their oppressions but also to my own . . . . (p. 132)

Helms and Cook's (1999) description of Euro-American racial identity development indicates that the cognitive factors that allow us to act in oppressive ways rely on distortions of reality. We must deny or distort information or to perceive groups dichotomously as "good" or "bad" (see chapter 7 for a more detailed discussion of racial identity). Whenever effective adjustment includes perceiving reality accurately, people who blindly accept oppression and privilege will be damaged by it. Furthermore, as argued throughout this chapter, the effects of oppression extend beyond the ones who are most obviously hurt by it, including bright, motivated, and successful college students (Cheryan & Bodenhausen, 2000; Steele, 1997, 1998).

Conclusions

North American culture and perhaps all cultures are oppressive, in that economic or social opportunities are available to some members and not others. Expectations about who or what the members of a cultural group are ("Will they be aggressive? Will they perform poorly academically, or will they be good dancers and athletes?) constrain some from pursuing their dreams. These expectations are also responsible for coercing others to follow less-preferred paths. Clearly, the dominant social group in the United States acts oppressively toward African Americans, Latinos and Latinas, and Native Americans using this narrow definition of the term. Oppression is something that must be acknowledged and addressed in therapy.

However, our society is often coercive and oppressive even to people in power, not only to economically oppressed groups. For example, Steele (1997) has demonstrated that even bright and privileged African American students show performance deficits when race is raised as an issue. Many recent writers have argued that while our culture has made significant strides in increasing the range of options and opportunities for women, it has not made similar changes for men (cf. Garbarino, 2000; Pollack & Levant, 1998). Men are still expected to avoid "feminine" pursuits, restrain emotional expressiveness, and value autonomy over relationships and intimacy. Boys are more likely to be diagnosed with ADHD and oppositional defiant disorder, perhaps a kind of social control, when their behavior does not match female norms or expectations. Asian Americans are supposed to be strong academically, highly motivated, and good at mathematics and the sciences. Jews are supposed to be hardworking and good with money. When we use this somewhat more inclusive definition of "oppression," any stereotype that prevents a group from meeting its full ability by limiting its ability to see or pursue options can be oppressive. Even Euro-American men can experience oppression. When positive stereotypes create anxiety about failing to meet expectations (Cheryan & Bodenhausen, 2000), yet another negative consequence of privilege arises.

Rather than argue about who is oppressed, we should instead focus on ways to reduce oppression and address its consequences. Our interventions, as we'll see in later chapters, can take several forms. These include challenging the stereotypes and valuing individual, cultural, and group strengths. It also means accepting goals that diverge from cultural standards. Cultural change initiated and symbolized by slogans such as "Black is beautiful" or "The personal is political", and advocacy groups such as the Gray Panthers and the Black Student Union have helped many people meet these goals outside of therapy.

When we accept or fail to challenge oppression, we imply that our clients' anger and pain are unjustified (cf. Raine, 1998). Contextually unaware therapies blame people for their victimization or oppression. Oppression and our clients' feelings about it are also dismissed thoughtlessly when we say things like, "Isn't it time to get past all of this?" When we block healthy outlets for venting feelings, anger can turn inward and manifest itself as self-mutilation, eating disorders, and unprotected sex. It can also direct itself outward in destructive acts like theft, fire-setting, assault, and rape. By identifying oppressive forces and accepting our clients' anger, self-hatred, shame, guilt, and fear in their full, dynamic range, we allow our clients to process their feelings and cope in healthy and adaptive ways (Greene, 1985; T. Robinson & Ward, 1991). As discussed in chapter 7, healthy coping includes accepting and exercising appropriate control over oppressive factors without ignoring others' rights and viewpoints.

VALUES AND WORLDVIEWS

It's always with a bit of chagrin that I read my students' evaluations of me at the end of the semester. Although the vast majority of my students speak of me as being respectful, fair, encouraging of critical thinking, calm, and supportive, there is sometimes one person who believes I cannot teach my way out of a paper bag. Each student has been in the same class and has seen the same stimuli. What accounts for these differences? I would guess that I meet the needs of some students better than others, perhaps because of what they value and what they believe a university education should be. Perhaps they want more structure or don't like psychology. Perhaps they see me and my teaching in a negative light because they are depressed, hopeless, doing poorly in my class, or don't like school in general.

Our values and stance on the world are like the shade of eyeglasses, coloring our view of events in our lives. They determine what we pay attention to, how we interpret that information, and what we remember (Kenrick et al., 1999). Becoming aware of our clients' culture and values is not an unnecessary and frivolous luxury; rather, it facilitates treatment by increasing the therapist's understanding of the client's needs, concerns, goals, and adjustment (Ridley et al., 1994). This chapter examines important approaches to identifying valuing systems and common differences in values that are especially important to therapy.

WHAT IS VALUING?

Valuing is as natural as breathing, as silent as a heart beating, and just as easily overlooked, especially for the dominant group. Why do many Euro-Americans, for example, find it easier to describe stereotypes of African Americans, Hispanics, or Asian Americans than of other Euro-Americans? Could it be because they see themselves as "just ordinary"? Group members tend to assume that the way they are is "normal" and that normal is the way things *should* be. This premise can cause problems for Euro-Americans in therapy unless this assumption is recognized and challenged. It often isn't as difficult for members of minority groups to identify stereotypes about their own group and about the dominant group. They have to be aware of the Other in order to protect Themselves, and they are often exposed to a picture of themselves from the dominant group's viewpoint (Zayas & Solari, 1994). Although having few interactions with minority group members is fairly easy for members of the majority group, the reverse is significantly more difficult.

Nonetheless, values direct people's emotions, thoughts, and actions. Recently, the youngest child of a family in therapy reported being molested by a neighbor boy who was 12 years his senior. The therapist had stayed with the family throughout the reporting process, while the police and Child Protective Services interviewed the family and child. By 9:00 p.m., the family was finally alone. The children were exhausted, but the dad wanted to take the family out to a movie. Around the conference table with her staff, the therapist reported this part of the story with an expression of distaste. She believed that the dad wanted to run off to see his girlfriend and that if he had been a good dad, he would have stayed home, read stories to his children, and tucked them into bed.

Are there other ways of looking at the father's behavior? Rather than being a bad parent, could he have been well-intentioned but was using a different strategy of reducing stress than the therapist wanted? Perhaps the question should have been "How would we know if, and in what ways, this strategy worked for the father, child, and family?" The therapist's goal, then, is to increase awareness of his or her own values in order to more effectively recognize and challenge them in the course of therapy.

Becoming aware of one's own values often happens under unusual conditions. When a person runs up stairs, the blood pressure rises, the breathing is loud, and the heartbeat is heard, things that are otherwise stable and silent. Similarly, in order to see the values of an individual or group, the "unusual" has to be probed. While some people may often be unaware of their values, they can begin to make inferences about them as they make everyday decisions about their lives.

Barriers to Recognizing Values

When asked about their values, many people will give a sanitized or dressed-up version (DeMaio, 1984), as in "I believe that freedom, free speech, and our environment are important." However, the verbal report is unreliable, because it changes as a function of how the question is asked. What makes the difference are the other choices available, whether the choice is free or forced, and who is listening. These can influence the responses, often significantly (Schwarz, 1999).

On the first day of class, I ask my students to talk about their values with other classmates. Their reports to the class about their most important values invariably include loyalty, honesty, and family relationships. Why don't I get responses that include less socially acceptable values such as hedonism, doing as little as possible for maximal output, and sexual promiscuity? These values would be consistent with some of the behaviors they describe in their journals. If I were to ask them about their values later in the semester—when they knew me and their classmates better—would I get a wider range of responses? What if the power relationships weren't so skewed? What if they were talking late Friday night with friends?

If I were asked whether being truthful and honest were important, I'd answer that both are very important. However, others might get a different picture of me by watching my behavior. While I value honesty, I rarely drive the speed limit on the highway. In this example of a value conflict, other values, such as attempting to arrive at my destination in a timely manner (given that I generally leave late), take precedence over my *announced values,* or what I *say* is important to me.

While I value being truthful with myself and with others, I only share the parts of the truth that I believe others will be ready to hear, and even then I may only share when asked. I don't value banging my head against a wall; I see pushing people to do something when they aren't ready as a waste of time. In this case, my perception of a situation determines my behavior.

Try these experiments. Observe your reactions, as well as others' reactions, to your behavior in these experiments.

- If you always have the door open when you use the bathroom, close it. If you always have it closed, open it.
- Have a heated argument outside, especially where your neighbors can hear.
- Think about telling a friend your deepest, darkest secret. Or, if you tell your friend everything, try not telling.
- Use an expletive in front of your priest, minister, or rabbi.
- If you don't generally hug, hug your parents or your children the next time you see them. If you do hug, don't.
- Pick a topic that is taboo in your family and talk about it at the dinner table. How do you and your family react to your bringing it up and breaking this taboo?

What part of each experiment caused your response? Did you have stronger reactions to some experiments than with others? How dependent upon your own values were your reactions? These experiments will help you begin to identify your values. For one week, extend this work by journaling about things that cause you to react strongly.

Sometimes, a person can fairly clearly identify another person's values, such as when falafel on pita bread is chosen over bologna on white bread. However, even with simple situations like this, drawing an accurate inference can be very difficult. Does Melody avoid meat because she wants to restrict her fat intake, because she refuses to be associated with killing animals, because she prefers eating food lower on the food chain, perhaps because she enjoys complex flavors, or because she simply wants to make her physician and family happy? More information is needed to find the right answer. But, humans are notoriously unreliable reporters of their own behaviors. Even when asked about why she doesn't eat meat, Melody may not give an accurate report (Nisbitt & Wilson, 1977).

By listening to people and observing their moods, behaviors, and interpersonal elationships, a picture of who they are can emerge, although it may be a picture that is modified by ifs, whens, and wheres, as in some of the previous examples. By observing how the emotional responses of one person relate to our own or to others' behavior, we can expand this picture.

Recognizing Others' Values

Similar issues arise when the values of others are considered. What others say (their *announced* values) may not match what they actually do (their *committed* values). This may be true for any number of reasons. Therefore, assessments of others' values will depend on context. How do they say what they say? What happens to their eye contact, paralanguage, and verbal context? What stories do they tell? Do their stories support their announced values? Although Sammi reported being a good and caring parent, she rarely spent time with her children and, when asked about them during a custody assessment, she could not identify their friends or what they enjoyed doing.

Discrepancies between announced and committed values can be due to other factors. Sammi had been caring for her dying mother and had been living in another state for the past year. She reported—and her children confirmed—that their relationship had been very close before this separation. Each person spoke about this period tearfully and anticipated a return to what had been "normal" previously.

What happens in the here and now during a therapy session is also an important, even essential, clue to a client's values. During the joint interview with Sammi and her children, her eyes frequently flitted back to her children. Her two sons, especially the four-year-old, played calmly in her presence and spontaneously showed her the progressive steps of their drawings. When her six-year-old began to get irritable, Sammi calmly stopped the interview to focus on her son's needs and was able to quiet him rapidly. If anything, the verbal report of her knowledge of her children significantly underestimated her parental abilities. In fact, when she became more comfortable in the interview, she was able to report much more about her children's interests and activities.

WHAT IS A WORLDVIEW?

When we talk about worldviews, we refer to the *pattern* of values and perceptions of the world that color our view of the world (Ivey et al., 1997). Much like a pair of rose-colored glasses, our worldview filters the information we receive from our world, determines the information we pay attention to (and what we don't), and assists in the way we perceive the information.

Different people often perceive the same event in different ways. In the movie *Rashomon* (Kurosawa & Minoura, 1950), a woman, her husband's ghost, a bandit, and a bystander each describe the woman's rape and her husband's murder in different ways, and they disagree about whether or not the sex was consensual and about who killed her husband. In the movie, the woman, her husband and the bandit claim culpability for the murder. The movie implies that people cannot be objective observers of their own lives and that their values and worldview influence the way they view themselves, their actions, and the world around them.

Our worldview influences whether we see the glass as half full or half empty or even whether it contains fluid at all. This is true whether an argument is a minor spat or becomes the initial stages of World War III. When we watch a mother and her young son hug, we compare the interaction to our own expectations of normative behavior, which is a part of worldview. Is the relationship close? If we value intimacy, we may conclude that the mother and her son are physically and emotionally close, and we may expect that a boy in such a relationship will be more in touch with himself emotionally, have higher self-esteem, and be a good nurturer to his children. In short, we would view this relationship positively. On the other hand, if we believe that boys need to be encouraged to individuate from their mothers and that physical closeness makes this process more difficult, we may see the relationship as enmeshed and emasculating.

Our worldview is a way of organizing and distilling huge amounts of complex material into simple and understandable forms, which allows us to respond to the world more rapidly and efficiently. Imagine the feeling of having to pay attention to every piece of information that was received every minute of the day. The sound of the rain on the window, the temperature of the room, the feel of a book, the sound of pages being turned, and one leg on the opposite knee with one foot on the floor. The amount of in-

Think about a time when you were in either a very good or in a very poor mood. What events and interactions did you pay attention to? What events seen by others as meaningful did you dismiss as unimportant? Did you interpret experiences differently than the people around you? If so, how? Spend a moment thinking about this before going on to the next paragraph.

If you are like most people, you probably see more bad things when you are in a bad mood and more good things when you are in a good mood. Some of these bad things may have caused your mood or, more accurately, been related to beliefs that caused your mood. However, you probably focused more on ambiguous events and perceived them negatively, such as the red light you didn't notice when in a good mood but ended up swearing at it when you were stressed and angry.

formation sensed at any moment is overwhelming. So, we perceive only part of it and use a still smaller portion. In the best of all worlds, the strategies we use to organize our experiences will be both simple and effective, without them having negative consequences for us, our friends, strangers, or the community as a whole.

Our worldview serves as a filter, accepting information that makes sense and discarding information that does not fit. Because they reject and distort irrelevant information, worldviews can be especially resistant to change (chapter 6 covers factors that influence changes in worldviews and factors that therapists can take advantage of in therapy). We actively seek information that *confirms* our expectations, that *interprets* ambiguous events and behaviors in ways that support our beliefs and values, and that *recalls* events that support our worldview (Kenrick et al., 1999). For example, when pro-Israeli and pro-Arab students watch an identical newscast about the Israeli-Arab conflict, they perceive the presentation differently and will tend to see it as being hostile to their view (Giner-Sorolla & Chaiken, 1994). Each group pays attention to those statements and behaviors that reinforce their viewpoint, while dismissing information that is contradictory. Because worldview can make experience parochial, the conscious use of critical thinking skills can increase one's empathy and the ability to adapt to the world (Halonen & Santrock, 1997).

SIGNIFICANT ASPECTS OF WORLDVIEW

Although worldviews take many different forms, some aspects are particularly important to the therapy process. The discussion in table 5.1 is especially indebted to Ibrahim (1985), Koltko-Rivera (1999), and D. W. Sue and Sue (1999).

Ontology: Explanations of Phenomena

Psychology and psychotherapy are scientifically based and rationally oriented fields, and interventions often make sense when they are connected to scientific theories and supported by empirical studies. Therapeutic approaches that do not have a rational or empirical underpinning are often met with skepticism. Many practitioners prefer explanations that make sense, can be explained logically and empirically, and are parsimonious. Nonetheless, some clients view the world through different eyes. Some believe in spirits, magic, the power of prayer, or non-Western approaches to healing. They accept that some things are outside of logic and too distant from their ability to observe them, and they may not wish to explain issues parsimoniously. These views influence their perceptions of the causes of

TABLE 5.1	SEVEN DIMENSIONS OF WORLDVIEW THAT ARE ESPECIALLY RELEVANT TO COUNSELING
Ontology	Does the universe have a spiritual dimension or is the best description of reality based upon events with a material and rational explanation?
Mutability	Can people change or is their behavior due to a permanent part of them, such as a trait?
Trust	Are other people trustworthy or can you expect that they will hurt you either intentionally or unintentionally?
Authority	Is it more natural to relate to people in an authoritarian or an egalitarian manner?
Group	Which comes first: What I want (individualism) or what my reference group wants (collectivism)?
Responsibility	Who got me where I am today: me (internal locus of responsibility) or forces outside of me (external locus of responsibility)? Are the forces outside of me benevolent, malevolent, or mere chance?
Control	Is the power to control what happens to me within me (internal locus of control) or is what happens to me a matter of luck, destiny, or other forces such as social prejudice (external locus of control)?

Note: From Ibrahim, 1985; Koltko-Rivera, 1999; Oyserman, Coon, & Kemmelmeier, 2002; D. W. Sue & Sue, 1999.

their problems—and of potential solutions (see table 5.2). Whenever there is a conflict in worldview, people run up against an unnecessary impediment to therapy. Francisco (1999) described this when she talked with her therapist about energy work:

> Her language is a problem for me right away—energy field, vibration levels, right intention. I thought I was getting *massages*. I sense that our conversation is as frustrating for her as it is for me. On her part, it's like trying to describe television to someone who doesn't accept the idea of electricity. (p. 145, italics in the original)

This conflict between worldviews is not insurmountable, however. Francisco (1999) and her therapist, for example, were able to work very well together. In another example, Charlene, an incest survivor, was raised in an impoverished family and had grown up in a fundamentalist church setting. Although her religious beliefs were still very important to her, she had not gone to church in several years because she believed that her history of abuse had made her "dirty" and "bad." Furthermore, she believed that she could not be forgiven for what she saw as her "sins." I do not believe that survivors should be blamed for their abusive history, and we discussed this. Charlene's actions as a 10-year-old trying to cope with an older and more powerful uncle were completely understandable—except to her. While we initially attempted to discuss her history of incest from this point of view, the approach was only marginally successful.

TABLE 5.2	LANGUAGE THAT INDICATES AN ONTOLOGICAL VIEW OF BEHAVIOR

Spiritual	Materialistic
• Mechanistic explanations and theories are ignored, especially when they conflict with spiritual ones.	• The world is expected to follow natural and predictable laws.
• The world is not expected to make sense. Faith and intuition are important guides for decision making. Example: "It just is."	• The world is expected to make sense. Logical and rational processes are valued. Blind faith and intuitive processes are often considered foolish. Example: "But how does it work?"
• The person frequently refers to spiritual or religious sources for decision making. Example: "My priest says . . . ." Note: Spiritual views may influence a few, but not all parts of life, such as views on conservation but not premarital sex.	• Spiritual or religious sources are rarely referred to for the decision-making process.
• Spiritual metaphors are more compelling than mechanistic ones.	• Mechanistic metaphors are more compelling than spiritual ones.

Note: An ontological stance can be independent of expressed religious affiliations.

As a result, we shifted to a discussion of how her actions could be seen from her religious viewpoint. We talked about the Old and New Testament views of God and forgiveness in an attempt to introduce flexibility into a tyrannical system. As it turns out, although she had generally adopted an intolerant Old Testament stance on forgiving herself ("An eye for an eye . . . "), Charlene believed that forgiveness for others was quite possible—a religious attitude closer to the New Testament. By becoming aware of this and having her beliefs challenged, she was able to move to a much greater level of self-acceptance.

My own spiritual beliefs are very different from Charlene's. But had I ignored the importance of her viewpoint and failed to address religious issues in therapy, I would have thrown away an important key to therapeutic change (Worthington, Kurusu, McCollough, & Sandage, 1996). We can respect our clients and their worldviews without subscribing to their beliefs (D. W. Sue & Sue, 1999). My own religious beliefs were irrelevant to this conversation *except* if they prevented me from listening to and understanding Charlene's story or *if* they reduced my credibility as a therapist.

Because she knew that I was not a fundamentalist Christian, my approach was necessarily different than if we had shared religious views. I began, "You know I don't know the Bible as well as you do, but I wonder what you think God says about forgiveness." Because Charlene thought of herself as something of a local expert, I adopted a one-down position. This stance was more genuine than faking expertise in a religious viewpoint that

I did not know well, and it was, incidentally, more empowering for Charlene. When she was the one enunciating the viewpoint, she became more committed to the ideas she described. Her description of the Bible and her use of words and paralanguage also allowed me to assess her views in a more lively fashion, such as when she said, "Jesus ran into a lot of problems with His followers because He forgave and ministered to the unforgivable. Sometimes, I pretend I am Mary Magdalene and that He could forgive me as easily . . . ."

Even though Charlene's views came from fundamentalist Christianity, a similar intervention style can be used with clients of different worldviews and religious philosophies (e.g., Muslim, Jewish, or Hindi). Therapists need to listen to clients' worldviews, assess the points of flexibility, and develop intervention strategies that will be acceptable within the context of the clients' existing attitudes and beliefs. Clients' views of the world are the key to identifying how they see their problems and to finding solutions they will be receptive to. Solutions for Charlene were couched in spiritual language, because it was her native tongue. Clients like Francisco (1999), however, require a more mechanistic language.

Mutability: Obstacles to Change

Our beliefs about our ability to change are important influences on our ability to actually change. Generally, change is faster when we believe change is *possible* than when we see the behavior as a central and unchangeable part of ourselves. For this reason, traits—essential and unchangeable aspects of ourselves—may be easy qualities to assess, but conceptualizing behavior as unchanging can be an obstacle to change.

People who see behavior as immutable are more likely to use stabilizing language when talking about the problem, as in table 5.3. Their language emphasizes continuity in time, internal causes, and biological explanations. In contrast, clients who see discontinuities, exceptions, and environmental causes and those who believe that they have identified the problem and are hopeful about their ability to overcome it, are more likely to be able to change rapidly in therapy (Walter & Peller, 1992).

Note the way in which therapeutic interventions across a variety of therapeutic viewpoints address this tendency to think of our behavior as unchangeable. Cognitively oriented therapists like Ellis (1994) and Beck (1991) challenge self-talk that uses stabilizing words like "always" and "never," dichotomous thinking, and the tendency to accept responsibility for failures while rejecting successes. Both teach helpful ways of thinking about self and about the "problem." Behavior therapists assess environmental controls of behavior—antecedents and consequences—while looking for ways to change the controls. Therapists emphasize learning histories

TABLE 5.3	LANGUAGE THAT INDICATES STABLE AND UNSTABLE VIEWS OF BEHAVIOR	

Stable	Unstable
• Stable view of problem. Example: "I'm always depressed."	• Unstable view of problem. Example: "I'm often depressed by the end of the day."
• Trait language. Example: "It's just that I am a hopeless parent."	• Environmental attributions. Example: "I'm little to no help with the kids when she criticizes what I do."
• Genetic or biological explanations. Example: "Depression is an illness. I can't help it."	• Learning explanations. Example: "It's a bad habit; it's just easier to do it this way."
• Self as hapless object. Example: "What do you want me to do about it? Her moods are just impossible to live with."	• High degree of self-efficacy. Example: "If I've learned anything, it's that I can do anything I set my mind to."

rather than physiological causes, and they design interventions that build self-efficacy and promote the belief that challenges can be met and overcome successfully. Many of Milton Erickson's tasks (J. Haley, 1993) work at least partly by building self-efficacy (Bandura, 1997). Berg's (1994) and de-Shazer's (1988) exception questions, such as "I know you have trouble most of the time, but when are you most likely to get along?," help clients recognize instability and learn that change can be accomplished when these exceptions are made more frequent. Finally, person-centered therapists emphasize that unconditional positive regard and the hopeful view of the future that it engenders are necessary to the change process. Hopefulness implies an expectation that things can and will change. This attitude transcends therapeutic viewpoints and seems to be one of the factors necessary for change (Rogers, 1957).

Trust: The Nature of Human Relationships

Trust underlies and colors the course of most interactions with strangers, partners, and friends. It is also fundamental to the therapeutic relationship itself (see table 5.4). For some people, trust facilitates the relationship. For others, however, trust interferes.

Some of our reactions to others are situationally elicited. It's hard to trust someone's motives when he or she does something unexpected, as when a politician makes a 180-degree turn from a previous stance and endorses another. In fact, many of us expect politicians to lie to get our vote, so we attempt to determine what they *really* think. Trust is also undermined by inconsistent verbal and nonverbal messages and inconsistencies over time, such as when one hears "I love you" before engaging in sex, but

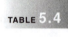

TABLE 5.4   LANGUAGE AND BEHAVIORS THAT INDICATE HIGH AND LOW LEVELS OF TRUST

Low Trust	High Trust
• Has relatively large personal space. Is intolerant of violations of this space.	• Has relatively smaller personal space. Is more tolerant of intrusions into personal space.
• Is suspicious or intermittently accepting of others' intentions.	• Is consistently accepting of others' responses without unnecessarily questioning their meaning or intentions.
• Is fairly reactive to mild rudeness or forgetfulness and often reads the worst into most situations.	• Is more tolerant of mild rudeness without taking things personally.
• Requires greater amounts of relationship-building from one meeting to the next. Requires greater amounts of information about the other party. May not ask for the latter, but may become uncomfortable in its absence.	• May ask for information in order to facilitate development of relationship. Trust is often situationally appropriate, rather than provided gullibly or withheld inappropriately.
• Frequently uses language suggesting disruptions in the therapeutic alliance, including "You say . . . ," "Yes, but . . . ," or "You don't understand . . . ."	• Puts greater emphasis on attempting to understand other viewpoints when disagreements occur.
• Language is characterized by disruptions, staccato speech, stutters, hesitations, and increased nonreflective silence.	• Language is relatively smooth. Silence seen as thoughtful and reflective rather than as an angry attempt to distance.

doesn't receive a phone call later. Conversely, people who are perceived as being genuine, open, and consistent in their interpersonal relations may inspire greater levels of trust (Emmons & Colby, 1995).

Our ability to trust is situation-specific and cross-situational. People with secure attachment styles respond in a trusting manner more frequently and across more situations than do those with anxious-ambivalent or avoidant styles (Mikulincer, 1998). Those who are especially suspicious, cynical, or paranoid may behave in this manner even with the most trustworthy of people. Clients with a history of abuse, especially those who learned the hard way that they will be hurt by the ones they love, may have the most difficulty trusting. In fact, many have learned that good times predict abusive episodes, as when Sam's Uncle Abram played a tickling game with him before fondling his penis.

Euro-Americans generally take on a trusting attitude toward those who maintain relatively small interpersonal space, good eye contact, an open and relaxed posture, and a congenial smile. In contrast, people who are not trusting require greater personal space, especially with strangers, and are more tense in their eye contact and posture. For example, while doing a genogram Jalyssa (a very trusting person) moved her chair closer to Sam (a person who found trusting difficult). She did this so Sam could see what was being written, but the move startled him. His eyes opened wide, and he sat bolt upright. Then, he moved his chair farther back.

How does this reaction affect the therapeutic relationship? Disclosures depend on trust (C. E. Thompson, Worthington, & Atkinson, 1994)—a concept discussed at greater length in chapter 9. People who see the world as discriminatory or oppressive are less willing to take risks, and they have poorer outcomes in therapy (Nickerson, Helms, & Terrell, 1994; Terrell & Terrell, 1984; C. E. Thompson et al., 1994; Watkins & Terrell, 1988). Disclosing potentially shameful aspects of ourselves is a risk. Whether or not we disclose, when we do, and how we present our story depends on the reaction we expect to receive from the listener. If we expect a negative reaction, we will be less likely to disclose the *content* and perhaps the *reason* we entered therapy in the first place. Or, we may do so only when a safe escape is possible. Sam, for example, waited until the end of his first session to disclose his Secret. Before disclosing, though, he made Jalyssa close her eyes and look away. Then, he blurted that he had been molested and attempted to leave the room. Jalyssa delayed this exit by asking him to look at her face and to see if she had responded negatively. Then, she briefly discussed her beliefs about incest and survivors. A client's interest in disclosing is related to whether or not he or she expects to be understood. Thus, C. E. Thompson and his colleagues (1994) found that African American women whose pseudotherapists addressed cultural issues were more likely to elicit self-disclosures, which was probably because the women recognized that their pseudotherapists understood the role of context in their lives.

Van den Bos, Wilke, and Lind (1998) suggest that procedures perceived as fair may be especially important when information about an authority's trustworthiness is lacking. While Van den Bos and his colleagues don't draw this conclusion, people who have a difficult time assessing trustworthiness on their own may especially need a setting with procedures that promote fairness. Initial paperwork, such as consent forms with information on the nature of the therapeutic relationship and on clients' rights and responsibilities, can be particularly helpful in meeting this goal. However, this often will not be enough. An atmosphere of fairness and trustworthiness may need to be fostered constantly throughout therapy.

Authority: The Nature of Helping Relationships

People enter therapy with expectations about the nature of therapy itself, about how they will be treated, and about what they will do in the course of treatment. The general belief is that when clients' expectations are accurate, clients are more likely to be happy with the therapeutic process and more likely to return (see exceptions in Hardin, Subich, & Holvey, 1988;

TABLE 5.5	LANGUAGE AND BEHAVIORS THAT INDICATE PREFERENCES FOR AUTHORITATIVE OR EGALITARIAN RELATIONSHIPS

Authoritative	Egalitarian
• May request feedback on decisions, beliefs, and behavior. Accepts feedback received.	• May request feedback on decisions, beliefs, and behavior. May reject or modify feedback received, especially if he or she did not contribute to the decision-making process. Example: "Yeah, but . . . ."
• May become irritable or "resistant" when therapist does not adopt an authoritative stance in sessions.	• May become irritable or show signs of "resistance" when given less autonomy than preferred in sessions.
• May need to be prompted significantly to express opinions. Often seems to pay greater attention to expert opinions than to his or her own. Often frustrated by therapists' attempts to increase clients' responsibility for their own decision making.	• May spontaneously express opinions or do so after minimal requests. May return to sessions having extended previous week's ideas or homework beyond that discussed.

Note: Be sensitive to the fact that refusals to express opinions, especially contradictory ones, may reflect respectfulness rather than an acceptance of authority. (This is particularly true of traditional Native Americans.)

Renjilian, Perri, Nezu, McKelvey, Shermer, & Anton, 2001; Yau, Sue, & Hayden, 1992). See table 5.5 for more on language and behaviors. Therapies differ significantly—from those that are relatively directive to those that are relatively nondirective and from those that are active and filled with advice-giving to those that are nondirective and advice-avoiding. Some therapies set up a hierarchical relationship in which the therapist assumes a more powerful stance. Others foster an egalitarian or even a one-down relationship between therapist and client. Some focus on making active behavior changes, while others focus more on increasing behavioral insights. One therapeutic approach may suit some clients better than others (A. Lazarus, 1993).

Individual differences in preferences within a cultural group do exist, and clients from different cultural groups have, on average, different expectations and goals for therapy. African American clients, for example, tend to prefer action-oriented and directive therapies (D. W. Sue & Sue, 1999). Sharone, an African American mother of four, was irritated when her therapist focused on why she had a difficult time imposing limits on her children. Their sessions became a mix of angry accusations and passive or non-responsive moments. Sharone was relieved when, after their fifth session, her therapist went on maternity leave. The therapist she transferred to helped her identify a simple token economy to apply when addressing problems with homework and chores. She was surprised when her therapist helped her identify after-school programs that could help her bridge the gap between the time school let out and when she returned home at the end of the workday. That gap was something Sharone had complained about to her first therapist to no avail. Her second therapist adopted a more action-oriented approach that was closer to her own expectations for therapy.

In contrast, upper middle- and middle-class Euro-American clients tend to expect and prefer more insight-oriented therapies. Advice is seen as disempowering and disrespectful, even when apparently asked for.

> MARCIA: *I'm so overwhelmed lately. I just don't know what to do. I wish you would just tell me what to do.*
> JON: *You have been floundering lately. Can you break your problems down into smaller pieces and let's take them one step at a time? Work would be a good place to start. (Feedback, closed question, advice)*
> MARCIA: *Work is bad, but it's not most important. It's almost like no one's listening to me. Everyone's always telling me what to do.*

Marcia rejected Jon's intervention with her "yeah, but . . . " comment ("Work is bad, but . . . "). In fact, Marcia seems to complain indirectly about his actions. Imagine if Jon had instead adopted the same goal—identifying strategies to decrease stress—but had assumed that Sharone was capable of arriving at her own solutions.

> MARCIA: *I'm so overwhelmed lately. I just don't know what to do. I wish you would just tell me what to do.*
> JON: *You have been floundering lately. We've been talking a lot about the things that cause you stress. What have you been thinking about our conversations? (Feedback, brief summarization, open question)*
> MARCIA: *Well, I feel like we keep going back to talking about work. Every time people need something done, I agree to do it and then I get so stressed! I seem to think that I've got to do what other people want, so they will like me. I don't have to do things so people will like me, do I?*

Native Americans, on the other hand, tend to see an active and directive style of intervention as rude and ill-mannered. The token economy intervention that was so appreciated by Sharone would be seen by Native Americans as coercive and manipulative (Paniagua, 1998). On average, Native Americans value being harmonious with nature, and they see active approaches as ill-considered attempts to control and change that harmony (D. W. Sue & Sue, 1999).

Group: Autonomy, Individualism, and Relationships

Euro-American culture is relatively individually oriented and emphasizes the needs of the individual above those of the group (see table 5.6). Euro-Americans value autonomy, independence, and fairly strong interpersonal

Look at a problem in your life. Identify as many advantages and disadvantages as possible for each potential solution before reading further. How many of these advantages and disadvantages take into consideration your own needs and wishes? How many consider the needs and wishes of your extended family or community? What do you learn from reviewing your lists?

TABLE 5.6   LANGUAGE AND BEHAVIORS THAT INDICATE RELATIVELY COLLECTIVISTIC VERSUS AUTONOMOUS STANCES

Collectivistic	Autonomous
• Expressions of individual needs are seen as selfish and self-centered. Example: "All he can think about is himself!"	• Appropriate expressions of individual needs are seen as self-affirming. Failures to assert individual needs are labeled pejoratively as weak or passive.
• The person frequently makes decisions relative to the needs and values of others in the family or group, even when the decisions are made at the expense of individual needs. Example: "My family needs . . . ."	• Although family needs are considered in the course of decision making, individual needs are assumed to take greater priority. Example: "I want to . . . ."
• Individual accomplishments are seen as less important than group accomplishments. Example: "My children did . . . ."	• Although successes of family members are seen as important, individual successes *and* failures are central to the self-esteem. Example: "In the last week, I . . . ."
• Success *and* problems are seen systemically as part of an interaction among group members. Successes are more likely to be relational and anonymous, such as a relationship or a group project (e.g., a quilt).	• Both success and problems are seen as a function of individuals. Example: "It's all his fault!" or "I did it!" Successes result in an individually identifiable product such as money, leadership, or an individual's artwork.
• Boundaries are less important than connections.	• Strong personal boundaries are valued.
• People are expected to listen to the opinions and decisions of those who are wise and have more experience.	• People are expected to make decisions for themselves rather than to rely on the decision making of authority figures.

boundaries and are more likely to look down upon groups that are less autonomous and independent. This group has traditionally valued the male role above the more relationship-oriented role of women. These values can also be seen in our culture's views of great art and literature like the works of Mary Cassatt and Käthe Kollwitz, who until recently had been omitted from art history books and disparaged for their focus on the "small" topics like mother-and-child relationships (Chadwick, 1990). History is often presented in the context of wars—clearly a group-oriented event—and has been obsessed with large and heroic decisions rather than the daily and mundane ones that make up the vast majority of life.

More individualistic cultures assume that the needs of the group will be satisfied when individual needs are met. Collectivist cultures take the opposite stance and generally assume that individual happiness follows group happiness. Many Asian Americans and Latins take a group-oriented approach, at the expense of individual needs (Hofstede, 1980). Parents are expected to sacrifice for their children, and adult children are expected to sacrifice for their parents and younger siblings. Asian folktales often focus on the "selfish" person who is either punished or confronted with lessons about contributions to make to the group (cf. Fang, 1995). These differences are also reflected in the advertising styles of popular magazines in individually oriented cultures (e.g., the United States) and more collectivist cultures, such as China (Han & Shavitt, 1994).

Western therapies often take a relatively individualistic stance and typically pay little attention to the individual's impact on family members. Zhang (1994) describes the response of other therapists-in-training toward a woman who was overwhelmed with caring for her elderly parents. Zhang's classmates—presumably born in the United States—believed that the woman should become more autonomous and begin to think and do things for herself. However, Zhang, who was born in China, appreciated the woman's respect for her elderly parents, although he suggested that her parents should become less selfish and recognize their daughter's needs. Because Western therapies tend to focus on the individual client's needs regardless of the client, it is conceivable that the therapists in Zhang's class would have conceptualized this case differently had the woman's mother or father been the client.

Family therapies focus on the "connections" between individuals and view interactions systemically and structurally. However, they often tend to promote the valuing stance that individuals should be encouraged to individuate and become autonomous from the family (Zhang, 1994). Even when looking at families, Euro-American therapists will often conceptualize families in terms of nuclear units instead of as extended networks, which is characteristic of many other cultures (Zhang, 2003f). Also, these therapists can often ignore the supports that extended families provide and suggest boundaries between parents and grandparents should be strengthened rather than seen as a useful resource.

Locus of Responsibility

Behavior therapy, Gestalt therapy, and family therapy are unconcerned with why clients have developed their problems and instead are more interested in what maintains the client's behavior now. Psychodynamic therapies are a notable exception. These frequently focus on the past at the expense of the present and future. Many clients, however, are often very interested in "why." They want to know whether or not a problem is their fault, someone else's fault, a result of chance or bad luck, or related to external circumstances. For many people, these questions determine how, when, and upon whom they should place blame for their current problems. But the questions also help clients begin to identify the changes that need to be made, so clients can avoid falling into the same old trap in the future.

Think about a problem at work, at school, or in your love life. What do you see as the cause(s) of this problem? Do you tend to give external explanations about "other people," "luck," or "prejudice" being the cause or internal explanation about your own "laziness," "lack of assertiveness," or "fear of relationships"? Think about your response to another, but different, kind of problem. Is your response style stable or does it depend on the situation?

For one week, consider the explanations you use with others, including clients. Ask yourself, "What type of explanations do I use?" Remember that people are more likely to use external and unstable explanations for their own problems and internal and stable explanations for others'.

TABLE 5.7	LANGUAGE THAT IDENTIFIES LOCUS OF RESPONSIBILITY	
External Locus of Responsibility	**Internal Locus of Responsibility**	
• Attributes events to chance or to external factors. Example: "It just happened" or "He did it."	• Attributes events to actions set into motion by the speaker. Example: "I made it happen" or "It's all my fault."	
• Perceives emotions as having an external cause. Example: "He made me depressed."	• Perceives emotions as having an internal cause. Example: "I upset myself."	
• The search for responsibility is external. Example: "How did my being the only female in the room affect what happened?"	• The search for responsibility is internal. Example: "What did I do?"	

In general, therapists tend to adopt an internal locus of responsibility, where the responsibility for the problem is assumed to reside within the person. This can be heard in the questions therapists use (see table 5.7). Depending upon the theoretical framework, questions may be, "What did you do first?" (behavioral), "What were you thinking then?" (cognitive), or "What was the relationship like in the past versus the present?" (psychodynamic). Loci of responsibility are also reflected in cultural idioms like, "You got yourself into this mess, now get yourself out," "Pull yourself up by your bootstraps," and "It's every man for himself."

Nonetheless, many clients have external loci of responsibility. They enter therapy feeling buffeted by life and will often see themselves as victims of things that happen to them. Magdalena, an impoverished Euro-American woman, entered therapy complaining of depression. Within the first week of her treatment, she was beaten by her partner and lost several teeth, had a gun held to her head, lost her job, and had her mortgage foreclosed. In the course of a few days, she'd endured more major stressors than most people experience in an entire year or more. She inappropriately blamed herself for all sorts of things—particularly the abuse she was subjected to as a child—and she felt little responsibility for or ability to control her current stressors.

Although Magdalena probably had more responsibility for her current problems than she admitted, she had fewer degrees of freedom than do many people. Being impoverished, she had few real options for housing, jobs, and education. Even when she had options, they were often usurped by people with power over her, such as her caseworkers and her husband who told her how she *should* handle problems rather than encouraging her to identify solutions.

Magdalena saw the events in her life as being caused by a malicious God and an unfair society. From her point of view, these were certainly not her responsibility and, of course, were outside of her control. Many people have similar attitudes, and they attribute problems and events to malevolent forces in the universe, chance, and even benevolent forces ("I'm just lucky, I guess"). Seventeenth-century Calvinists believed that they had neither responsibility for nor control over their entry into heaven, and they attributed this to celestial powers. However, they did believe that good living would *demonstrate* their status among the chosen few. Some modern-day Christians see prayer as their means of controlling an apparently absent-minded, but benevolent God. Nonetheless, as with the Calvinists, they view luck as being bestowed by God instead of it being the responsibility and result of their own actions. Nathan, for example, an exceptionally bright and hardworking man, spoke of his plans for the future—a job, student loans, spouse, and children—as being dependent upon God's will.

An internal locus of responsibility may make considerable sense in many situations, but it can be inappropriate or pathogenic in others (Raine, 1998). For example, asking a woman with a history of child abuse what she did to cause the abuse would be highly blaming. This type of assumption may have been common 25 years ago, but it is a measure of how far the field of psychology has come that therapies now assume that responsibility for the abuse lies with an adult or older child. Modern professionals are also less likely to excuse domestic violence or to ask people who have been beaten by their domestic partners what they did to cause it.

A value conflict gets created when therapists have an internal locus of responsibility and their clients have an external locus of responsibility. This is especially true for lower-class and minority clients. Therapists may blame clients for problems that are better attributed to prejudice, discrimination, and poverty. We are not all free. In addition, when we see clients attributing problems to other causes, we may conclude that they are unwilling to change. As the next section shows, this can be an inappropriate conclusion.

Locus of Control

The therapist-client conflict described in the previous section comes, at least in part, from failing to distinguish between loci of responsibility and loci of control. While responsibility generally refers to the causation of *past* behavior and problems, control refers to the ability to intervene in the *present* and *future* (see table 5.8). Nathan saw himself as being low in both control and responsibility—both being in God's hands. However, control and responsibility can be independent of one another. One can have an external locus of responsibility ("The problem was caused by heterosexism and homophobia"), yet also an internal locus of control ("I will do what I can to change my world and hold my head high"). Having an internal sense of control is often advantageous, regardless of whether responsibility is attributed internally or externally (D. W. Sue & Sue, 1999).

TABLE 5.8   LANGUAGE THAT IDENTIFIES LOCUS OF CONTROL

External Locus of Control	Internal Locus of Control
• Events are perceived as unpredictable. Example: "I never know what I can do . . . ."	• Events are perceived as predictable. Example: "He's always irritable when he needs to work long shifts. I just remember this and try to be especially understanding . . . ."
• Events are caused by external factors with little or no influence from internal ones. Example: "It just happens . . . what can I do?"	• Events are somewhat or entirely caused or controlled by internal factors. Example: "He's unfair, but I can study differently next time."
• Control, such as it is, is at the whim of external factors. Example: "What can they do to make things different?"	• The search for control is internal. Example: "What can I do different this time?"

Note: Language is in the present or future tense and does not imply anything about the initial causation of the event.

An internal locus of control and a high sense of self-efficacy, in fact, are strong predictors of successful change and its maintenance (Bandura, 1997; Harackiewicz, Sansone, Blair, Epstein, & Maderlink, 1987). Many therapeutic interventions can be seen as attempts to increase self-efficacy and move locus of control in a more internal direction. With clients who take an external locus of control and ask others to change, as in "Things would be okay if she would just stop hassling me," Walter and Peller (1992) ask, "What do you want to be doing differently?" Their question avoids issues of past responsibility and urges individual control of present and future events. Creating hierarchies for systematic desensitization can be seen as an attempt to create small successes in order to increase the likelihood of other small victories, increasing self-efficacy. Berg (1994), de Shazer (1988), and others ask about other successes either with the same problem, "When isn't this a problem," or with other similar problems, "How did you handle quitting smoking?" The reinforcements associated with token economies, as well as the more mundane social reinforcements of change that are common in therapy, build both self-efficacy and hopefulness.

Internal Responsibility/Internal Control   Having an internal locus of control enables clients to have the confidence to work toward potentially difficult goals. Although some general advantages to an internal locus of control exist, each combination of levels of control and responsibility has its own advantages and disadvantages (D. W. Sue & Sue, 1999). The dominant culture of the United States is very achievement-oriented and individualistic. We believe people can and should "pull themselves up by the bootstraps." When someone hits a bump in the road, we may say things like,

"You can do it!" Members of the dominant culture tend to believe that the world is fair and just and that we earn what we get (and vice versa).

The United States' dominant beliefs about control and responsibility are characteristic of people with internal loci of control and responsibility. Clients and therapists who adopt this stance are independent, high in individual responsibility, and achievement oriented. Oprah Winfrey demonstrates an excellent example of this viewpoint when she says, "Excellence is the best deterrent to racism or sexism" (as cited in *Columbia World of Quotations*, 1996). However, when people with this viewpoint confront real barriers, they may blame themselves inappropriately. They tend to believe that the world is fair and just and that failures are their fault alone.

Because people in this group are strongly individually oriented, they may have a difficult time shifting viewpoints and understanding the relational and contextual approaches of other cultures and worldviews. This can be a significant barrier with clients who do not see themselves as responsible for their problems or able to change the situation.

Internal Responsibility/External Control   D. W. Sue and Sue (1999) talk about clients in this group as being marginalized and having accepted the dominant society's values about being responsible for their own fate, but believing that they have little control over their future. This is an especially difficult position, since they may inappropriately blame themselves for their inability to overcome the real barriers in their lives. For example, Lane, a lesbian, was attacked in a parking lot at work and wondered what she had done to cause the confrontation. When she identified the assault as the work of a homophobe, she worked to fit in and be "better" according to the dominant culture's standards.

Although people with an internal locus of responsibility and an external locus of control can be culturally flexible, chameleon-like, and able to succeed both within their own culture as well as in the majority culture (D. W. Sue & Sue, 1999), they may also end up feeling like they don't fit in either culture and are not truly accepted by either one. African Americans who are successful within the majority society are often referred to pejoratively as "oreos," both by their own race and by Euro-Americans. They may denigrate themselves for not being successful in the ways they would wish (e.g., in culturally accepted ways) and may attribute their failures to laziness or stupidity (see Ramírez, Maldonado, & Martos, 1992). Perlow and Latham (1993) reported that feeling helpless and without personal control will increase acts of aggression against people who have even less power, such as stressed and underpaid employees against residents of a mental health facility.

Members of this group can bang their heads against the glass ceiling without recognizing its presence. Their therapists can also make the same mistake. When clients believe they are responsible for their own fates, therapists can fail to challenge this belief even though it is inappropriate. Failing to do so, however, can lead to a perpetuation of the self-hatred and alienation that the client may already feel. D. W. Sue and Sue (1999) suggest that therapy with these clients should have two goals: (1) to assist them in recognizing and coping with the political forces that have been problematic in their lives and (2) to help them recognize positive attempts to acculturate without rejecting their cultural heritage.

For example, Lane acknowledged the prejudice and discrimination in her society and began to attribute the attack to prejudice rather than to something bad about her. She coped with the attack in a self-affirming way rather than with depression. Moreover, she recognized the amount of homophobia and physical self-hatred that she had internalized in her childhood and began to make conscious decisions about who she was instead of unthinkingly incorporating a restrictive definition of the successful woman she had found in her family and her culture. As she explored the images she had absorbed, she started to make conscious decisions about her beliefs. She began to define her worth independent of her weight, her ability to match commercial ideals of beauty, and her willingness to accept traditional gender roles. Ironically, she had long-held liberal ideals for others, but not for herself. She had been blinded by her apparent tolerance in other areas of her life and assumed that she held the same ideals for herself.

External Responsibility/Internal Control   Mary McLeod Bethune said, "The drums of Africa still beat in my heart. They will not let me rest while there is a single Negro boy or girl without a chance to prove his worth" (as cited in Simpson, 1988, p. 110). This is the kind of activist statement made by people who have an external locus of responsibility and an internal locus of control. These people recognize the barriers, but they also see their ability to control their destiny and overcome the challenges. Because of their strong self-efficacy and awareness of societal injustice, they are more likely to be involved in social-change movements. On the other hand, this group can be very challenging in therapy, especially with majority-group therapists. Clients may dismiss their therapists as members of the oppressing group or as simply being unknowledgeable about the problems they face, regardless of the therapists' true abilities (D. W. Sue & Sue, 1999; C. E. Thompson et al., 1994).

> SUZANNE: *You say that you've had people who don't trust you and block you because you're black. I wonder whether it might also be something about how you approach unfamiliar situations. (Paraphrase, interpretation)*
>
> DARYL: *What you know? You a educated white woman. People bend over backwards when you come in the room.*

Rather than having trust and self-disclosure come readily, a Euro-American therapist like Suzanne may have to earn it by demonstrating an understanding of the issues facing a minority group and the privilege associated with being a member of the majority group (C.E. Thompson et al., 1994). Beginning her paraphrase with "You say . . . " suggests that she does not believe his perception of events. Responding defensively to him with, "What do you mean? I had to work as hard as anyone else to get here," would only further undermine her credibility and make it more difficult for the two to form a strong therapeutic alliance, even if her self-disclosure was accurate. A better response might be, "You're right. Because I'm an educated white woman, people just assume I'm safe. It's not fair."

Regardless of whether Suzanne's initial interpretation made sense, clearly she did not have the therapeutic relationship to use it at that point. She had acted before Daryl felt listened to and understood. Before attempting to shift Daryl's view of his world, she had to help him recognize that she understood him.

> SUZANNE: *You've had people be distrustful of you and block you just because you're black. (Paraphrase)*
> DARYL: *Yeah, I walk down the street and people clutch their purses.*
> SUZANNE: *That sounds frustrating and alienating. It'd be hard to feel accepted and understood when people react like that. (Reflection of feeling, feedback)*
> DARYL: *Yeah . . .*
> SUZANNE: *(Tentatively) I wonder whether some part, maybe some small part, might be something about how you approach unfamiliar situations. (Interpretation)*
> DARYL: *Hmmm. Like when I came in here that first time?*

In the first exchange, Suzanne ignored the real barriers that Daryl faced when she emphasized internal responsibility to the exclusion of external responsibility. By underestimating these barriers, she adopted a viewpoint at odds with Daryl's worldview. Daryl was more likely to accept external barriers such as poverty, prejudice, and discrimination as sources of problems rather than internal explanations of laziness, paranoia, and aggressive responses. However, once she acknowledged these and his reaction to them, she could question his role in the problem, which he could then accept.

Particularly with this sort of client, a contextual and systemic view of problems may be particularly effective (Atkinson, Maruyama, & Matsui, 1978; Atkinson, Casas, & Abreu, 1992; Gim, Atkinson, & Kim, 1991; C. E. Thompson & Jenal, 1994; C. E. Thompson et al., 1994). The problem does not occur in isolation, but is co-determined by the individual and the environment, including family, community, and culture. From this perspective, external forces may support or be antagonistic toward clients' actions. Although this viewpoint is acceptable to external responsibility/internal control clients, it challenges the culture's firmly held belief in the supremacy of the Autonomous Self, a self with free will that can act independently on the world without forces to moderate these actions (Minuchin & Nichols, 1993).

External Responsibility/External Control   People with an external locus of responsibility and external locus of control believe they live in an environment in which there is little opportunity for success, recognition, or achievement, and that they have little ability to change the rules. D. W. Sue and Sue (1999) describe two typical types of responses to this worldview: (1) giving up and (2) learning to placate and please those in power.

Learned helplessness—giving up—develops in an environment in which people are unable to earn reinforcements, regardless of their actions (Alloy & Seligman, 1979; Seligman, 1968). After a period of acting unsuccessfully on their environment, they may give up and fail to respond even in situations where they are capable of being successful. Imagine Luellen in a third-grade classroom where her teacher is unresponsive to anything positive she says or does. Regardless of how well Luellen does, her teacher fails to praise her ideas and even grades her papers poorly, perhaps because the teacher believes children learn best when their ideas are criticized. Eventually, Luellen stops trying and continues to stay shut down even when she is moved to a new classroom with a more responsive teacher. Seligman (1975) describes learned helplessness as being very much like, and even causal of, depression. Performance that was easily achievable when Luellen entered her third-grade class is now seen as impossible. Before Luellen can again see herself as successful, the bar may need to be lowered to a level where she can see herself as able to achieve.

Flexibility of Stance   People who perceive a loss of control and see themselves as helpless in their world, cope less effectively with stressors and their health suffers (S. C. Thompson & Spacapan, 1991). On one hand, residents of nursing homes who are given some control fare better (Rodin, 1986). The positive effects of control seem to be especially true with moderate or severe stressors rather than with trivial ones. Studies strongly suggest we should assist our clients in discovering ways to maximize their sense of control, particularly when the stressor is nontrivial.

On the other hand, it is unlikely that any stance is healthy in all situations. What is "healthy" may depend greatly on the nature of events that are causing the problem and on one's real ability to influence it. Accepting responsibility for things that are beyond one's control such as abuse, poverty, or racism may simply lead to frustration, self-blaming, hopelessness, and poorer adjustment (Reed et al., 1993).

This is consistent with research on Rorschach responses from children who have recently reported a history of abuse (Shapiro, 1989). Paradoxically, those who identified some responsibility ("I shouldn't have worn that skirt," or "I shouldn't have said that.") were *less* depressed than those who saw themselves as blameless. Perhaps this is because those who identified *some* blame also identified ways of coping with this significant stressor and saw things to do to prevent it in the future (increased control). Those who saw themselves as blameless seemed to feel that they were in an unpredictable, uncontrollable world.

Isaac felt like he was in a world spinning out of control. He was a middle-aged executive traveling home from work when a drunk driver crossed the center line and hit him. Isaac had been driving at the speed limit and wearing his seat belt at the time. The depression and post-traumatic symptoms that followed the accident shocked him. Clearly, Isaac saw himself as not responsible for the accident, but in drawing this conclusion, he also abdicated control over controllable parts of his life. He began thinking, "That could have been me. It could happen again at any time." He reported feeling like he was "falling" whenever he thought about the accident and often felt nauseous at these times. When he started driving again he would castigate himself for going too slow and when getting too close to the shoulder, all of which intensified his fears.

His recognition that the other driver was at fault was appropriate and helpful. However, with control in the other driver's court, he felt powerless. We reframed his "overly cautious" behaviors as coping mechanisms for regaining control of his world. He began to look for other things that he was doing to keep safe, and he valued these. In making these changes, we moved to an external locus of responsibility, but a more internal locus of control, a stance that was consistent with his history as a Jewish male with parents who had survived the Holocaust.

CONCLUSIONS

The way clients talk about and present themselves gives us clues about their worldview. This, in turn, helps us understand and approach our clients' dilemmas. Many other aspects make up worldview, and the dimensions described in this chapter are of particular importance to the therapeutic process (Ibrahim, 1985; Koltko-Rivera, 1999; D. W. Sue & Sue, 1999). However, as seen in table 5.9, these values are not as simple and dichotomous as might be expected. Rather, they are complicated and they interact with one another in complex ways.

Mervyn (from chapter 2) believed in action as table 5.9 shows. He saw himself in a world where chance ruled, yet he continued to believe in his

TABLE 5.9   SIGNIFICANT ASPECTS OF MERVYN'S AND RASHELLE'S WORLDVIEWS

Mervyn	Rashelle
Ontology	
• Tends to take a rational view of the world, although believes that God intervenes in "unusual" situations. Believes God is testing him.	• Tends to take a semirational view of the world. Expects the world (and her religion) to conform to natural rules, although she does not really understand these rules and has a difficult time seeing when the world does not conform.
Mutability	
• Believes change—even rapid change— is possible even while he feels "stuck." He especially refers to his ability to go "cold turkey" when quitting smoking.	• Tends to doubt her ability to change and half-accepts the idea that "racial traits" prevent her from being successful.
Trust	
• Does not particularly expect that he will be heard or understood by anyone. Feels "alone"—like a lone fighter against the world.	• Has an easy time trusting extended family and friends, although trusts authority figures superficially.
Authority	
• Expects that authority figures will work with him in a rapid and egalitarian manner, giving him suggestions and allowing him to develop and extend these suggestions.	• Expects that authority figures (when benevolent) have knowledge and expertise and will tell her what to do. Believes most authority figures will not act on her behalf.
Group	
• Believes his first responsibility is to his family, although he does not expect this to be reciprocated.	• Believes her first responsibility is to her extended family and has a difficult time doing things that she sees as putting her own wishes above the group's.
Responsibility	
• Believes current problems are his fault.	• Attributes problems to systemic problems of oppression and privilege.
Control	
• Believes things can be better if "I can just figure out what I'm supposed to do."	• Does not believe that she can do anything to make things different or better.

own ability to create and resolve problems. He was a Calvinist at heart and believed in his own ability to act on the world and to change it through his own hard work, even as he doubted others' willingness to help him. Once a good working relationship was developed, we were able to brainstorm solutions in an egalitarian fashion. Because he saw himself as an active contributor to the therapeutic process, he frequently returned to sessions having gone far beyond the goals we had set in our previous meeting. In addition, he had little familial and community support, although he wanted more but was afraid to ask. We identified simple strategies to increase his support within his family, at work, and from his church. Because he had experienced so little support for so long, he was satisfied with relatively small increases.

Rashelle (from chapter 4), on the other hand, saw herself as part of a benevolent system, surrounded by malevolent forces beyond her control (also table 5.9). While Mervyn had internal loci of responsibility and control, Rashelle tended to have external loci of responsibility and control. She subscribed to mainstream goals and values, but perceived few opportunities for achieving them. She was lucky to have been referred to Sherene, her therapist, with whom she quickly developed a strong therapeutic alliance. Sherene straddled both of Rashelle's worlds, because she was an African American who was also successful in the school system. Sherene modeled healthy coping strategies and empowered Rashelle to believe that she could also be successful in a way that was consistent with her values. In addition, she assisted Rashelle in identifying ways to challenge the system to make it better for all culturally different peoples. Rashelle started an informal mentoring group, strengthened the library's resources on ethnic and racial minority authors, and began an internship program with African American-owned businesses.

Although there are no "right" ways to think about oneself in the context of problems, some are very useful. By taking advantage of the strengths in Mervyn's worldview, his treatment was expedited and he developed new ways of identifying and strengthening his support systems. His treatment was egalitarian in nature and action-oriented. Although Rashelle accurately identified oppression and prejudice in her environment, she saw them as insurmountable. Sherene, therefore, chose a relatively supportive, yet directive approach with Rashelle, and she emphasized empowering interventions. At the end of treatment, Rashelle continued to adopt an external locus of responsibility for life's problems but believed that she was capable of addressing them.

Recognizing each client's worldview is a respectful approach to clients *and* to the therapy process. Communicating our understanding of the problems and of the person is often sufficient for successful therapeutic change (Rogers, 1957). When empathic understanding is not enough, our understanding may indicate how to approach therapy in a rapid and efficient manner.

WHEN WORLDVIEWS CLASH

"Just a spoonful of sugar helps the medicine go down, in a most delightful way . . . ." (R. Stevenson & Walsh, 1964)

Mary Poppins, the title character in one of my favorite childhood movies, suggests that we should sugarcoat potentially distasteful interventions to get our clients to move in the direction we hope they will go. (Mary Poppins wanted Jane and Michael to clean their room.)

While Mary Poppins' goals were only minimally aversive, consider the extreme and certainly questionable therapies in the movies *A Clockwork Orange* and *One Flew Over the Cuckoo's Nest*. In *A Clockwork Orange*, aversive conditioning techniques are used to protect society from a man convicted of rape and vicious assaults, but these also prevent him from enjoying the classical music he used to love. In *One Flew Over the Cuckoo's Nest*, electroconvulsive therapy and frontal lobotomies are used to control a psychiatric patient who had been operating outside the norms of his society. Clients are sometimes clearly aware of the potentially coercive aspect of medication and therapy, as was my client Martha, who described the antipsychotics she'd been placed on during a short hospital stay in this way: "They are punishment pills to guide me in the direction they want me to go."

D. W. Sue and Sue (1999) would agree with Martha's concerns and the sentiments expressed in *A Clockwork Orange* and *One Flew Over the Cuckoo's Nest*, arguing that:

> [W]hile mental health practice enshrines the concepts of freedom, rational thought, tolerance of new ideas, and equality and justice for all, it can be used as an oppressive instrument by those in power to maintain the status quo. In this respect, mental health practice becomes a form of oppression in which there is an unjust and cruel exercise of power to subjugate or mistreat large groups of people. When used to restrict rather than enhance the well-being and development of the culturally different, it may entail overt and covert forms of prejudice and discrimination. (p. 7)

The potential for abuse is a viewpoint that Szasz (1963) would agree with and is exacerbated by the difficulty in identifying clearly accepted criteria of mental illness with high inter-rater reliabilities. He argued that "Looking for evidence of such illness is like searching for evidence of heresy: Once the investigator gets into the proper frame of mind, anything may seem . . . to be a symptom of mental illness" (p. 709). Surely, this must be why Madanes' student's client, a man not responding to antidepressants, was hospitalized (see discussion in chapter 3; Madanes, 1999.) If you are looking for mental illness, you will see it. When you remember his context—his father's recent death and the threatened loss of his job—his depression becomes understandable, albeit still problematic.

Szasz's (1963) viewpoint seems to be confirmed by Rosenhan's (1973) research on psychiatric workers' abilities to reduce the severity of their diagnoses following a patient's admission to a psychiatric hospital. The researchers were admitted after reporting vague symptoms that did not fall into any psychiatric category. No symptoms were reported following admission. Nonetheless, in the period before managed care, the researchers' psychiatric health was not readily recognized by staff and, in fact, all but one pseudopatient was diagnosed with schizophrenia. The average hospital stay of the researchers who had no obvious symptoms was 19 days.

One interpretation of Rosenhan's (1973) findings and Madanes' (1999) story is that *unusual* behaviors such as hearing "thud," taking notes, and having nonresponsive depression are more likely to be seen as pathological

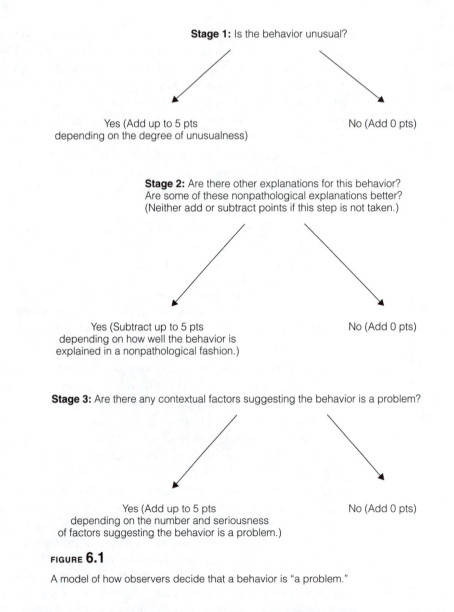

Stage 1: Is the behavior unusual?

Yes (Add up to 5 pts
depending on the degree of unusualness)

No (Add 0 pts)

Stage 2: Are there other explanations for this behavior?
Are some of these nonpathological explanations better?
(Neither add or subtract points if this step is not taken.)

Yes (Subtract up to 5 pts
depending on how well the behavior is
explained in a nonpathological fashion.)

No (Add 0 pts)

Stage 3: Are there any contextual factors suggesting the behavior is a problem?

Yes (Add up to 5 pts
depending on the number and seriousness
of factors suggesting the behavior is a problem.)

No (Add 0 pts)

FIGURE 6.1

A model of how observers decide that a behavior is "a problem."

when viewed in a context that creates an expectation of pathology; in this case, a psychiatric hospital (see figure 6.1). Having fewer factors reduces the probability that behaviors will be identified as problematic. For example, throwing one's hat high in the air is an unusual behavior under most situations and would generally cause raised eyebrows *except at graduation!*

The second step of figure 6.1, when we search for other nonpathological explanations for this behavior, is probably the most problematic and most readily missed. Most people tend to identify a single interpretation for a person's behavior. For example, when Sojah didn't smile and say hello to Magrete, Magrete concluded that Sojah was angry with her, even though she couldn't understand why she would be. There are, of course, many other reasons why Sojah did not say something, including that she didn't see Magrete, that she believed Magrete hadn't seen her, or that she was depressed and may have assumed that no one wanted to spend time with her. Unfortunately, when we skip Step 2, as Magrete did, or address it in a cursory fashion, we are more likely to make mistakes.

When we tend to identify values, beliefs, and behaviors that differ from our own as "problematic" (D. W. Sue & Sue, 1999), we will be more likely to have trouble working with culturally different clients. More accurately, we will have difficulty working with people outside our cultural understanding, which may include other cultures. These problems will be especially marked when we miss seeing the behavior's context or underestimate its impact. Alex, a Euro-American man without children, was very concerned when he interviewed the Han family, whose young children continued to share the marriage bed. Alex's supervisor challenged his initial concerns about incest and enmeshment, noting that this behavior was traditional in many Asian societies (D. W. Sue & Sue, 1999). She did, however, ask whether there were any other evidence that may point to incest other than the parents and children sharing a bed.

Our therapeutic goals occur in a context that is influenced, even constructed, by our values and worldview (G. Greenberg, 1997; McGuire, Nieri, Abbott, Sheridan, & Fisher, 1995). When we believe being open with our feelings is healthy, we encourage emotional expression. When we believe that feelings should be shared with a select few, we are more likely to encourage stronger boundaries. Deciding to focus on or avoid negative thoughts is a decision influenced by culture (D. W. Sue & Sue, 1999). Therapists with strongly homophobic attitudes are more likely than non-homophobic therapists to break confidentiality about HIV/AIDS status and to recommend involuntary hospitalizations for clients not using safe sex techniques (McGuire et al., 1995). As a result, becoming aware of our own values and their impact on our clients is especially important because imposing these values may be harmful, especially for clients outside of the dominant culture.

CLASHING WORLDVIEWS

One of my favorite cartoons depicts Calvin (from the *Calvin and Hobbes* comic strip) going downstairs, much as in Marcel Duchamp's painting, *Nude Descending a Staircase* (see figure 6.2). His mother stands at the

Calvin and Hobbes by Bill Watterson

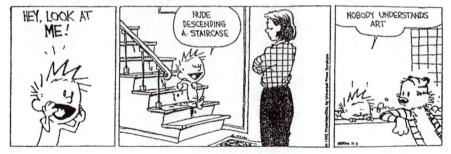

FIGURE **6.2**

Calvin's view of art clashes with his mother's. (*Calvin and Hobbes* © 1993 Watterson. Reprinted with permission of Universal Press Syndicate. All rights reserved.)

bottom of the staircase with her arms crossed and a disapproving expression on her face. Calvin responds with, "Nobody understands art."

Calvin's action (perhaps performance art?) questioned the definition of art and whether it is the exclusive object of one group and not another. His mother, on the other hand, simply saw a naked child escaping the bathtub and trailing water down the stairs. His worldview, which values living spontaneously in the here and now, differs from that of his exasperated and tired mother's, which emphasizes order, rules, and quiet (perhaps because these were in short supply in their home). When two worldviews clash, as here, rather than identifying one another as "different," the one with power (in this case, Calvin's mom) frequently identifies the other as "bad" or "crazy." The one without power may either accept this judgment, as some gays who have internalized society's homophobia, or may see it and the person (or group) who is making the judgment as "unreasonable."

The most extreme examples of this phenomenon are political prisoners like the poet Ezra Pound, who was put in a U.S. psychiatric hospital for 13 years because of his political views during WWII. Other examples include the Soviet novelist Alexander Solzhenitsyn and other Russian dissidents who were put in hospitals and gulags (Seligman, Walker, & Rosenhan, 2001; Solzhenitsyn, 1962/1963). Being different and seeing the world differently *was* crazy. Because of our mistrust of differences, our society readily justifies engaging in questionable practices including failing to treat African Americans who had syphilis (from 1932 to 1972, 399 African American males were denied treatment in the infamous Tuskegee Syphilis Study), sterilizing people with Down's syndrome without their consent, or stripping convicted felons of the right to vote. This last group, perhaps not coincidentally, includes a disproportionate number of African American males. The majority of both rural and urban arrests are Euro-American, and nearly half of those in jail or in prison are African American (Wilson, 1999, in Jackson, 2000). Also, African Americans are more likely to be convicted and given longer sentences. Each of these affected groups is relatively powerless.

Less extreme stories are also examples of this problem. Jackson (1999) criticized his son's teachers' attempts to refer him for treatment of Attention Deficit Hyperactivity Disorder (ADHD). He described his son as bright, curious, active, and misunderstood by the system: "The problem was not the son, but the teachers." Jackson's son is now a member of Congress.

SEARCHING FOR CONSISTENCY

Heider (1946) argued that people prefer internal states of harmony and consistency. We want to agree with people we like and disagree with those we dislike. When we disagree with someone we like, we search for ways to resolve the cognitive dissonance (Martz et al., 1998). Maintaining consistency is an important motive that advertisers take advantage of, paying highly admired people like Michael Jordan enormous amounts of money to endorse products. The fact is that we are more likely to prefer and buy products endorsed by people we admire (Kadlek, 1997; Kenrick et al., 1999).

Cognitive dissonance, or an awareness of the differences between disparate worldviews, is uncomfortable for many (Festinger, 1957). During any interaction where dissonance exists, an attempt to decrease it will also exist (see table 6.1). Dissonance is greater when the other party is more attractive or powerful. Power is certainly a frequent component of therapy,

---

TABLE 6.1 **FACTORS THAT INITIATE, AMPLIFY, OR REDUCE DISSONANCE BETWEEN WORLDVIEWS**

Dissonance begins with awareness that one's worldview significantly conflicts with another's:

Dissonance is greater when:

- The other group is more powerful or attractive.
- There are significant costs to maintain the viewpoint.
- The other worldview cannot be avoided.
- The dissonant values are seen as personally important.
- Self-esteem is low.

Dissonance is reduced through changes to remove unpleasant arousal including:

- Changing opinion of the other group
- Changing perception of costs of worldview.
- Avoiding the other worldview, thus experiencing dissonance.
- Changing values and worldview.
- Affirming your own positive attributes or values in an unthreatened realm.

Note: From Aronson, Blanton, & Cooper, 1995; Kenrick et al., 1999.

even an aspect that therapists attempt to manipulate in order to maximize the change process—by hanging their diplomas, displaying expertise, and using mailings that foster an image of professionalism (Frank, 1961). Dissonance is also greater when there are costs to maintaining the viewpoint and when the other viewpoint cannot be avoided or is seen as personally important.

When two divergent worldviews come together, conflict is inevitable, especially when the area of difference is something each person or group identifies as important. This can be seen at the international level (e.g., Russia versus the United States), national level (e.g., pro-choice versus pro-life movements), or in interpersonal relationships (Bill Clinton versus Newt Gingrich). Sometimes, the conflict is physical and may be maintained in full force for years. Often the cognitive dissonance is resolved by one party diminishing the other, one person avoiding an area of disagreement, or an individual changing his or her viewpoint (Festinger, 1957). See table 6.1 for examples of greater and lesser dissonance.

Maintaining two opposing views side by side (agreeing to disagree) is difficult but under special conditions, it can be possible. Our response depends on the salience of the other viewpoint, its personal importance, and the costs associated with either maintaining or changing the viewpoint. We may be unaware of some group differences or they may be seen as relatively trivial. For example, we may be unaware of the fact that many Asians use chopsticks when eating and, when we become aware of this difference in dining habits, we may conclude that it has no personal impact; that it doesn't matter. Likewise, becoming aware of prejudice toward and persecution of ethnic Albanians by Serbs may have a significant impact on our behavior and attitudes when we or people we care about are members of either group. The specific nature of this impact will depend upon our own values. If one is a Serb and has tended to objectify ethnic Albanians, his or her negative attitudes may become more pronounced and rigid. On the other hand, even if one is a Serb and values human rights, he or she may need to do things like protest the war to reduce the resulting dissonance.

Power further affects this dynamic. When one group (A) is more powerful than another (B), B will have fewer options for resolving the conflict. Immigrants, for example, often experience a culture conflict shortly after they immigrate but have little power in their new home. They may resolve this conflict by denigrating the majority group and its ways, but more commonly (because of power differences) may avoid it by living in ethnic enclaves or attempting to assimilate to American culture. Note that by living in ethnic enclaves, they have equalized the power inequity, which gives them the freedom to put down the "foreign" way (see table 6.1).

Each decision comes with a cost. The energy invested in denouncing another group or viewpoint and defending one's own could be used more efficiently (see Lorde, 1984a; D. W. Sue & Sue's, 1999, for a discussion of cultural identity). Distorting and avoiding reality decreases the ability to perceive the world accurately and respond efficiently. This is true for groups in power and those that are not.

FEELINGS AND ATTITUDES ABOUT THOSE WHO ARE DIFFERENT

Next week, notice your reactions to differences in worldview and behavior around you. How do you respond to these differences? When do you accept them? When do you deprecate them? What sort of pattern to your reactions do you notice?

A quick, and unfortunately true, story is about the rumor of a rapist at large that circulated through a small town one spring. In the town, a teenager went door to door selling candy for his track team. This boy was not very bright or attractive, he had poor social skills, and he was from a very poor family. He was, however, a nice boy with good intentions. When he sold candy at the first house, he was so excited that he threw his arms around the woman and gave her a hug. She pulled a gun on him (remember the rapist?). He apologized profusely and went to the next house, where he again threw his arms around the woman after she bought a piece of candy. At this point, a police car pulled up, and officers charged him with assault.

The boy probably would not have gotten into this predicament had he been more bright or socially gifted (in our society, it's not the norm to hug strangers). But I can't help but wonder whether the story would have played out differently had there been no rumor of a rapist. We should also ask how much of this scenario can be attributed to classism. After all, the boy was unattractive and poorly dressed.

The boy's name was protected because he was a juvenile, but in a small community there's no way to stop rumors from circulating. The school heard about the charges and attempted to throw him out because he was a sexual predator. He became enamored of a girl in school, which was certainly a common event, but when he began sending her love notes with "You have pretty hair," and such and he hugged her in the hall, he was called a "pervert." The level of the discourse declined even more.

I wonder how many girls will receive provocative notes and get groped in high schools without this type of a reaction from teachers and others. Why was this relationship seen as nonconsensual? How does this relationship's context influence how it was perceived?

A running theme throughout this book is: We see the best intentions in people who are like us, and we see adverse intentions in people who are different from us, especially if their difference is considered negative (Martz et al., 1998). We are more likely to see positive intentions in those who are different from us but who may be of a higher status. Consider President Clinton and ask yourself these questions: Why were many of us so tolerant of his behavior with Monica Lewinsky? Why did his approval ratings reach all-time highs during the scandal?

Our tendency to view the intentions of people "like us" as good and the intentions of those who are different as bad has the potential to seriously impact our work with clients who differ in race, ethnicity, class, affectional orientation, physical ability, and the like. In every interaction we have with clients, our job requires that we make numerous judgments about their behavior and motivations. Our values have the potential to be coercive, as can be seen in these examples:

- The Hernandez family was referred for treatment after their three-year-old was found down the block without her father, who was a single parent. The family was also reported to Child Protective Services for neglect. Although Mr. Hernandez was clearly not a vigilant parent, the child's older siblings (ages 8 and 10) were with this child. Because his was a very dark-skinned Latin family in a largely Euro-American community, Mr. Hernandez accused his neighbors and the agency of being racists when they made the referral and started an investigation.

  At about the same age, my daughter had run off to a neighbor's house before I knew she was even gone, so I wondered how issues of race and class influenced the decisions—either protecting me or causing others to be especially vigilant about his behavior.

  Being a single father may also have played into the referral. Can a single dad be a good parent? Is our skepticism about a single dad's ability to be an effective parent one reason for funny and poignant movies like *Daddy Day Care; Me, Myself, and Irene; Big Daddy;* and *Mrs. Doubtfire?*

- Mrs. Maki canceled three family sessions in a row because her work schedule as a janitor changed. The Maki family's therapists wondered whether she believed that therapy was important. They believed that if she thought therapy was important, she would make attendance a priority.

  However, therapy appointments might not be a priority when keeping them may cause one to lose a job. Making appointments in the middle of the day is a luxury not always available to people who work menial jobs. Could they accept her behavior as an exemplar of how much she cared for her family? Did they understand that she did not have the same freedom on the job as they have?

- T. J.'s parents Josephine and Mildred were trying to deal with his acting out behavior in the home. Their therapists wondered whether T. J.'s problems stemmed from the lack of a positive male influence at home. The therapists were straight and, perhaps because of this, they had a difficult time understanding the impact of sexuality on families.

The therapists also believed that young males *should* have a father figure in their home. They saw mothers as potentially emasculating, especially when several women live with a child. What might have been different had the therapists wondered instead about the boy's having difficulty dealing with the homophobia of his classmates? What if the therapists had wondered whether he was questioning his own sexuality during a period when other teens were largely unaware of the options? Did they wonder whether the family was experiencing more stressors than other families, as do many gays and lesbians who live in areas where they are a significant minority? Could this behavior be unrelated to their sexuality?

In each of these cases, the behaviors described serve as exemplars for the therapists and others about context. The focus behaviors prime expectations. When the Hernandez child ran down the block, it primed the stereotypes of his Euro-American neighbors who saw it as an example of neglectful parenting, inadequate supervision, and perhaps an inability to parent three young children successfully. When my daughter ended up at her friend's house four blocks away, a different schema was tapped. Because those involved knew me to be a psychologist, their assumption was that I was a good parent but with a very slippery child. With this assumption, my friends intervened differently than Mr. Hernandez's neighbors did.

Our expectations prime the way we perceive situations. Because the schedules of typical professionals are often very flexible, they may assume that people doing shift work are just as flexible, if not more so (especially if such jobs are not considered as important). However, Mrs. Maki may have been unable to change her schedule because of financial considerations or because her boss may have mentioned to her that she was "expendable." Similarly, T. J.'s "straight" therapists did not understand the full impact that having gay parents might have on a young person. Because they lived in a superficially tolerant community, the therapists underestimated the degree to which homophobic tirades could catch a person off guard just as much as a sucker punch could. These professionals failed to see the ways in which Josephine's and Mildred's sexuality affected their lives outside their bedroom. And, they didn't ask.

RECOGNIZING AND CHALLENGING POTENTIALLY COERCIVE VALUES

Steingarten (1997) describes his reaction to earning a position as a food critic at a major magazine and focuses on his concerns about how his idiosyncratic responses to food might compromise his work:

. . . I, like everybody I knew, suffered from a set of powerful, arbitrary, and debilitating attractions and aversions at mealtime. I feared that I could be no more objective than an art critic who detests the color yellow or suffers from red-green color blindness. At the time I was friendly with a respected and powerful editor of cookbooks who grew so nauseated by the flavor of cilantro that she brought a pair of tweezers to Mexican and Indian restaurants and pinched out every last scrap of it before she would take a bite. Imagine the dozens of potential Julia Childses and M. F. K. Fishers whose books she peevishly rejected, whose careers were snuffed in their infancy! I vowed not to follow in her footsteps. (pp. 3–4)

Unfortunately, our own values and preferences can block our ability to evaluate a situation objectively, while "questions about power are always hidden in the plain light of psychotherapy" (G. Greenberg, 1997, p. 267). Although not all decisions and values are equally good, we must find some way to openly and objectively respond to the valuing dilemmas that our clients bring us each day. We need to ask, "How can this different world-view or lifestyle be a valid and useful approach to the world? How would I know whether and when it might be problematic?"

This is the challenge that Shimrat (1997) gives to the psychotherapy community. She sees therapy as a controlling device, one to which many cannot readily consent. Furthermore, this mechanism of control is used to coerce the minority into the valuing system of the majority:

Psychiatric treatment seeks to help (or make) people conform to social norms. It aims to produce successful, productive people who can function and fit in. But what if success, productivity, and "normal" functioning can sometimes be achieved only at the expense of creativity and critical thinking? What if social norms need to change in order for the world to become a better place? What if change is better than stagnation, and nonconforming people are an important source of change? (p. 2)

Steingarten (1997) worked to overcome his food preferences and aversions by exposing himself to novel and nonpreferred food on a regular basis. Similarly, we can begin to overcome parochial valuing systems by listening carefully to friends and clients who are different from us, reading a wide range of works, and watching movies frequently. As we do so, we must listen to other worldviews and values and pay attention to how they differ from our own. As Diller (1999) describes, effective immersion in other cultures can range from brief activities such as visiting rallies, attending celebrations, and eating at ethnic restaurants to more sustained ones like learning a language, volunteering in the community, and traveling to clients' countries of origin. This is not a year-long set of activities to pencil in, but a lifelong journey of discovery.

Simply exploring differences will not be sufficient to recognize and challenge parochial values. We need to ask whether a behavior, belief, or value works, and then we need to consider what its costs and benefits are for the person and his or her system.

COERCIVE EFFECTS OF THERAPY

Tell the same story, perhaps a description of a mistake in your life, to several people. They could be your best friend, your parents, your therapist, and a stranger. Does your story change with each telling? How? Why does it change? (modified from Bogart, 1999)

Madanes (1999) concludes that therapy is a subversive act but only discusses its positive impact. I am more pessimistic about its nature. Our values have consequences on others, from relatively trivial (e.g., how we tell or hear a story) to significant ones (e.g., what treatment goals we identify, what interventions we use, and how we employ these). These consequences can be relatively benign in nature, significantly healing, or iatrogenic. While our work can reframe the world and allow a person to view himself or herself in a new and healthier way, we can just as easily accept the status quo and undermine our clients, particularly those who come from a very different context. If, as this book advocates, we should be aware of the importance of context in our clients' lives, we will also need to become aware of how *we* are part of this context and how *we* positively and negatively contribute to our clients' changes.

Just as the telling of your story depended on who is listening, your clients' telling of their stories will be affected by your responses. While reviewing the literature in a telling picture of the role of influence in the therapy room, Frank (1961) concluded that affirmative grunts increase the use of certain words (and probably the discussion of those ideas), and punishment decreases these. Although most of the research Frank reviewed did not occur in the therapy room, it does appear that therapists' social influence is greatest when therapists have more power and prestige, when clients have a positive relationship with their therapists, when clients care about their therapists' perceptions of them, when clients are anxious or compliant (rather than defensive), and when the task is ambiguous.

In the next three sections, we will discuss the specific kinds of changes that occur in therapy and some ways that the therapeutic relationship can, paradoxically, be coercive, even while being helpful. Overtly antagonistic relationships are clearly problematic, such as those in which two people do not like each other, they do not respect one another's point of view, or they see the other as bad (as with abusive parents or forensic work). However, the often-hidden conflicts that are part and parcel of normal interactions also have significant iatrogenic potential (Bachelor & Horvath, 1999).

Socialization to Therapy

During therapy, a number of changes occur in the way the client talks. As we have already discussed, Frank (1961) suggests that these changes are due to minimal reinforcers (e.g., "uh huh") that encourage certain ways of talking about the "problem."

A client story "does not remain a freestanding reflection of truth, but rather, as questions are asked and answered, descriptions and explanations are reframed, and affirmation and doubt are disseminated by the therapist, the client's narrative is either destroyed or incorporated—but in any case replaced—by the professional account" (Gergen & Kaye, 1992, p. 169, cited in G. Greenberg, 1997).

Presumably, "the professional account" is one that supports clients' healthy growth and change. This is fine as long as both parties agree on what is healthy.

In addition, clients begin to speak their therapist's "language." Minuchin and Nichols (1993) describe this process:

> I know a family is changing when some of its members begin to use my language. After I have challenged interruptions, I hear a mother tell her children not to interrupt. Family members become attentive to a scapegoated member after I have found her communications significant. (p. 41)

Gergen and Kaye's (1992, cited in G. Greenberg, 1997) and Minuchin and Nichols' (1993) examples are not coercive, but the potential for coerciveness exists if, as a result of the power differential between therapist and client, the client feels *compelled* to reject or overlook some values and stories and adopt others. However, Minuchin and Nichols (1993) note that the changes occur in both directions with their own being part of a mimetic process:

> . . . while I am joining them, the family members are also joining me. I am pulled by their demands, and they modify my behavior. Unwittingly I adopt the family's style. (p. 46)

Identification of the "Problem"

What is identified as pathological depends upon the context and the observers' values and beliefs about clients and their problems. Sherri, for example, loved to read. In fact, she read nearly one book a day for most of her childhood. When her son didn't read as much or as often as she had, she thought that something was wrong, and this thought became the source of frequent fights despite his being an otherwise bright, attractive, and socially adept child. The greater the disparity between the client's and therapist's culture and values, the greater the problems we can anticipate. This is, at least in part, due to our tendency to equate "different" with "bad" (Ingram & Kendall, 1986). We act as though there is one and only one "right way of being" in the world. However, when therapists' assumptions about clients and cultural groups are faulty, therapy will be negatively impacted.

Stereotypes and faulty assessments may bias how a client is viewed, conceptualized, and treated, as is seen in Bogart (1999). Bogart asked her students to describe what they thought was wrong with a man who never married and continued to live with his mother. She reported that they began to "eagerly suggest dependency schemas, unresolved Oedipal conflicts, separation-individual issues, and so on" (p. 46). While the man's behavior may be symptomatic of a whole series of problems, it is not clear how this brief scenario might be inherently pathological. Instead, their rapid diagnostic and pathologizing responses seemed to be caused by the nature of the context (e.g., the counseling classroom) and the observers' Western values (see figure 6.1, p. 112). Her students pathologized his behavior in the absence of any clearly identified problems; it would have been different had her scenario included information that he drank heavily, was afraid to leave the home or make friends, and was frequently depressed. Can we still admire his loyalty to family, his continuing support of his mother, and his valuing of interpersonal relationships? See, for example, Zhang's (1994) similar case and his challenge to the highly individualistic assumptions of U.S. culture. While these assumptions are characteristic of Euro-American culture (Helms & Cook, 1999), they are not the only approach within Euro-American culture or the only way to be happy in it.

Identification of Treatment Goals

As Bogart (1999) and Zhang (1994) clearly conclude, our values influence our identification of the "problem." They also influence what we see as treatment goals. Hays (1995) describes a Muslim woman who recently immigrated to the United States from Tunisia. She was referred to a feminist therapist because of her increasing loneliness and unhappiness. Her therapist saw her problems as stemming from her emotional and financial dependence upon her husband, neither of which the client saw as problems. In fact, the woman perceived her relationship as being good and even saw her contributions to the relationship as being equal to those of her husband.

This woman's treatment goals (Hays, 1995) and those of her therapist were quite different. Each led to different kinds of interventions. The woman's might lead to a referral to a social skills group in order to decrease the barriers that were making it difficult to make friends and be happy in the United States. Her therapist, however, might suggest cognitive restructuring of beliefs in order to challenge the client's dependency. Can this therapist work from her client's set of values and accept her definitions of the problem and of relational health?

We often act as though our inferences are both drawn objectively and irrefutably. Nevertheless, labeling a behavior as dysfunctional is a value-laden decision influenced by our own imperfect observations and our own culturally based inferences about these observations (Wood & Mallinck-rodt, 1990). Even Newton's observations of the basic laws of acceleration, which are often admired for their objectivity, were inferred from an imperfect data set contaminated by confounding variables (L. S. Greenberg, 1995). Similarly, although Euro-Americans value assertiveness, this trait can be very problematic in Eastern cultures. Confucius, for example, observed, "He who walks with his head held high hits his head."

Although some observations will be identified as "dependent" in all cultures, others will be influenced by the culture's values about normal behavior. The farther away we are from simple observations, the more subjective and unsubstantiated our inferences become. The less aware we become of contextual factors, the more likely we are to have problems with the nature of our inferences. Unfortunately, these errors can lead to the kinds of disagreements in goal identification described by Hays (1995). They can also play a part in the valuation of these goals as this story illustrates:

> I'm thinking of the Jesuit priest who spent 40 years with the Arabs and never made one convert. He was a bit of a figure of fun at anthropological conferences. Bob asked him at one such conference how many converts he had made in his time with them. He said proudly, "None. But I have shown those Bedouin that a Christian is every bit as much a man as they are" (J. Rumsey, personal communication, August 31, 1999, by permission).

Clearly, the Jesuit's goals were markedly different from Bob's (or Bob's assumptions of the Jesuit's goals). This discrepancy in goal identification may also happen when apparent similarities between therapist and client exist, as with Mañuela and Teresa who were both Latinas. Although Teresa is generally doing well with her life, she still has several potential blind spots that may be problematic in her work with Mañuela (see table 6.2).

1. Because Teresa is an acculturated Latina and has earned a graduate degree in psychology, she values insight and openness more than Mañuela is likely to. As a new immigrant with more traditional values, Mañuela is more likely to reject therapeutic demands for openness in favor of traditional taboos against violating familial boundaries. Teresa is likely to see Mañuela as shy, passive, and repressed. Mañuela, however, is likely to expect disclosure to occur in the context of a friendship, something they may have difficulty achieving given the normal counseling process.

Teresa clearly has internal loci of control and responsibility and may underestimate the real barriers that a new immigrant faces, especially if she focuses on their superficial similarities.

Mañuela, because she tends to see fewer opportunities for personal control and responsibility, may have a greater need than Teresa for a formal community support system (and Teresa might be less likely to recommend it).

TABLE 6.2   MAÑUELA'S AND TERESA'S PSYCHOSOCIAL HISTORIES

Mañuela	Teresa
Problem	
Current symptoms	
She is stressed, mildly depressed, and ambivalent about her marriage and her future. She is significantly distressed about her inability to create a good support system for herself in the United States.	N/A
Beliefs about symptoms	
She believes her reactions to her marriage and the domestic violence are normal and appropriate, but she also thinks that she should be able to adapt to the situation. She tends to blame herself for her inability to make friends in the United States and acknowledges that she had a significant number of close friends in Chile.	She has strong, negative attitudes about domestic violence, but also tends to believe that violence occurs within a system, with the whole system condoning or preventing violence.
Personal history of psychological disorders	
She reports no problems with anxiety or depression before her marriage.	She has had several significant episodes of depression. The first of them began shortly after the death of her best friend and shortly before her departure for college.
Family history of psychological disorders	
She reports that the women in her family have a history of mild depression (dysthymia) and that the men frequently drink too much.	There is no significant history.
Current Context	
Recent events	
She immigrated from Chile three years ago to marry a man she barely knew. She recognizes that they have significant differences in goals and values. His parents, with whom they live, tend to side with him against her. She has been having difficulty making friends and feels isolated, especially because her thoughts of divorce are counter to cultural imperatives.	Life is going more smoothly than in the past. Her children are getting older and more independent, and she is able to focus more on her career.
Physical condition	
She reports suffering minor brain damage and tinnitus after incurring a severe concussion during a domestic violence episode. She attributes problems with concentrating to the concussion. Her health is otherwise unremarkable.	Her health is generally good, although she has experienced stress injuries from running. She was very thin as an adolescent and as a young adult. Although of average weight for her height, she is worried about getting heavier and thicker through the waist—and she hates worrying about this!
Drug and alcohol use	
She reports no past or current use of substances. Past incidents of domestic violence occurred when her husband was drinking fairly heavily.	Occasionally, she drinks socially, but has no significant history of recreational drug use or abuse.
Intellectual and cognitive functioning	
Is bright and verbal, although she identifies some problems in attention and concentration. She attributes these to neurological damage caused by domestic violence injuries. She has completed college and is considering getting a master's degree.	Bright and hardworking, she has a master's degree in social work.

(continued)

TABLE 6.2   *(continued)*

Mañuela	Teresa
Coping style	
She tends to get overwhelmed easily, but she asks for help when stuck. She is persistent in working to solve problems.	She is assertive and direct in resolving problems. When this does not work, she runs (sometimes several miles a day) or works in the garden. She occasionally drinks socially.
Self-concept	
She sees herself as "smart" and "hardworking," although she blames herself for the problems she has in making and keeping friends. She is pessimistic about the future and about her ability to make "good" decisions.	She sees herself as "smart," "attractive," "competent," and "hardworking," especially in her professional life. She is pleased that, after an awkward childhood and adolescence, her life has been getting "on track" during the last ten years.
Sociocultural background	
She is a recently arrived, dark-skinned, working-class immigrant from Chile caught between two cultures. She describes herself as neither "traditional" nor "American." She doesn't understand "upper-class" Latins and their focus on material things. She also thinks that upper-class Latins are "rude." On the other hand, she blames herself for these problems.	She is an American-born Latina of Cuban descent. She identifies herself as Cuban American, but an American first. She is comfortable in both Latin and Euro-American groups. She enjoys a wide range of music and art that is not particularly associated with Latin America. Her mother is worried about her drifting away from the family and from Cuban ways.
Religion and spirituality	
She attends a Catholic church with many acculturated Latins. She studies the Bible in her church and sees this primarily as a way to make friends and improve her English. This has been only marginally successful, and she feels rejected and frustrated in this church.	She was raised a Catholic and says this is somewhat important to her, although she rarely goes to church. She disagrees with several major stands of the Church, especially concerning divorce, abortion, and marriage for clergy, and gets annoyed by most priests. She tends to find more "spiritual connections" in her daily walks and in her talks with friends.
Resources and Barriers	
Individual resources	
She is bright, and she values family, education, and hard work. She is persistent in seeking out resources for herself.	She is bright and hardworking and is creative and efficient in solving problems and doing several things at once. She makes friends easily.
Social resources	
She has several acquaintances, but they are only partially supportive. Each relationship starts when she is either being a helper or is being helped. She sees people as backing away from her when she discloses her history of abuse and is confused about how to self-disclose to people she likes. She is upset about her inability to create the kinds of friendships that she had in Chile.	She has several very close friends. Unfortunately, most of them live out of town. She has been strengthening other friendships.
She believes that education is the avenue to future success; that is, a good job and respect within her community. She doesn't understand her husband's refusal to further his education. She has gone to the emergency room on three occasions when he has been physically abusive. They have no children, although he pressures her to become pregnant. She believes it will be impossible to leave him if they have children together.	She enjoys her family, but at a distance. Family members are 400 to 500 miles away. They are supportive of her during her weekly calls home, but she does not share with them any "controversial" aspects of her life.

(continued)

TABLE 6.2 **(continued)**

Mañuela	Teresa
His parents (with whom they live) think she's lazy because she's not a better homemaker. They want her to quit work to "make babies" and take care of her husband. Her parents are still in Chile and do not support her leaving the marriage. They believe that she will be unmarriageable if she divorces.	She is married and has two children (ages 8 and 10) about whom she cares very much. Her relationship with her husband is less intimate than she would like, but they have a good collaborative relationship. She says that she doesn't think she would get remarried if her husband were to die before she does. Her relationships with her children are sometimes bumpy, but generally are good.

Work

While she has some minor problems at her office job, she sees them as "normal" and not worth worrying about.	She enjoys her work very much, although she complains about there being too much of it!

Community resources

She attends a Latin church, but is uncomfortable there and does not know of any Latin community center. Her physician recommends that she leave her husband because the abuse "will only get worse." She is very ambivalent about this recommendation, especially since it clashes with cultural messages and her family's wishes.	Both of her children attend a Catholic school that she likes. The children are involved in after-school sports, music, and scouting. They have had the same adult babysitter for several years.

Community contributions

She tutored a friend while in college and felt good about this experience. She describes no current community contributions.	She is required to volunteer at her children's school and frequently helps her son's scout troop. She actively mentors other beginning therapists in her community and frequently agrees to speak for local groups and organizations. She takes an active role in several other volunteer settings.

Mentors and models

She admires several acquaintances, all of whom are in helping roles.	She admires Cesar Chavez's commitment and dedication. Her high school math teacher mentored her and stayed in touch for several years after her graduation.

Obstacles and opportunities to change process

While she would like to leave her marriage, she faces significant cultural and religious injunctions against this. She is afraid that she will be rejected by her family and other Latins. She expects to never get married again or to have children. Nonetheless, she is an assertive woman who likes to take action.	She tends to expect that "good things happen to good people," despite knowing better. She tends to look at internal elements of control and to underestimate external contributing factors. As a result, she can take a blaming stance in therapy. However, her optimism is often an asset in therapy.

Therapeutic relationship

She tends to take a respectful, one-down stance in therapy and expects to receive advice from Teresa.	She expects that their relationship will be relatively egalitarian, with Mañuela taking an active role in determining the direction of therapy.

As an educated Latina with an internal locus of control, Teresa prefers a nondirective approach to solving her own problems and doing therapy. She is likely to become irritated by Mañuela's requests for increased directiveness and help, although these are often culturally normative.

While Mañuela is distressed by her inability to connect with others and to be supported by family members, Teresa tends to be more autonomous and tends to tolerate greater distance from her friends and family. She may, as a result, underestimate the importance of Mañuela's need for Teresa.

Because of her more autonomous and independent stance, Teresa may have greater difficulty understanding Mañuela's resistance to leaving an abusive relationship and defining herself as independent from her husband and family. Teresa may also underestimate the importance of familial and religious taboos against separations and divorce held by Mañuela.

Because Teresa is fairly direct and assertive and Mañuela often acquiesces to her and asks explicitly for guidance, Teresa may underestimate Mañuela's obstacles to change. It is significant to note that, despite her physician's recommendation and the domestic-violence workers' explicit suggestions to leave her husband, Mañuela has never done so. Part of her acquiescing response in therapy can be attributed to cultural demands for *respeto* (respect for authority figures and their earned wisdom).

Identifying these sources of potential conflict should be an important part of supervision and consultation and should allow us to recognize and challenge our therapeutic blind spots.

Because therapists are more powerful, clients tend to make shifts in their therapists' direction. This can occur while the client is unaware that other viable options exist. As divergent thinking decreases during stress, anxiety, and depression, we can expect clients to overlook some of their options. We must make special attempts to increase their awareness of their options and assist them with their ability to choose those options that best fit them and their values.

NEGOTIATING DIFFERENCES

To this point, we have talked as though the differences between therapist and client are not negotiable. Can they be resolved? If so, how? We need to listen carefully and empathically and intervene in ways that are respectful of our clients' worldviews and avoid those interventions that are disempowering (D. W. Sue & Sue, 1999). Working *with* the current of change, rather than against it, increases our probability of success in the long run (Walter & Peller, 1992).

Several authors (G. Greenberg, 1997; Ivey & Ivey, 2003; Ivey et al., 1997; Wood & Mallinckrodt, 1990) have suggested approaching these conflicts by first acknowledging the therapist's position and power and then relying upon basic listening skills such as paraphrasing, encouraging, reflecting feelings, making summarizations, and questioning. Initially, therapists use paraphrases and summarizations followed by a basic checkout ("Is that close?" or "Am I hearing you correctly?") to determine whether

---

If you are currently doing therapy, spend some time looking at the values inherent in your treatment plans and interventions. Do a psychosocial history of yourself and compare it with that of your clients. What do you discover? If you are not currently doing therapy, pay attention to your daily interactions with others. What values do you see? To what extent are you pushing your values onto others? Are your valuing decisions helpful to them or not? How?

Play devil's advocate. What is the downside of your valuing behaviors? What is the cost of investing in these values rather than in others? What is gained?

their understanding is accurate and also to communicate their understanding to the client. Following this, the therapist may help the client identify other ways of looking at the problem. This often includes some self-disclosure of the therapist's viewpoint. Finally, and most importantly, the therapist communicates a here-and-now acceptance of the client's values and decisions (those that aren't self-destructive, of course). This process is seen in the following dialogue:

> TOMMI: *Darlene, if I understand you correctly, you're thinking about dropping out of school because you're feeling overwhelmed right now and you don't see any way you can get caught up. Am I on track? (Summarization, checkout)*
>
> DARLENE: *Yes. I'm afraid that, if I keep going on like this, I'm going to be in over my head and will never get back out.*
>
> TOMMI: *Okay. I agree that if we don't do anything different you're going to be in over your head. However, you don't see anything you can do different, and I think there's a lot you can do. It's still early in the semester. (Self-disclosure, confrontation, information)*
>
> DARLENE: *I . . . I suppose it's still early. But I can't stand it when I don't get As. There's no way I can pass now.*
>
> TOMMI: *It is uncomfortable, but I think it's too early to tell whether you can get an A, and I think you can stand it if you get a B. What can we do that will help you do as well as you want and need to do? (Reflection of feeling and confrontation, open question)*

Not all values and decisions are equal. In this example Tommi chose to accept Darlene's feeling ("I can't stand it when I don't get As"), while simultaneously refusing to accept that there was one and only one way of addressing this problem. Although Darlene could drop out of school, she could also get tutoring, join a study group, challenge the necessity of As for self-acceptance, and identify more successful ways of studying. Each of these behaviors is potentially consistent with Darlene's own valuing stance.

There will be times when clients have less flexibility in how they are able to approach a problem. An example is when a particular solution has a special cultural meaning. Wood and Mallinckrodt (1990) suggest that an example of this is when a therapist works with people from other cultures on issues of assertiveness (see table 3.3, p. 52). Euro-Americans often value expressing themselves clearly and directly, albeit respectfully. Reservation-born Native Americans, however, often have strong prohibitions against directness, and they often use storytelling, teasing, and hinting to express an opinion (Tafoya, 1990). In addition, they view direct eye contact as disrespectful or as a challenge being made. Native American clients struggling with issues of assertiveness may need to develop culturally appropriate ways of expressing their opinions. Alternatively, they may need to identify situations in which it is acceptable to use Euro-American methods of assertiveness, such as with people raised outside the reservation (Brokenleg, 1996; Wood & Mallinckrodt, 1990).

In these examples, a client's goals are consistent with the therapist's, even though the client may choose different methods for reaching those goals. Sometimes, the client's goals are very disparate from the therapist's own values and goals, and therapists may initially identify these as self-destructive. Examples of this include:

- A Euro-American professional woman who chooses to drop out of school or leave work to become an at-home mom.
- A Latino college student who chooses a major that will best contribute to the family's financial needs and help his younger siblings get into school (D. W. Sue & Sue, 1999).
- A man who holds very fundamentalist religious views and refuses to leave an emotionally abusive relationship because it could create a schism in his family and cause him to be excommunicated from his church.

In these cases, the traditional goals of Euro-American males, such as autonomy and individualism, conflict with the more relational goals of each cultural group. In these cases, it is especially important to clarify goals and examine the perceived advantages and disadvantages of each behavior and do so from the client's point of view (Oz, 1995). Of course, if a client is thinking very narrowly, the therapist may need to help the client identify all potential costs and benefits.

This work must often be unfailingly open, honest, and direct and have a level of self-disclosure that is unusual, even uncomfortable, in other therapeutic approaches. Therapist self-disclosure is often necessary:

> The therapist must be prepared to say why he or she subscribes to this ideology, what principles justify the claim that [the behavior] is to be eliminated from the client's interior landscape and, by extension, from the social world. And therapists must be willing and able to acknowledge the limitations and contradictions as well as the strengths of their ideologies. (G. Greenberg, 1997, p. 266)

Tommi, for example, handled the dilemma like this:

TOMMI: *Darlene, I know that you are feeling overwhelmed right now and that you think As are necessary, even essential, for maintaining your sense of self-worth. I'm sure you can tell that I disagree with your point of view. I think there are other things more important in life, like friendships, enjoying life as it is, and learning rather than just getting grades. I feel that you are selling yourself short when you ac-*

cept nothing less than an A. This decision about school is yours, but I want you to be able to make it with your eyes open and be aware of other possibilities. (Summarization, self-disclosures)

As this example shows, it is not that this approach to therapy is nondirective, but that it acknowledges both points of view and puts them on the table for discussion and even disagreement. Tommi's viewpoint will be present and influential no matter what happens, but Darlene has the opportunity to reject it in a thoughtful and conscious manner when Tommi identifies her values and concerns and, of course, makes them salient.

Moreover, being open and honest in therapy moves Darlene from a one-down position as she put herself in during the first exchange to an egalitarian stance in the second. There, Tommi implied, "Here's what I believe. What do you believe? Let's join in making this decision together."

Failing to Identify Options

Clients generally come to therapy in crisis, and they often think dichotomously ("I can either go on like this forever or I can kill myself"). As a result, part of our job in therapy is to assist clients in identifying other options and to help them brainstorm other approaches to a problem. These solutions or approaches to the problem will be influenced by our own worldview and theoretical approach. This can be seen in our discussion of Mañuela and Teresa.

Consider the situation Mañuela is in. She described her husband as abusive, and she has ended up in the emergency room on several occasions. She feels alienated from friends and family by physical and cultural barriers, not least of which is that she runs up against strong taboos against any thought of dissolving her marriage. She is feeling paranoid, depressed, and lonely and doesn't see any happy future for herself. What options does she have in resolving these problems?

Because therapists hold considerable influence with their clients, especially the ones in crisis, Mañuela will probably look to Teresa for hints about how to handle her dilemma. Teresa, an educated and successful Latina, has different options available to her than does Mañuela, and she has very different priorities of values, despite the fact that they share a relatively similar ethnic background (see table 6.2, p. 125). Has Teresa pursued available options from Mañuela's point of view? When Teresa tells Mañuela that she thinks leaving her husband is a good idea, Mañuela will be more likely to pursue this idea and may even ignore other possibilities. However, does Mañuela really accept this option? Will she do what she needs to do to make it work? What are the potential costs of the options she identified (Oz, 1995)? What are the benefits? What obstacles prevent change?

Those of us who have experience working with people who have known domestic violence firsthand expect that women will often leave in a crisis but will later go back home. The greatest probability of long-term success occurs when we follow our clients' lead in identifying problems and their solutions rather than attempting to impose our own (Prochaska, 1999; Walter & Peller, 1992).

Really Listening to Someone with a Different Worldview

Challenge yourself to become aware of how your worldview is different from someone else's. Also, think about how it is similar. Write about the differences and the similarities. What, if anything, was a surprise to you?

Really listening to someone who has a markedly different worldview will always be difficult. Being able to listen to another viewpoint without being judgmental or dismissive requires patience and significant empathy. Kenrick and his colleagues (1999) suggest a threefold process for handling difficult situations. First, practice, practice, practice! As we will discuss later in the book, this theory is both knowledge-based and skills-based. Both the understanding of others and the ability to use this skill will increase with exercise. Engaging in a variety of behaviors as disparate as listening to a waitress, watching a foreign film, reading a novel, and watching politicians of a different political party will improve empathic listening skills and the ability to recognize and respect different worldviews. However, simple exposure is not enough.

Remember that improvement takes practice. Think about your athletic or music practice in high school. Can you devote the same amount of time to increasing your skills in listening and empathy?

Second, because we are more likely to encounter problems with staying fair and objective when our capacity for responding is stressed, we need to minimize the stressors and distractions in life. Sort coins (pennies, nickels, dimes, and quarters) into piles while singing the ABCs. Begin again without singing. Most people find it much easier to sort coins without distractions. Be aware of your stress level and handle it proactively by talking to a friend, meditating, or walking in the woods. Any simple, well-practiced task is easier to perform well when you're under stress. A second benefit of practice is that it makes skills more automatic and less susceptible to interference from cognitive load and stress.

Finally, work *less* hard to control your behavior. Wegner (1994) notes the paradoxical effects of paying attention to our behavior and of attempting to control it when we are stressed. For example, insomniacs who try to go to sleep ("I must go to sleep. I must go to sleep!") actually take more time to fall asleep than those who try less hard. People under stress attempting to avoid making sexist remarks made even more sexist comments than members of the control group not given this instruction! Certainly, I am not recommending that you ignore the issues raised in this book. Just as your nonverbal listening skills probably declined sharply as you were beginning to work on them, they will improve as they become habitual (Ivey et al., 1997). Your ability to be fair and empathic while listening to someone with a different worldview will grow and develop as well.

CONCLUSIONS

Problems seem to result most frequently at the intersection of two cultural worldviews (gay versus straight, male versus female, Black versus White) especially when they involve differences in the power and status of the two groups. Following the killings at Columbine High School, Milloy (1999) questioned how the police and media would have interpreted the event had the killers been black. Milloy suggests that, "Had the killers been black, the parents would no doubt have been hauled off in handcuffs in front of television cameras, and everybody who knew them would be under suspicion" (p. C01).

Furthermore, different explanations for this massacre were offered than in similar cases where the culprits were African American. When suspects were Blacks, their parents were blamed for failing to instill values in them. The judicial system promised more arrests, convictions, and hard time for juveniles in adult institutions. In the aftermath of Columbine, "a culture of alienation" is blamed, and talk of gun control; improving school curricula; and regulating violence in movies, television, video games, and the Internet grows. "It's not just that it looks like excuses are being made for the killers at Columbine; it's that some of them are the same ones that were so roundly rejected when used to explain violence among Blacks" (Milloy, 1999, p. C01).

As we have discussed all along, the group with more power and with which the dominant group identifies is more likely to be afforded less pathological and more contextualized explanations. The largely white media saw Harris' and Klebold's behavior as a result of their alienation at school and their exposure to violent media. If these students had been Blacks, they would have been seen as bad, violent, and out of control, each an internal or trait explanation of the same behaviors.

When explanations conflict in the therapy room, and especially when the therapist's explanations are coercive and blaming, there is likely to be a significant dampening of the therapeutic process. Ethnocentrism, cultural encapsulation, diminished empathy, misdiagnosis, and treatment selection errors have been identified as consequences of cultural insensitivity (Ridley et al., 1994). The underutilization of mental health services by ethnic minorities as well as their premature termination from treatment have also been attributed, at least in part, to problems in cultural sensitivity (D. W. Sue & Sue, 1999). Therapy depends on a relationship in which therapists can be hopeful about their clients and, by extension, clients can be hopeful about their future. Trait language (e.g., "shy people" as opposed to "people who are shy" or even "she ran into problems talking to people on the first day of class") can be blaming and stabilizing and can be harmful to clients (*Ohio Public Images,* nd).

We may differ in viewpoints, but we must respect others' worldviews (D. W. Sue & Sue, 1999). We must learn to listen carefully and empathically and to intervene in ways that are respectful of different worldviews. We must also avoid comments and solutions that further disempower clients. The exchange between Darlene and Tommi shows that working with the current, rather than against it, increases our clients' probability of success in the long run (Walter & Peller, 1992). Wachtel (2002) describes the following in his analysis of cultural issues as they apply to psychoanalysis:

> Changing the approach to fit a new cultural context does not mean "watering it down." Alloys, after all, are quite often stronger and more resilient than a single "pure" ingredient. . . . [W]e are not simply accommodating a rather perfect product to unfortunate necessities, but are being afforded an opportunity to gain some perspective on what we have assumed is essential or intrinsic to our task but may be simply a cultural artifact—or even an impediment. (p. 204)

Problems Resulting from Group Membership

I went to two meetings recently. In the first, one faction brutally attacked the other and questioned their integrity and competence. The "losers" crawled away to lick their wounds, feeling like their viewpoint hadn't been heard or understood. Later that same day, I went to a second meeting. Although its agenda was equally contentious, both groups walked away feeling heard and understood and believed that they had accomplished something important.

TABLE 	**WHAT INTERFERES WITH THE ABILITY TO DEVELOP PARTNERSHIPS?**
Dichotomous thinking	We may see life in terms of "either-or" rather than "and." Who's right when we see things differently?
Failure to listen	We may work against others' viewpoints when we feel we aren't being listened to or understood.
Historical factors	We may have personal or cultural histories that lead us to expect that we will not be heard by others in general or, more specifically, by people or groups in power.
Power	We may be afraid of giving up power in order to listen to and validate someone else's viewpoint. This may include giving up control over events or outcomes of relative importance.
Beliefs	We may believe that an authoritarian and directive stance is more successful in our dealings with employees and consumers—believing that things will be smoother or more productive—and may not be aware of any other kind of model.
Frustration	The frustration within the system and lack of coordination may reflect the client's or family's frustration.

Note: From Bean et al., 2000.

What was the difference? The groups in the first meeting believed there would be winners and losers and that they could only win by defeating the other side. In the second meeting, several people consciously stopped to listen to the other viewpoint and assumed that the other side was being reasonable, and neither group gave up its own views. Although some members avoided conflict by swallowing their disagreements, both factions eventually validated one another's viewpoint and worked to incorporate *all* viewpoints into a resolution.

Listening to another viewpoint without sacrificing one's own "voice" is often difficult (see table 7.1). Our voice can be compromised by our (Bean, Jones Bean, Slattery, & Becker, 2000):

- Style of thinking about problems.
- Fears about giving up power.
- Beliefs about how we should resolve problems.
- Frustrations about the problem and the problem-solving process.
- Perception that we are not being heard.

Being able to listen successfully to another racial or cultural group requires us to be willing to sacrifice some power. *Listening* means really *seeing* the other person for who he or she is, rather than only as a member of another group. Opening our eyes to context helps considerably in making this possible. Understanding context requires that we step outside our dichotomous thinking patterns to recognize the good guys and bad guys on both sides of the fence. Finally, while admitting that people sometimes will take advantage of you, take the time to distinguish between those who are *very* likely to and those who are *less* likely to do so. The problems described here may be reality-oriented or due to historical factors, but the causes of them are not as important as the search for solutions. A number of solutions will be discussed throughout the next three chapters.

Although work with culturally different clients can suffer from the same types of problems as that with clients from the dominant group, this work has new problems. These problems can come largely from the therapist's side, from the client's side, or from both. Race and other group issues will not stay out of the therapy room just because the client and therapist prefer to avoid them. Culturally different peoples struggle with their identity and can be very mistrustful of in-group members and vice versa (see Hegi, 1997). When therapists miss these factors, they may excuse oppression and prejudice, intervene unnecessarily, or generalize inappropriately from their own experience. In contrast, counselors who are culturally responsive are generally rated as more credible and more culturally competent than counselors who ignore culture (Atkinson et al., 1992; Gim et al., 1991; Propst, Ostrom, Watkins, Dean, & Mashburn, 1992; C. E. Thompson et al., 1994).

Good communication across groups is possible, but it requires a special ability to hear others' values and worldviews (Helms, 1984; Propst et al., 1992). Therapeutic responses must help groups and individuals feel that each one of their issues is being heard in all of its complexities and ignoring racial and group issues can cause us to miss the "big picture" (Quindlen, 2000). This means that by only seeing race and group as the "problem," we may be disempowering clients. This can encourage them to slough off personal responsibility for their problems (Greene, 1985). Seeing only the differences between races or minimizing them can be equally dangerous to the therapy process (Saba & Rodgers, 1990).

THERAPISTS' CONTRIBUTIONS TO PROBLEMS

Therapists contribute to problems in a variety of ways. As therapists begin to identify contributions to problems, they can then begin to reduce or prevent them. This section will address both problems and initial solutions.

Translating Language and Ideas Across Worldviews

Reading words and accepting them as objective statements of fact is easy. But, most words and sentences have layers of meanings that can facilitate or inhibit communication. My daughter's violin teacher praised her work on

Pay attention to systemic interactions for a week. How does your behavior affect the behavior of the person you talk to (and vice versa)? What barriers to working together do you see (These barriers can be either contemporary or historical). How does your behavior reinforce or challenge these barriers?

Try changing your behavior and see what happens. For example, if your listening skills are initially good, act frustrated and irritable or try listening poorly. What happens? Be fair to your partner in this interaction. When you're finished, take some time to explain what you were doing and why.

the viola by saying, "She doesn't know that people can't play a viola like a violin." (It *is* difficult to play the thicker viola strings in the same rapid and effortless way that one can play the violin.) My daughter, who was already frustrated with her playing, felt publicly humiliated. Communication occurs in a context.

Real empathy and understanding depend on our ability to step outside our individual and cultural frameworks and to respect and accept others'. This already-difficult process is further complicated by cultural and linguistic differences, as seen in this ludicrously translated interview (Zhang, 1999):

> ASIAN WOMAN (IN CHINESE): *My husband and I work two jobs each just to pay back what we owe to the people who paid our fare to this country. We are almost never home early because of that. However, I always leave enough good food and clean clothes for our son. But he meets all kinds of bad people in his school. They say now he is part of a gang. What can we do?*
> TRANSLATOR (IN ENGLISH): *She said she and her husband work all the time and have little time for the son. The kid may have joined a gang and got in trouble in school.*
> SOCIAL WORKER (IN ENGLISH): *It seems that you work too much and have neglected your son. Is that correct? (Paraphrase, checkout)*
> TRANSLATOR (IN CHINESE): *You are to blame for your son's problem because you work too much.*
> ASIAN WOMAN: *Well . . . Yes, I am to blame. (pp. 118—119).*

Each translation moved the mother and social worker slightly further apart. The translation process could have been successful, but it failed here because the mother was unwilling to correct the social worker's paraphrase—perhaps because of cultural imperatives to respect authorities or because of her own sense of guilt and because the social worker and translator did not check out their assumptions carefully.

Do these problems go away when we attempt to be objective? Ursula LeGuin (1994) argues in her short story "Dancing to Ganam" that people continue to have difficulty even when being objective. In her story, Dalzul travels to Ganam, a distant planet where the inhabitants seem primitive and innocent. Dalzul joyfully immerses himself in the culture, but rather than attempting to be objective in his observations (as he had been trained to be), he recommends to his fellow travelers that they "Process later. . . . How often does one get to be a child?" (p. 131). Unfortunately, the explorers do not understand the culture even when they understand its words. They translate the ideas of Ganam into those of their home culture with disastrous results (death). Although those who attempt to remain objective and skeptical about their limited understanding of Ganam are better off, they too grossly misread the intentions of Ganam's inhabitants.

Fontes and Piercy (2000) argue that similar misunderstandings happen when we translate surveys and other psychological measures across cultures. Culture serves as a framework for how questions should be answered. Should grief be expressed and, if so, how? How long should one grieve? How close should children be to their parents? When (and how) should children be encouraged to individuate? Should sisters be encouraged to individuate differently than their brothers? Because these questions are answered in a cultural framework, assessing someone in a different cultural context may cause us to pathologize normal and healthy behavior. On one hand, Costa Ricans expect relatively long periods of grieving. On the other hand, Euro-Americans often are uncomfortable with all but the shortest periods of mourning. Laotian children usually stay very close to their mothers and begin to individuate at about three unless another sibling comes earlier (Zaharlick, 2000). Nowadays, Euro-American girls are expected to be more independent, autonomous, and assertive than they were at the beginning of the last century.

Observe a disagreement from its beginning to its resolution. How do the parties differ in their descriptions of the conflict throughout this period? How do their descriptions change after they make up (if they ever do)? Do they emphasize different facts at each point? Do they perceive the facts of the disagreement differently? At what points are they more or less accurate, from your point of view? What beliefs undergird their initial conclusions? How do these beliefs change as the disagreement proceeds from beginning to end?

Rather than simply measuring one culture's behaviors by another's cultural yardstick, we should ask whether the behaviors work on balance (Oz, 1995). What are the disadvantages of grieving for an entire year? What positive function does grieving serve? Are there other options that will meet the person's needs better? Do these options work as well for other important parts of the person's system? Although short-term costs and benefits are generally identified easily, longer-term costs and benefits are often ignored but should also be considered.

Objectivity in Diagnosis and Treatment

In its standardized description of disorders, the Diagnostic and Statistical Manual (DSM, American Psychiatric Association, 2000) suggests that the diagnostic process is an objective one. If this is true, then the DSM *should* work equally well across different cultures and times. However, many disorders are defined subjectively, not operationally, and the definitions are not always consistent from one culture and time to another. What, for example, is "inappropriate, sexually seductive, or provocative behavior" (Histrionic Personality Disorder, American Psychiatric Association, 2000, p. 714)? Certainly our definition is both situationally and culturally determined. The same behavior that is acceptable in a bar on Friday night is unacceptable in a job interview. Behaviors and ways of dress that are currently conservative would have been extremely provocative during Hester Prynn's time (Hester is the tainted heroine of Hawthorne's *The Scarlet*

Letter). Culture alters our internal yardstick and influences our definition of if, why, and how behavior can become problematic.

A number of researchers have reported that race and gender influence our willingness to diagnose a person with a particular diagnosis. Ford and Widiger (1989), for example, report that therapists diagnose men differently than women. Even when the same symptoms are reported by both, men are more likely to be diagnosed with antisocial personality disorder, and women are more likely to be diagnosed with histrionic personality disorder. These differences are in line with base rates, which include our predictions about the probability that a person with the diagnosis would be found in the person's gender based on its frequency of occurrence within the population as a whole.

Steinpreis and her colleagues (1999) reported that when two identical academic résumés (one from a female and the other from a male) were reviewed, the "male" résumé received more positive responses. This preference for male applicants appears to be most true for "marginal" résumés, since a much stronger résumé for tenure was responded to equivalently, regardless of its gender identifier.

Different stimuli that have the same characteristics are often evaluated differently (Ford & Widiger, 1989; Steinpreis et al., 1999), but Atkinson and his colleagues (1996) also reported that race influences diagnoses as well. When responding to vignettes, Euro-American therapists were more likely to use severe psychiatric disorders such as major depression, dysthymia, and borderline personality disorder to diagnose patients than did their African American colleagues, who were more likely to diagnose the symptoms with an adjustment disorder. It seems that even when we sincerely attempt to be "impartial" or "fair," our culture's values continue to influence our actions and to interfere with our ability to be objective (Steinpreis et al., 1999).

Values influence (1) how people interpret behavior from among different groups, (2) how people of different groups diagnose a single group, and (3) how therapists make treatment recommendations. Yi (1998), for example, described her experience with a Euro-American woman who was being treated unfairly at work and was considering suing her employer. Yi, without thinking, blurted out, "Well, maybe this is [just] our individual differences, but a lawsuit would not be something I would be thinking about" (pp. 257–258). She reported that, upon reflection, she realized that her strong aversion to her client's proposal came from the difference between their cultural backgrounds. Yi's reaction came from an Asian value system that prefers interpersonal harmony even if it might incur significant personal sacrifice. She believed injustice should be resolved by appealing to moral obligation. Her Euro-American client, however, had internalized values of the dominant culture that individual rights should be asserted and interpersonal problems should be resolved even when it meant invoking contractual agreements. Although there was nothing inherently wrong in either approach, both Yi (1998) and her client were prevented by their cultural blinders from seeing other possible resolutions for this situation. Becoming aware of their own cultural values as well as the wider range of options available allowed both Yi and her client to make a wiser decision.

How did a cost-benefit analysis affect Yi's (1998) decision? Yi's client came to therapy seeing the benefits of filing suit against her employer and the costs of keeping quiet. Yi, in contrast, perceived the costs of filing suit for her client's relationships with her employer and others in her social network. Both tended to focus on their own goals first and foremost (e.g., assertiveness versus interpersonal harmony and indirectness). After discussing this value conflict, Yi and her client began to identify other options for resolving this problem, and the client decided eventually not to sue her employer. Instead, she spoke to the general manager of her company, who in turn exerted pressure on her boss to pay her for previously uncompensated time and services. While this problem was apparently resolved, it continued to haunt the therapy process: Yi reported that her client continued to believe that Yi, too, wanted her client to "keep quiet and not complain" (p. 258).

Although assessing culturally different clients can be problematic, goalsetting can be equally problematic. Just as diagnostic decisions reflect values, so do our goals. In the last example, Yi (1998) adopted a more collectivistic stance than her client. In such cases of mismatch, treatment goals should be mutually decided with clients, and the racial and cultural environments in which they are living should be taken into consideration (Helms & Cook, 1999). Jointly developing treatment goals and strategies is good therapeutic practice, even when therapist and client have similar values and beliefs.

Therapeutic Stances with Culturally Different Clients

Greene (1985) describes four therapeutic stances that interfere with the therapeutic process when working with culturally different clients (see table 7.2).

- The racist stance
- The color blind stance
- The paternalism stance
- The unquestioning acceptance of client's perspective stance

Greene suggests that a racist stance comes from a conscious or unconscious belief that Whites are superior to members of other groups and that many minority-group problems are outgrowths of this inherent inferiority. People taking this stance ignore contextual issues and assume an internal

Observe yourself talking or playing with children over the next week. What are your goals in the interactions? Do you assume that the children will be good or not and that they are capable or not? How do you think they can perceive this?

Did your stance with them help you meet your goals? Did the amount they talked or the content of their conversations change? If so, how? Did their moods shift? How? Did they become more (or less) responsible and cooperative? If you were more successful at some times than others, what were you doing differently in these conversations?

TABLE 7.2   FOUR STANCES THAT THERAPISTS CAN TAKE TO INTERFERE WITH THE THERAPEUTIC PROCESS OF CULTURALLY DIFFERENT CLIENTS VERSUS A MORE ADAPTIVE APPROACH TO RESOLVING CULTURAL ISSUES

	Description of Process	Therapist's Actions
Racism or prejudice	All problems are internally caused. Often, this is related to the therapist's feelings of superiority and of "blaming the victim" (client). "Different" may be seen as "bad" and strengths ignored. Environmental factors contributing to problems may be overlooked.	"What did you do to cause this?" "Well, you know how *they* are. It's unlikely that you can do anything for him." "They're just in here to qualify for disability payments."
Color-blindness	All people are alike, and color doesn't matter. Often, interventions are applied without considering the effects of environment, racism, or prejudice. Assessments may ignore important racial and cultural factors, and therapists may collude with clients in ignoring these.	"I treat everyone alike . . . and I ignore racial or cultural factors that contribute to the problem . . . ." (Not necessarily something therapist recognizes.) "I use [fill in the blank] therapy with everyone, and I ignore the research suggesting that there are real differences in preferences for therapeutic styles." (Not necessarily something therapist recognizes.)
Paternalism	All problems are attributed to racism and discrimination. Intrapsychic factors are ignored. Rather than encouraging responsibility and independent responses to problems, the paternalistic therapist may unknowingly encourage dependence.	"Your boss is just another racist bastard out to get you. I know your boss. Let me see what I can do to fix this."
Unquestioning acceptance of client's perspective	A variation of paternalism, this view encourages clients to act out their anger and frustration about racism against others without considering others' viewpoints or rights.	"Your neighbors are racists. Get in touch with your feelings and act."
Acknowledge and challenge to accept appropriate control	This view encourages acknowledgment of real problems and oppression, while also encouraging change of situational or individual issues that can be changed or controlled. Others' rights and viewpoints are considered without excusing discrimination."	It sounds like your boss is making decisions based on gender rather than competence. How can you address this in a way that your point will be heard in order to make the change that you want?"

Note: From Greene, 1985.

locus of responsibility ("What did you do to cause this?"). Of course, most therapists have internal loci of control and responsibility and recognizing one's own control and responsibility is often useful (D. W. Sue & Sue, 1999). However, we must be careful to foster healthy control rather than adopt a blaming stance ("You should have known better than to be in that neighborhood at night"). Similarly, we may take a narrow and prejudicial approach toward culturally different clients and infer negative intentions (as with Luisa in chapter 1) or assume an inability to profit from preferred interventions ("Blacks just don't do well with psychoanalysis or other long-term treatments").

In their attempts to be fair and avoid being labeled a "racist" or "politically correct," white therapists may adopt a color blind stance (Greene, 1985; Helms & Cook, 1999). Though ignoring race and other group issues may be useful and appropriate in the context of employment decisions, it is not effective in therapy. It can prevent therapists from seeing the context that explains otherwise unexplainable behavior and may serve as a regressive force in therapy (Helms, 1984). Also, this stance can be an ill-conceived attempt to avoid conflict, but healthy conflict is at the heart of good therapy. Recognizing the oppression and color barriers that cause, maintain, or exaggerate symptomatic behavior is often very helpful.

The tendency to take a color blind stance is intensified by a nearness to our own values. Because values are so much a part of the fabric of society, we may be unable to identify them as choices, as in "That's just the way it is!" We may also assume that race and cultural issues are unimportant psychological or behavioral patterns, and we may do this without remembering that many were developed by white therapists with their privileged white clients in mind without considering the specific needs and concerns of culturally different clients (Greene, 1985; Guthrie, 1997). Therapists with low multicultural competencies, in particular, attempt to ignore race and group issues, believing that being fair means providing the same treatment to all clients, regardless of culture or race (Sodowsky, Taffe, Gutkin, & Wise, 1994). Finally, because members of groups in the numerical minority are more likely to have contact with multiple groups, they may have an easier time recognizing that there are choices in behavior, beliefs, and values and may more readily identify racism and oppression than therapists in the majority group.

Avoiding issues of race and group membership, even with good intentions, is less effective than taking more culturally responsive approaches (Atkinson et al., 1992; Gim et al., 1991; Helms, 1984; C. E. Thompson & Jenal, 1994; C. E. Thompson et al., 1994). Such avoidance also ignores the data suggesting that groups often have real and valid preferences for particular therapeutic approaches and interactional styles (Paniagua, 1998). Race and ethnicity—their own and those of their therapists—have meaning in clients' lives. When therapists ignore racial and group issues, we obscure our view of clients and the real issues at hand (Helms, 1984).

The paternalism stance and the unquestioning acceptance of client's perspective stance are Greene's (1985) last two stances, and both are disempowering. While these approaches acknowledge the roles of prejudice and oppression in a client's experience, they also assume that the client is incapable of resolving problems on his or her own in a mature fashion. In the case of the paternalism stance, the therapist attributes all problems to racism. This, however, prevents clients from examining their own role in their problems, as majority-group clients would presumably be encouraged to do. Well-meaning, therapists may act to resolve their clients' problems sometimes out of a need to be nice or helpful or out of a need to make up for past injustices. But they end up disempowering clients and fostering dependence.

In the stance involving an unquestioning acceptance of their clients' perspective, therapists will acknowledge racism but may foster the belief that their clients' history of racism and oppression absolves them of the responsibility to take into account others' feelings and needs (Greene, 1985). For example, Yitzhak, a therapist with grandparents who were killed in the Holocaust, was angry at the religious intolerance he experienced in his own life. He tended to encourage the righteous anger of his African American clients and not hold them accountable for their actions in the same way that he would hold Euro-American clients accountable for theirs.

In contrast, a more successful stance in therapy is one where therapists see their clients' humanity as well as the context for their clients' behavior. While acknowledging contextual factors, therapists are able to treat clients in an empowering fashion. They encourage clients to become active participants in the change process, and they help clients accept control or responsibility when appropriate. These are the tenets that undergird the interventions described this book. Therapists behaving in this manner frequently have a racial identity that is at least as advanced as that of their clients (Helms, 1984). When one of Yitzhak's clients finally acted out her anger in a way that put her in jail, he was forced to challenge his stance. He came to realize that he was behaving in a disempowering manner, even though his intentions were to acknowledge the oppression in his culturally different clients' lives and be supportive of their struggles. He began working to help his clients recognize their anger and express it in more adaptive ways.

> Think of a time when you were warned about a person, place, or situation. For example, "That professor (or job, restaurant, etc.) is terrible (or unfair or prejudiced)." How did your expectations influence the situation?

CLIENTS' CONTRIBUTIONS TO PROBLEMS

My mother used to say that it takes two to cause a problem. Although therapists are clearly responsible for some difficulties in therapy, clients also play a role. When we recognize potential problems in therapy and accept control rather than responsibility for them, we can identify ways to reduce or prevent them. This section will address both these problems and initial solutions to them.

Cultural Mistrust and Resistance

A variety of problems in therapy, especially increased premature terminations, lower expectations for therapy (Atkinson, Morten & Sue, 1998; Liddle, 1996; Nickerson et al., 1994; Terrell & Terrell, 1984; Watkins & Terrell, 1988). The association between racial dissimilarity and negative counseling-related outcomes has been attributed, in part, to African American clients' mistrust of white therapists and to their concern that they might be misunderstood or treated in a stereotypical or oppressive fashion (C. E. Thompson et al., 1994). Terrell and Terrell (1981) argued that because African Americans as a group have a long history of race-related mistreatment by Whites, they may have developed a generalized suspicion or mistrust of Whites. They expect dominant-group therapists to attempt to impose "White" techniques and values upon them, to blame them for the effects of oppression, and to attempt to make them White (D. W. Sue & Sue, 1999). This mistrust (as well as Whites' mistrust of African Americans) can taint new relationships.

Perceiving prejudice in these ways tends to increase minority-group identification and minority-group hostility toward the dominant group (Branscombe, Schmitt, & Harvey, 1999). Highly mistrustful African Americans are more likely to terminate therapy sessions prematurely and to expect less from counseling than those with lower levels of mistrust (Nickerson et al., 1994; Terrell & Terrell, 1984; Watkins & Terrell, 1988). Mistrustful African American college students see Euro-American therapists as less credible and less able to help them than African American therapists (Watkins, Terrell, Miller, & Terrell, 1989). Conversely, Gim and her colleagues (1991) report that Asian American college students view Asian American therapists as more credible and competent.

Not surprisingly, disclosure rates are also related to cultural mistrust. African American female pseudoclients were more likely to disclose to other African Americans. Clients high in mistrust were least likely to disclose, even to other African Americans (C. E. Thompson et al., 1994). However, African American pseudoclients were more likely to disclose when their therapists paid attention to issues of culture than when they did not.

Ridley (1984) attributes the problems of requesting therapy, terminating early, and making minimal information disclosures during therapy to a healthy cultural paranoia stemming from African Americans' history of oppression.

> In light of this legacy, the goals and situational context of traditional psychotherapy appear to be especially incongruous with the disclosing tendencies of many black clients. By disclosing, black clients again render themselves vulnerable to racism and oppression. Yet, the process of

disclosure is facilitative of the client's therapeutic movement. [On the other hand,] by not disclosing, black clients protect their self-esteem. (p. 1237)

Rather than being maladaptive, cultural mistrust and apparent resistance to therapy can be effective mechanisms for coping with racism and environmental stressors (Boyd-Franklin, 1990). Both may keep culturally different clients safe from both physical and psychological attacks and serve as a kind of defensive pessimism. Risa, for example, hoped that things would be different but found it difficult to believe that her therapist Kristen would believe her or believe in her. As a result, Risa held back and watched until she began to see Kristen as different. The therapist's job, then, is to be open to individual and cultural strengths, to recognize the advantages of our clients' solutions, and to challenge those strengths at the points where they begin to be maladaptive.

Cultural mistrust and resistance may serve as barriers even in therapy conducted by African American therapists. Because most therapists are well-educated and middle- or upper middle-class economically, culturally different clients may assume that African American therapists have accepted the oppressive values and stereotypes of their white counterparts (Greene, 1985). Just as not disclosing to white therapists may be perceived as an act of maintaining self-esteem, it may also be seen the same way with black therapists.

Ridley (1984) suggests that the assessment process differentiate between those clients who are mistrustful across a range of situations, such as those diagnosed with paranoid schizophrenia or paranoid personality disorder, and those who are especially mistrustful in situations where racism is seen or suspected. While it is unhealthy to be paranoid across situations, being mistrustful in the face of racism can be healthy and adaptive, especially if racism and oppression are correctly identified and responded to. To the degree that therapists fail to make this distinction, more racial and cultural minority clients will be identified falsely as having paranoid disorders and schizophrenia, a finding that has been repeatedly reported in the assessment literature (Trierweiler et al., 2000).

THERAPISTS' AND CLIENTS' CONTRIBUTIONS

We have one important rule in our house: Our daughters cannot be in a bad mood at the same time that we are. Some of the worst episodes in our lives together stem from the time prior to this simple rule. Sometimes, we'll remind one another of this rule and get back on track with laughter. We've learned that each of us can contribute to problems, and that each of us can prevent or resolve them. Similarly, both client and therapist can contribute to problems in therapy. It's bad enough when a therapist or a client acts out in therapy, but things are much worse when both are involved.

Racial Identity Development

Spend a few minutes thinking and writing about several significant racial events in your life such as meeting your first international student, being prevented from doing something because of your race, or being the only member of your race at an event. How did you view the event then? How do you view it now? If your picture changed, describe how the two views are different. Compare your responses to Helms and Cook's (1999) descriptions of racial identity as shown in tables 7.3 and 7.4. What do you see?

Part of being competent to work with a diverse population of clients is being aware of your own beliefs about race, class, ethnicity, and affectional orientation and considering when and how these beliefs might affect clients. Competence also involves knowing how people from other groups might react to you. A therapist's racial identity and attitudes can lead to infantilization of clients, protective gestures, or subtle kinds of prejudicial decisions (Greene, 1985; Helms & Cook, 1999; Sodowsky et al., 1994). In addition, clients' racial identity and attitudes toward the therapist can lead to outright rejection, skeptical acceptance, or even unthinking acceptance, regardless of whether therapist and client share important values or demographic values. Becoming aware of racial issues and one's own racial identity is an important part of a therapist's multicultural competency development (Helms & Cook, 1999; Ottavi, Pope-Davis, & Dings, 1994; D. W. Sue & Sue, 1999).

Racial identity is a social construction that develops in people over time, and it develops later than initial understandings of gender. Children begin to use gender to organize their approach to the world at around 18 months (Kohlberg, 1966). African American preschoolers generally describe themselves in terms of skin color rather than race. Because young children are concrete thinkers, they may even deny being Black ("I'm coffee colored"). Skin color may not be mentioned at all; rather, gender or religion may be focused on instead, and children may have difficulty seeing race even when it is pointed out to them (Kerwin, Ponterotto, Jackson, & Harris, 1993; M. A. Wright, 1998). By adolescence, however, race is often a central part of self-concept and usually is mentioned by black and biracial youth in their descriptions of themselves.

Racial Identity Development for People of Color   Several authors have developed models of racial identity for people of color (Helms & Cook, 1999; D. W. Sue & Sue, 1999). A single generic model will be described here: People of color often face similar issues in the United States and where greater advantages are acquired based upon lighter skin color. In general, these models have described people at higher statuses as also having (1) more awareness of the role of race in their experience, (2) a greater ability to recognize the arbitrary nature of racially determined decisions, and (3) an increased probability of using personal rather than societal stereotypes. In these respects, the models are similar to others that describe developmental processes that are limited by cognitive development (e.g., Belenky, Clinchy, Goldberger, & Tarule, 1986; Gilligan, 1982; Kohlberg, 1966, 1981; Piaget, 1960). Helms and Cook, in particular, predict that a more "mature" racial identity will be associated with more flexible and abstract thinking. They do not see racial identity as following a set of lockstep stages, but rather as styles of thinking about race that are more or less prominent at different points in time.

Helms and Cook (1999) describe people of color in conformity as being relatively oblivious about race and its implications (see table 7.3). People with conformity status prominent tend to be relatively accepting of society's prejudices about their race and more accepting of the status quo. Rather than challenging society's messages about who they are, they tend to conform to expectations and distort or ignore information that contradicts stereotypes. People at this ego status may prefer a dominant-group therapist, someone whom they are readily able to identify as competent and capable ("Why did you put me with this black guy? I deserve a good therapist, too").

Over time, however, most people have experiences that challenge the fairness and accuracy of the stereotypes to which they have been exposed. They may see competent and hardworking people of color who have had opportunities blocked from them, and they may see white people of equal or lesser competence who are afforded privileges that are not available to people of color. These experiences can be very confusing for those at the dissonance status, and these people may begin to integrate this contradictory information into their worldview (Helms & Cook, 1999). Rather than dealing with these contradictions directly, they may become anxious and may attempt to ignore or repress the information ("Don't tell me! I don't want to know!"). Unfortunately, attempts to ignore prejudice and oppression are rarely completely successful. People in this status may continue to prefer majority-group therapists in their attempts to avoid the anxiety raised by their experience with and acknowledgment of the presence of racism.

Eventually these contradictions become overwhelming. Rather than idealizing Whites as those at the conformity status did, people at the dissonance stage tend to uncritically idealize other members of their own racial or cultural group and ignore or criticize the successes of Whites (Helms & Cook, 1999; D. W. Sue & Sue, 1999). Like previous statuses, the style of thinking about racial issues present at the immersion and emersion statuses tends to be dichotomous (e.g., good guys versus bad guys), and people may actively engage in cognitive activities that maintain this distinction. Because their anger is often directed at Whites, they generally prefer working with a therapist of their own race. When therapy does involve Euro-American therapists, people at these statuses may become hypervigilant about possible racist attitudes and behaviors and may even react

TABLE 7.3	EGO STATUSES AND COGNITIVE STYLES ASSOCIATED WITH HELMS' RACIAL IDENTITY SCALE, AS GENERALIZED FOR CULTURALLY DIFFERENT GROUPS

Conformity

External standards for self are accepted and may devalue one's own cultural group in favor of the one in power. Societal prejudices are accepted. People may attempt to conform either to dominant group standards or to stereotypes about their own group.

> But there was a part of me that feared black power very deeply for the obvious reason. I thought black power would be the end of my mother. I had swallowed the white man's fear of the Negro, as we were called back then, whole . . . I thought to myself, *These people will kill Mommy* (McBride, 1996, p. 27, italics in original).

In their attempts to conform either to dominant group standards or to stereotypes about their own group, people with this status prominent devalue or ignore contributions made by their own group and the real role of historical or political factors. Similarly, they tend to ignore, distort, or excuse information that puts the dominant group in a bad light. Anger about racial issues is directed toward self and the members of their group. "Specialness" depends on similarity to the group in power and acceptance by its members.

Dissonance

People with this status prominent are increasingly aware of group history and discrimination and believe that it frequently seems "unfair." Nonetheless, they are equally uncomfortable about accepting themselves and their cultural group as valid and valued members of society.

> I cut the questions and ate the cake, though it never stopped me from wondering, partly because of my own growing sense of self, and partly because of fear for her safety, because even as a child I had a clear sense that black and white folks did not get along, which put her, and us, in a pretty tight space (McBride, 1996, p. 25).

Information about complexity of group behaviors and weaknesses is not well-integrated by the person, resulting in frequent confusion and ambivalence about self and cultural group as racial entities. Feelings of disorientation and dislocation are common and are frequently handled by repression of anxiety-provoking group information.

Immersion

Uncritical idealization of own racial or cultural group exists, with a concomitant denigration of the group in power. People with this ego status prominent may use the definitions and values of their own group to define and evaluate self. Loyalty to the group is valued, and decisions may be made on its behalf.

> Kind, gentle, Sunday school children who had been taught to say proudly, "I am a Negro," and recite the deeds of Jackie Robinson and Paul Robeson, now turned to Malcolm X and H. Rap Brown and Martin Luther King for inspiration. Mommy was the wrong color for black pride and black power, which nearly rent my house in two (McBride, 1996, p. 96).

People in this group initially may be hypervigilant and hypersensitive to racial stimuli and be uncritical of their own group. All issues may be seen in terms of racial or group dynamics. Dichotomous thinking about racial or group issues, such as "Blacks and Black culture are good, and Whites and White culture are bad," is common and members may tend to think "I can only be good if they are bad." Anger is directed toward members of the dominant group.

Emersion

While part of the same journey as the last status, a greater sense of discovery, sanity, security and group solidarity exists with others of their own race.

> "Yes, but is the Man you? Or are you the Man?"
> "Do you mean the *Man,* or the *Wo*-man !"
> "Who is the Man . . . ?"
> "But are you the *Main* Man . . .?"
> (Sung) *"When a maaan loves a wooomannnn!!"*

(continued)

TABLE 7.3   *(continued)*

These goof sessions, which almost always ended as earnest talks on civil rights, often went on until Mommy got home from work. (McBride, 1996, pp. 73–74, italics in original)

Positive emotions of security, pride, and positive connection with others of similar attitudes are present. People with this status dominant tend to be uncritical of others of their own group.

Internalization

People at this status have a positive commitment to and an acceptance of their own group, and they have internally defined racial attributes. At the same time, they attempt to assess members of the dominant group in a fair and objective manner rather than perceiving all Euro-Americans as the same or bad.

Given my black face and upbringing, it was easy for me to flee into the anonymity of blackness, yet I felt frustrated to live in a world that considers the color of your face an immediate political statement whether you like it or not. It took years before I began to accept the fact that the nebulous "white man's world" wasn't as free as it looked; that class, luck, religion all factored in as well; that many white individuals' problems surpassed my own, often by a lot; that all Jews are not like my grandfather and that part of me is Jewish too. Yet the color boundary in my mind was and still is the greatest hurdle. (McBride, 1996, pp. 262)

People with this ego status prominent attempt to see self and their cultural group in a flexible manner, making individual decisions about these issues rather than accepting cultural or societal dogma. They tend to think abstractly and to rely on intellectualization.

Integrative Awareness

People with this ego status prominent now have the capacity to value the collective identity as well as to empathize and collaborate with members of other oppressed groups. Self-esteem is good, as individual and cultural strengths and weaknesses are now accepted.

Now, as a grown man, I feel privileged to come from two worlds. My view of the world is not merely that of a black man but that of a black man with something of a Jewish soul. I don't consider myself Jewish, but when I look at Holocaust photographs of Jewish women whose children have been wrenched from them by Nazi soldiers, the women look like my own mother and I think to myself, *There but for the grace of God goes my own mother—and by extension—myself.* When I see two little Jewish old ladies giggling over coffee at a Manhattan diner, it makes me smile, because I hear my mother's laughter beneath theirs. Conversely, when I hear black "leaders" talking about "Jewish slave holders," I feel angry and disgusted, knowing that they're inflaming people with lies and twisted history, as if all seven of the Jewish slave owners in the antebellum South, or however few there were, are responsible for the problems of African-Americans now. Those leaders are no better than their Jewish counterparts who spin statistics in marvelous ways to make African-Americans look like savages, criminals, drags on society, and "animals" . . . . (McBride, 1996, pp. 103–104, italics in original)

Decisions may be made relative to general humanitarian issues and humanistic self-expression. The decision-making process is abstract, flexible, and complex. Positive attributes of self that are characteristic of other cultures are accepted and embraced rather than ignored or denigrated. Similarly, pictures of other people and groups are allowed to be as complex as is necessary to allow healthy intrapsychic and interpersonal functioning.

Note: Ego statuses may fluctuate over time. Although ego statuses can co-exist, generally one or two are more dominant than the others. From Fischer, Tokar, & Serna, 1998; Helms & Cook, 1999; Martin & Hall, 1992; Walters & Simoni, 1993.

adversely to relatively benign behaviors ("He always asks about problems. Does he think that's all we are?").

In the last two statuses, an increasing ability to integrate "grays" into dichotomous thinking about race comes into play. When the internalization status is prominent, for example, people will work both to accept themselves and other members of their group and will assess Whites in a fair and objective manner (Helms & Cook, 1999). Although it may have been previously difficult to be good if the "Other" was good, this is no longer a necessary contradiction in terms.

Finally, in the integrative awareness status an increasing awareness of the complexity of all peoples is present. People are increasingly aware that each group and its members have strengths and weaknesses and have been both beneficent *and* destructive. People in this status are able to think more flexibly and with greater complexity. People at these last two statuses may choose a therapist based not upon race, but upon his or her competence and other factors. They readily recognize the notion that strengths and competence transcend skin color. In addition to the cognitive flexibility that comes with more developed concepts of racial identity, African Americans who accept their "Black" identity and identify with the oppression of other peoples have the highest levels of internal control (Martin & Hall, 1992).

Racial Identity Development of Euro-Americans   The racial identity of people of color is certainly important to assess. But equally important is assessing the racial identity status of Euro-Americans, especially in mixed dyads; for example, when a Native American therapist works with a Euro-American client or a Euro-American therapist works with an African American client. Helms and Cook (1999) give a useful description of this model (see table 7.4). As with Helms and Cook's description of racial identity for people of color, ego statuses are seen as fluctuating over short periods of time, although the ego statuses generally grow more complex throughout the lifespan. Generally one or two statuses is dominant at a time.

People with a dominant contact status are relatively oblivious to the role that race plays in their lives or in the lives of those who are culturally or racially different (Helms & Cook, 1999). They cannot clearly recognize oppression or privilege in their lives or in the lives of others. When they do recognize the role that race has played in history, they generally see it as something confined to the past, with trivial implications for the present: "I'm not sure why we should have affirmative action programs. Slavery has been gone for more than 100 years."

Euro-Americans may, at different times, observe things that increase their awareness of the role of race and privilege in their lives, and they may challenge the religious or humanitarian ideals they hold dear (Helms & Cook, 1999). However, when the disintegration status is prominent, the recognition is an uneasy one and people may back away quickly from these issues and from the associated anxiety ("Well, sometimes people treat Blacks unfairly—and that's terrible—but it doesn't happen often. The media tends to overreport the bad things for their own purposes. I don't personally know anyone who is a racist.").

TABLE  **EGO STATUSES AND COGNITIVE STYLES ASSOCIATED WITH HELMS' WHITE RACIAL IDENTITY SCALE**

Contact

Euro-Americans at this status are satisfied with the status quo and are oblivious to the effects of race on their own life or on the lives of others. When racism is acknowledged, it is acknowledged in a superficial manner. Their own participation in racism is ignored, minimized, or excused.

> There are still comments like this: "Oh, this is over now. . . ." "This has been fifty years. . . ." "Look at what they're doing in *fill-in-the-blank* . . ." Even people of my generation—and that's what scares me—don't want to think about it too much. (Johanna, in Hegi, 1997, p. 63, italics in original)

In order to maintain the illusion that race doesn't matter and that racism, when it occurs, is a rare situation perpetrated by someone else, people with this status dominant feel the need to use significant denial, superficiality, avoidance, and obliviousness.

Disintegration

The illusion that race doesn't matter begins to shatter as they are faced with unresolved racial and moral dilemmas. Their belief that "life is fair" may conflict with evidence of discriminatory practices. Their loyalty to their own race may conflict with humanist ideals.

> From time to time, I would remind myself that I should know more about what was going on in the world, that I should get involved. Uncomfortable with my lack of political knowledge I would read newspapers, listen to the news. But after a while I'd grow disillusioned. It would become a duty. And I'd stop. Until the next time. (Hegi, 1997, p. 38)

Confronting these dilemmas often involves some suppression of contradictory observations, ambivalence, and vacillation in attempts to resolve the dilemma and to control the world in order to make it "right." Often people feel confused, distressed, or disoriented in response to race-related problems and may be unsure about whether or not the cost of acting in a non-racist way is worth the benefits.

Reintegration

When this status is dominant among Euro-Americans, they idealize their own group while denigrating others.

> I hate waiting on what we call dots. Indians from India. The dot on their forehead. Hate them for two reasons: they smell bad, and they do the same thing the Orientals do. Never offer you a fair profit. Certain cultures, used to bargaining for everything, come to this country and try to bargain unreasonably because they don't know where to stop. (Kurt, in Hegi, 1997, p. 190)

Adopting the racial attitudes and behaviors of the status quo relieves the anxiety of the previous status. Because this is "just the way it is," people at this status can abdicate responsibility for their actions. Idealization (of other Whites, for example), selective perception, and distortion of information about out-group members are commonly used.

Pseudo-Independence

Members of other groups are tolerated inasmuch as they conform to White standards of merits and reject their native culture. From this point of view, sending Native Americans to boarding schools to learn English and other Euro-American customs, for example, is seen as good. There is a recognition that there are "good" nonracists, as well as "bad" racist Whites. Racism is recognized in a superficial manner, however, and perceived as being the group's responsibility rather than its own.

> Look at all the people who denied that they were homosexual. I would have denied it. I have to be honest with you. Because I *did* deny it. Look, I denied it all these years, and *ja,* I consider myself fortunate that I can get away with it. I've heard the talk about people who are gay. Even the Jews discriminate against us. (Joachim, in Hegi, 1997, p. 167, italics in original)

(continued)

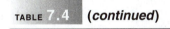 **TABLE 7.4** *(continued)*

Energy is expended to maintain the illusion of being a tolerant liberal. This requires selective perception and distortion as well as avoidance of negative information about oneself. Members of other groups are often given conditional positive regard. "For a Black, she's . . ." is one example.

Immersion
Throughout the journey that is occurring in this status as well as in the next ones, Whites are searching for an understanding of their own race, racist attitudes, racist behavior, and ideas of privilege. This re-education process is especially challenging at this point, but it can also be fulfilling.

> I was not encouraged to play with certain girls in my school because they had Polish names. It's so stupid. Living in isolation, I was hungry for friends. It was a matter of class—not a matter of accomplishment, intelligence or good qualities. It was not a matter of money, because I grew up in absolute poverty, but always with the idea that you can do better than that. You *are* better than that. I've very much tried to overcome this. I don't know how much I succeeded, because there are times, still, that I have to fight this certain arrogance in me as a German. (Marika, in Hegi, 1997, p. 201, italics in original)

This journey is associated with a hypervigilant and judgmental attitude about themselves and of others' racist attitudes.

Emersion
As part of the same journey in the last status, a greater sense of discovery, sanity, security, and group solidarity exists with other likeminded Whites who are rediscovering ways of connecting with themselves while minimizing their use of privilege and oppressive actions.

> I went into the Peace Corps because it fit what I believed in. I was part of that generation, and I got a draft deferment out of that. I went to Tunisia. We lived in the medina, and I learned Roman history. I met my wife in the Peace Corps at a riotous New Year's Eve party. She was like me—I mean, she read the same things. She was smart. (Karl, in Hegi, 1997, p. 115)

Positive emotions of security, pride, and positive connection with others of similar attitudes are present.

Autonomy
An internalized, positive connection to other groups has developed. People at this status have developed a flexible and analytical approach to seeing themselves and are capable of relinquishing privilege and racist attitudes and behaviors. They may or may not choose an activist stance, but they are likely to attempt to avoid oppression in all of its forms.

> This kind of evil or negativity is really something I have to see as part of human beings, which means part of myself . . . that's the hardest work, the hardest aspect. But ultimately that is what needs to be done—what Germans particularly need to do—to look at ourselves and say: *So what in me supports this? What attitudes in me are just down that line?* And that's of course painful. (Johanna, in Hegi, 1997, p. 63, italics in original)

Decisions may be made for general humanitarian reasons and humanistic self-expression rather than for defensive purposes. The decision-making process is abstract, flexible, and complex. Pictures of other people and groups are allowed to be as complex as necessary to allow healthy intrapsychic, interpersonal, and inter-group functioning.

Note: Ego statuses may fluctuate over time. While ego statuses can co-exist with others, generally one or two are more dominant than the others. From Helms & Cook, 1999.

When the reintegration status is dominant, Euro-Americans accept the status quo and the privilege they receive and do not examine the race-related issues that previously caused anxiety. At the same time, they denigrate members of other groups (Helms & Cook, 1999). They ignore or distort information to maintain Euro-Americans' relative status in society and to reduce the anxiety associated with the disintegration status. Kurt's quotation in table 7.4, ignores or distorts any information that does not fit his stereotypes about other groups. In addition, his interactions with minority groups likely elicit behaviors that he focuses on and that confirm his prejudices.

When the pseudoindependence status is dominant, Euro-Americans attempt to resolve the anxiety associated with racism in yet another way. Their actions reveal another, more subtle form of racism (Helms & Cook, 1999). Despite the fact that they had earlier attempted to identify all members of the out-group as bad, now they report that the group has many good and worthy members. However, they tend to see culturally different peoples as "good" only to the extent that they share idealized Euro-American behavior and values. As a result, Euro-Americans at this point may, with good intentions, propose and support social change programs, such as opposition to bilingual education, in order to make other groups more similar to Euro-Americans.

What begins as an intellectual challenge to the issues of racism when the immersion status is prominent becomes a positive and affirming experience during emersion (Helms & Cook, 1999). In each case, Whites begin to challenge their own and others' attitudes about race and privilege. They may initially be judgmental and hypercritical about racial issues, but they will have less difficulty and will experience more positive emotions as they work in groups with others who are like-minded ("We stayed up all night talking about civil rights, affirmative action, everything! We agreed on the problems and disagreed about the solutions, but we agreed that we could get there . . . .").

With a little luck and hard work, some people will be able to reach a place where they are able to accept themselves and members of other groups and be able to see individuals and groups in all of their complexities. The autonomy status is a flexible and complex ego status that avoids dichotomous thinking—something characteristic of most of the earlier statuses (Helms & Cook, 1999). Other statuses, especially disintegration, are characterized by anxiety about contradictions between moral imperatives and how these are carried out in the real and less-than-ideal world. People with a prominent autonomy status are better able to tolerate the anxiety associated with this conflict and are able to use it more productively. See, for example, Johanna's questions in the supporting quotation in table 7.4. Rather than backing away from difficult questions, Johanna embraces them and uses them as opportunities for continued growth.

Racial Identity Matches and Other Similarities

What factors play a role in your choosing a therapist? What factors affect your decision making about choosing an attorney, a dentist, a physician, or others? Which of these are most important? Which would be nice to have?

In their review of the literature on the effectiveness of therapy with ethnic minorities, S. Sue and his colleagues (1994) note the significant contradictions that were reported. Some African Americans, for example, report a preference for racial matches, while other African Americans prefer *not* to have a therapist of the same racial background. Clearly, other variables also contribute to whether a particular type of therapist is preferred.

Group mismatches can act as barriers to feeling understood and may play a role in the increased premature termination rates reported for many minority group members (Atkinson et al., 1998; Liddle, 1996). Some authors attribute at least a portion of these problems to issues of racial identity (Helms & Cook, 1999; D. W. Sue & Sue, 1999). Minority clients who are at the conformity status and value members of the dominant group more than those of their own group or other racial or cultural groups may have a difficult time feeling that they are being heard by members of their own group (Helms & Cook, 1999). Perhaps more importantly, they may have difficulty valuing the relationship enough to take advantage of it. African American clients at this status may work best with Euro-American therapists. On the other hand, people in the resistance and immersion statuses tend to deprecate everything about the dominant group and will have a difficult time feeling understood by a dominant-group therapist. They may work much more successfully with a therapist with the same racial background.

Religious beliefs may also influence therapy and the therapeutic relationship. Religious identity is more similar to the White identity development model (see table 7.4) than to the model for people of color. Most people initially believe that their religion is right and that other religions are wrong. They may later recognize the strengths of other religious leaders and philosophies, as well as of the people subscribing to other religious views. Just as in the discussion of racial identity, people who adopt dichotomous views of religion will be more difficult to engage and to work with than people who adopt more relativistic views of religion. Similarly, when authority is ascribed on religious grounds, cross-religion therapist-client matches will be more difficult to develop.

Although highly religious clients, particularly those from fundamentalist backgrounds, often prefer working with religious therapists (Worthington, Kurusu, McCullough, & Sandage, 1996), they can work successfully with therapists who have been trained to understand and to work sensitively with specific religious issues and perspectives (Propst et al., 1992). Clients' ability to work effectively with therapists of different religion backgrounds depends upon the salience and importance of clients' religious viewpoints and upon how they perceive others' religious and spiritual views (see table

TABLE 7.5   THE IMPACT OF RELIGIOSITY ON THE THERAPEUTIC RELATIONSHIP AND THE THERAPY PROCESS

Relevant Religious Values and Beliefs	Effects of Cultural Values on Therapy
Highly religious • Cope better with stressors and resultant stress than nonreligious clients do. • More likely to use religious attributions for causes of behavior and ways of understanding the world.	• Religious meaning-making can be a natural coping strategy to access. • Listen for religious attributions and use interventions consistent with their worldview such as discussions of sin, guilt, forgiveness, church attendance, and prayer. Sometimes clients' problems may come from their inconsistent applications of their own religious views.
• Prefer counselors who share their religious values, although they may believe that these counselors will be less expert. • Fear their values will be undermined in counseling and that they will be misunderstood or misdiagnosed. They prefer that counselors not challenge religious values.	• Counselor's religious values may be used as a litmus test for counseling, although clients will tend to rate *all* counselors favorably. • Disclosure of counselors' religious views can be problematic when views are very different than clients'. Listening and understanding their religious worldview is important. Religious clients may come to treatment only after other outlets have been exhausted. Some are hypervigilant about value conflicts and are at risk of premature termination.
Nonreligious or less religious • Religious meaning-making is not a natural coping strategy and coping is not as effective. • More likely to use nonreligious attributions for causes of behavior. • May prefer value matches with therapists, but these generally are not based on shared religious values. • Often see religion as irrelevant to therapy and may be confused or put off when therapists discuss religion.	• Although religious meaning-making may not be important, search for other strategies that are useful, including other kinds of meaning-making. • Discussing religion in therapy may be a barrier to developing a therapeutic relationship. • Consider how other aspects of worldview match, facilitate, or inhibit effective collaboration. • Prefer counselors who do not discuss religion or do not see it as the core of all problems. May feel coerced or misunderstood when religion is discussed.

Note: Most research on religiosity available in the West uses people of Christian faiths, especially Euro-American Christians. From Propst et al. 1992; Worthington, 1988; Worthington et al., 1996.

7.5). Success also depends on therapists' willingness to accept and respect other worldviews and to work within a given belief system.

Finally, other group variables influence therapist preference. Many of my female students, regardless of race, strongly prefer a female therapist and do not believe that a male therapist can understand them. This is consistent with the writings of many feminist therapists; a same-gender therapeutic relationship can increase therapists' understanding of their clients' lives and can create a more nurturing and empowering therapeutic environment (Enns, 1992). Female therapists can also model behavior, such as assertiveness, that can superficially appear gender-inappropriate. But, not all female therapists will have these skills, while some male therapists will.

As with other groups, a strong and useful therapeutic relationship is possible when women clients feel understood and when feminist issues, such as gender-related oppression, are recognized and integrated into therapy (Enns, 1992).

Furthermore, it can sometimes be empowering to have a positive therapeutic relationship with someone of an oppressive group, especially where oppression is identified and successfully challenged. For example, C. J., a lesbian with a history of physical and sexual abuse, was appalled when she was referred to a rather large and burly male therapist. She was reticent during her first several sessions until he empathically challenged her refusal to acknowledge her anger toward him and, more to the point, toward the uncle who had molested her (as well as toward her parents who had refused to believe her accusations). From that point on, she was one of his biggest advocates. It might have been *easier* for her to work with a female therapist and this certainly would have had its own advantages, but working with a male turned out to have its own unique benefits.

Other Variables Influencing the Therapeutic Alliance   Group match is important in work with culturally different clients. However, many researchers also emphasize the important role of other counselor characteristics such as reputation, competence, expertness, and cultural sensitivity (Atkinson et al., 1986; Atkinson & Wampold, 1993; Bennett & Bigfoot-Sipes, 1991; Gurung & Mehta, 2001; Liddle, 1996; C. E. Thompson et al., 1994). These variables interact with client variables such as previous experience, level of acculturation, racial identity, and cultural mistrust in a complex manner, affecting the nature of the therapeutic alliance as well as the process and outcome of the therapy.

In addition, therapist-client teams with moderate similarity tend to work more effectively with one another than those with significant similarity or low levels of similarity (T. A. Kelly & Strupp, 1992; Propst et al., 1992). African American, Euro-American, and Native American students report preferring therapists who are perceived as being more similar, especially those who have values, attitudes, or personalities similar to their own (Atkinson, Furlong, & Poston, 1986; Bennett & Bigfoot-Sipes, 1991). In fact, African American students report that these ingredients, as well as those influencing expertness (e.g., greater age and education), are more important than racial match (Atkinson et al., 1986). In one study, Native American students were more likely to prefer a similar counselor when they were seeking help for a personal issue but not when they needed help with academic issues, probably because of their expectation for greater empathy (Bennett & Bigfoot-Sipes, 1991).

Premature termination rates may also be related to the therapist's behavior. Gay, lesbian, bisexual, and transgendered (GLBT) clients are more likely to terminate therapy early and be dissatisfied with the nature of the treatment when their therapist engaged in any one of eight heterosexist and homophobic behaviors (Liddle, 1996). They also reported that the therapists with whom they were happier behaved in a group-sensitive manner (e.g., when their therapist asked about their partner or wondered about their interest in developing a group-sensitive support system in their community). African Americans and Asian Americans also seem to respond best to culturally sensitive therapists who share similar views and beliefs about their "problem" and their life (Gim et al., 1991; C. E. Thompson et al., 1994).

Finally, because of their relatively greater interpersonal orientation, culturally different clients tend to respond best to therapists who pull positive interactions and are able to engage them personally *and* professionally in the therapeutic process (S. Sue et al., 1994). In contrast, white therapists often bring a relatively greater task orientation into the therapeutic process and may not spend adequate time building a therapeutic alliance. This may be yet another cause of problems in interracial therapeutic relationships.

TRANSFERENCE AND COUNTERTRANSFERENCE

Choose a client or a group of clients and think about their typical reactions to you. How are their reactions helpful to therapy? How do they get in the way? How might your own typical responses be helpful or get in the way?

The nature of the therapeutic relationship accounts for as much as 30% of the variance in outcomes in therapy (Asay & Lambert, 1999; Lambert, 1992). Factors influencing this relationship include feelings of caring, empathy, warmth, and acceptance, as well as the ability to encourage risk-taking, mastery, and a strength-based stance (Hubble, Duncan, & Miller, 1999a). The ability to accomplish these tasks, however, can be compromised by issues of transference and countertransference.

Even when a client has no memory of being personally oppressed or even when the therapist has no memory of committing oppressive acts, histories of prejudice and oppression can influence the course of therapy (Helms & Cook, 1999). Being a member of a group with a history of oppression can color relationships both with other members of his or her own group and with members of other groups. Ignoring this history and the reality basis of the clients' continuing concerns can pathologize even normal or adaptive responses (see also Ridley, 1984). Therapists *and* clients may choose to ignore racial prejudice in order to protect themselves from the uncomfortable feelings raised by the continuing realities of racism and oppression (Greene, 1985; Helms & Cook, 1999; C. E. Thompson & Jenal, 1994). Recognizing and addressing continuing patterns of racism, oppression, and privilege take courage and persistence, but doing so is essential to successful therapeutic outcomes.

Role of Racial Identity

Transference and countertransference can take a variety of forms. Transference or countertransference might be suspected when therapists have to work too hard to prove themselves capable of being helpful or when they are idealized and seen as the perfect counselor, regardless of evidence to the contrary (Helms & Cook, 1999).

The need to work hard or to be idealized may be related to the client's racial identity status. People of color who have dominant immersion and emersion statuses may experience difficulty with recognizing Whites as competent helpers. But those people of color who idealize Whites and accept the status quo (conformity or dissonance statuses) may have a difficult time accepting another culturally different person as helpful and will often prefer a white therapist (D. W. Sue & Sue, 1999). Neither reaction is helpful; in fact, both interfere with the client's ability to critically listen to and integrate new information. Furthermore, therapy becomes disempowering when clients uncritically accept their therapists' ideas and suggestions. To the same degree, the therapeutic process becomes disempowering when therapists uncritically accept their clients' viewpoints.

As discussed earlier, therapists may have a variety of countertransferential reactions that interfere with the counseling process (Greene, 1985). The color blind stance is very similar to a therapist's racial identity in the contact status, a status that ignores the role of race. Racist and blaming responses are most typical of the reintegration status. On the other hand, the paternalistic stance and the unquestioning acceptance stance are approaches that we might expect in some of the later statuses, when therapists become aware of race, oppression, and privilege but are still struggling with how to address these issues successfully.

Although some statuses are more likely to be associated with certain kinds of mistakes, we can expect some of these mistakes across statuses. Racist responses may be made in even the most complex statuses when the therapist has not yet identified a source of oppression or privilege. For example, Marilyesa, an acculturated Latina, suggested to Javier that he would receive better reactions from others if his interactional style was less defensive. Although she correctly identified his contribution to his "problems," she overlooked the privilege in her own life that came from being light-skinned, well-educated, and verbally skilled. Javier's defensive reactions were often reality-oriented in his less privileged society. As this example makes clear, people of color can be racist and oppressive to the degree that they have internalized or acted upon the dominant culture's attitudes and prejudices (Helms, 2000).

Therapists at immersion and emersion statuses may ignore race because they do not know how to talk about it or because they believe it is unimportant. Dan, a young Euro-American intern working with his first African American family, was certain that race played roles in both the evasiveness of the Johnsons' interactions with him *and* in the nature of their presenting problems. However, he was not very self-confident or assertive and did not know how to address these issues. Unfortunately, his supervisor dismissed his concerns with, "Work with them just like you'd work with any other family."

Becoming aware of and challenging privilege and oppression is a journey, not an endpoint. Dan did not handle his discussion of race and privilege well, but he recognized this and searched for good supervision on these issues. The next time he was faced with a similar problem, he was more aware of the dynamics that needed to be addressed and was better prepared. Nonetheless, while we hope this journey will become easier with reflection and practice, it will still be difficult from time to time.

White and Affluence-Related Guilt

Guilt over assimilating, being affluent, or being a member of a group with a history of power can contaminate the therapy process if it prevents therapists from listening to clients or recognizing the real power of guilt (Helms & Cook, 1999). April, a Native American therapist, felt guilty about her professional success and she recognized the role that privilege played in it. She noticed her tendency to behave in disempowering ways in therapy situations, especially the tendency to try to solve her lower-class clients' problems for them. She began to pay attention to the feelings and behaviors that signaled this impulse, and she learned to interrupt them early in the process.

When guilt plays out as avoidance or the tendency to dismiss uncomfortable information, it can have an especially deleterious effect upon therapy. This problem is seen in the following interaction between an African American attorney and his African American therapist. The attorney Mr. C. sees Dr. Holmes' earlier client (a Euro-American) leaving a session:

> MR. C.: *What is that "honky" doing in the waiting room?*
> HOLMES: *Clearly, you feel that her presence is intolerable. What's bad about her being there? (Reflection of feeling, open question)*
> MR. C.: *That you're a goddamned traitor. You fraternize with the enemy! (He flailed about on the couch and cried inconsolably.)*
> HOLMES: *Your great distress makes me wonder about what other betrayals have hurt and angered you so. (Interpretation)*
> MR. C.: *(struggling for composure) My grandmother, she let my Uncle Joe get killed!* (Holmes, 1992, p. 5, as quoted in Yi, 1998. Therapeutic leads identified for consistency.)

Holmes' avoidance of her part in this problematic interaction, her rapid move from the here and now experience to historical ones, and her focus on individual issues at the expense of cultural issues led her to pathologize and trivialize Mr. C.'s concerns (C. E. Thompson & Jenal, 1994; Yi, 1998). If she had instead heard and validated his concerns with a different kind of statement (Saba & Rodgers, 1990), their alliance could have been strengthened and could have become more meaningful.

> HOLMES: *You sound very angry that I would work with people whom you view as "the enemy." It sounds like you question whether I can really understand you and help you grow as a Black man when I also work with Whites. (Reflection of feeling, interpretation.* Note that the focus of the interpretation is on the therapeutic relationship in the here and now and does not ignore the role of race in the interaction.)

Although Holmes attributed her client's early termination from therapy to Mr. C.'s intrapsychic issues, Yi (1998) instead wonders whether Mr. C. had ended therapy because of a pattern of disrespectful interactions if the quoted interaction was typical. In this case, Holmes had adopted a color blind approach (Greene, 1985), a stance that proved to be particularly destructive to Mr. C., who was probably generally functioning at either the immersion or emersion status. Because of her relatively greater power in this situation and because of the apparent absence of racial dynamics (both being African American), Mr. C. felt he had to give up his viewpoint rather than work through their problems. Furthermore, because Holmes seemed unaware of her own role due to her theoretical viewpoint or her guilt about her success she was unable to sustain a conversation about race in an empowering fashion, something that she might have been able to do with a non-African American client.

Idealization of Others

Therapists, clients, supervisors, and colleagues often idealize others who have "made it" despite life's odds against them (Helms & Cook, 1999). Although this may make it easier for therapists and clients to bond early in therapy, it can create difficulties when they try to raise and resolve the anger that is often a useful aspect of therapy. In addition, countertransferential issues may cause some therapists to excuse all problems and attribute them to racial dynamics, rather than to intervene as needed (Greene, 1985; Yi, 1998).

This idealization phenomenon may have been one reason for the contamination in the earlier interaction from Mr. C.'s point of view. Although many clients idealize their therapists and their own psychological "togetherness," Mr. C. seemed to value Holmes' ability to succeed as a black woman while maintaining Afro-centric values. When this vision of her was shattered, however, he cried ("You're a god-damned traitor. You fraternize with the enemy!"). Perhaps his reaction was because Holmes failed to understand his complex idealization of her as a therapist, as a black woman, and as a successful African American professional. Because she did not acknowledge the differences between their racial identities, she was unable to empathize with his challenge or to help him work through it. Without this support, he was unable to handle these issues and ended up terminating the therapy.

While clients may idealize their therapists' success in life, therapists can similarly idealize their clients' success, which in some ways can interfere with their ability to raise and confront issues in therapy. Holmes (Yi, 1998) may have idealized Mr. C. as a successful black attorney and underestimated his inability to feel threatened by Whites, the very people with whom he worked in the course of his own workday. Holmes may also have overlooked the degree to which Mr. C. conflated race and point of view ("If our skin color is alike, we must also think alike"). In overlooking these, she neglected opportunities to understand her client and to engage him in issues that he perceived as central. As a result, she failed to see him as a whole person (Krech, 1999).

Nonspecific Mismatches

Although the sources of transference are sometimes relatively easy to identify, they are often difficult to interpret in cases where race, class, gender, and other variables differentiate therapist and client (Helms & Cook, 1999), as in "How can you understand me? You're a white male and a married professional and I'm a black lesbian living in poverty!"

Perceived differences are often very different from real differences. The greater the *perceived* difference in the clients' eyes, the more the therapist must listen carefully, communicate empathically, and understand as fully as possible (see table 7.6). Manuela (compare to table 6.2, p. 125) draws both negative and positive conclusions that could impact the relationship unless Teresa recognizes Manuela's inferences and identifies ways to address them. It is also not useful when Manuela concludes that there is no way for Teresa to understand her life because of their differences in country of origin, class, history of immigration, and religion. Unless Teresa can see these apparent differences and demonstrate that she can be a useful therapist, Manuela will shut down.

Were Manuela to accept the apparent similarities and dismiss the differences between them, she may create an even more invidious trap in therapy. Will they accept apparent similarities in order to develop a work-

TABLE 7.6 HOW MANUELA COULD VIEW TERESA IN ORDER TO MAXIMIZE PERCEIVED SIMILARITY AND UNDERSTANDING OR TO MINIMIZE THEM

Manuela	Teresa	Focus for Maximum Similarity and Understanding	Focus for Minimum Similarity and Understanding
Cultural issues			
Female	Female	"We are both women."	"Teresa is a feminist who does not face my problems."
Latina from Chile	Latina from Cuba	"We are both Latinas."	"We are from different countries in Latin America, with different histories and cultural forces."
Recent immigrant	Second-generation American	"We have a recent history of immigration with out-group status."	"Teresá was raised in America in relative comfort with immigration being a distant memory."
Lives in an ethnic community	Lives in a professional community with few other Latins	"We share common concerns about being Latinas in the United States."	"Teresá's world is culturally divorced from my world and has few continuing ethnic ties."
Practicing Catholic	"Fallen away" Catholic. Both of her children attend Catholic school.	"We're both Catholic."	"Teresa does not value the Catholic Church and cannot understand the role of women as dictated by the Church."
Working class	White-collar professional	"We both value work."	"Her work is very different than mine."
Neurological damage stemming from domestic violence	No obvious health problems	"She looks healthy, but says she knows something about domestic violence and brain damage."	"What can she know about violence and its effects? She is probably treated like a queen by her husband."
Real or inferred living situations			
Married with no children. Husband is pressuring her to have children.	Married with two children.	"Familism is an important value for both of us."	"What does she know about being pressured to have children?"
Violent and distant marriage	Generally good marriage, although less intimate than hoped for.	"Every marriage has problems."	"My life is straight out of a *telenovela*. She is probably treated like a queen."
Values and goals			
Values hard work and education	Values hard work and education. Has been successful professionally.	"We both value hard work. Maybe I can end up where she is."	"She was probably fed from a silver spoon from birth."
Does not value exercise or physical fitness	Values exercise and runs seriously	"It would be nice to have the time to exercise."	"She is self-absorbed, another product of the United States' materialistic upper class."
Conflicted about the relative roles of the individual and family in decision making.	Values her family but makes decisions for herself	"Teresa may be a good model of how I can work this out in my own family."	"Her life has nothing in common with mine. She can afford to disrespect her husband."

Note: See table 6.2 for more complete contextual genograms.

Consider a time when you worked with a person of a different race. It can be in or out of the therapy room. When did things become difficult for either of you? What things complicated your working together? Did you resolve the problem(s) successfully? What did you do (or not do)?

ing alliance rapidly? Can they recognize and address differences to create real communication?

Just as the problem of reifying apparent differences can become a problem to address in therapy, so could dismissing the differences. Exaggerating apparent differences is similar to the actions taken in the immersion status (Helms & Cook, 1999) and can occur when one's own group is idealized and other groups—including other culturally different groups—are denigrated (see table 7.3, p. 149). Dismissing differences is most similar to the conformity response. As Helms and Cook conclude, neither stance—having to work too hard to be helpful or being seen as the perfect therapist—is useful for the client or helpful to the therapeutic process. Challenging each style can be an important piece of therapy and central to addressing many issues, especially those with interpersonal dynamics.

ADDRESSING GROUP DIFFERENCES SUCCESSFULLY

Membership in racial, gender, and class groups has meaning in our society. These meanings interfere with the therapeutic process, especially when they go unaddressed. Helms and Cook (1999) note that "whatever your unresolved issue is, it will suddenly appear in your therapy chair in increasingly extreme forms until you take steps to deal with it" (p. 26). Unresolved guilt can lead to avoidance or dismissal of problems, resulting in a paternalistic stance. Rather than allow countertransferential reactions to interfere with therapy, resolve them as much as possible outside of therapy, preferably before seeing your first client. This can be done by learning as much as possible about group issues, by requesting supervision when dealing with these issues, and by finding ways to address these needs on your own.

April, an outspoken Native American, knew she often felt guilty about leaving her family and reservation to become a therapist. She tended to underestimate the resources of people in disadvantaged groups, to give them more advice than she gave other clients, and to treat these clients in disempowering ways. When challenged on this issue by her supervisor, another Native American woman, April was chagrined, particularly since this was antithetical to her true goals for therapy. Over the next several weeks, she spent time listening to people inside and outside the therapy room and became more aware of the real strengths her clients brought to therapy.

Maddi, the daughter of wealthy parents, had a particularly difficult time working with people who struggled to make ends meet. She felt guilty that she had a nice home when many of her clients did not, and she frequently fantasized about ways to help them. She felt stymied because these thoughts were inconsistent with her theoretical point of view. She identified two ways of addressing this conflict: First, she increased her volunteering and her charitable donations within her community—especially with agencies that were addressing barriers in getting good housing and jobs (Helms & Cook, 1999). Second, she focused on how she could empower her clients (i.e., by helping them in more ways than just giving things to them).

Luke, a Euro-American male, was unaware of racial issues and had been complacent about them because "I rarely see clients where it's an issue." His consultation group, however, gradually helped him to understand that he does see people for whom group membership plays a role. His group criticized him because he tended to sidestep race in the places where clients brought it up. He and his consultation group worked together on his tendency to be color blind, and he gradually became more aware of the roles of group membership in creating privilege and oppression (Greene, 1985). When these ideas became concrete to him, he began to have a visibly greater impact on his clients.

CONCLUSIONS

On one hand, therapists can sometimes assume that their clients share their values and goals and ignore potential problems. On the other hand, clients may mistrust their therapists whether or not their therapists are culturally different. Both clients' and therapists' racial identities may contribute to these problems. Our countertransferential feelings about our own success and group membership can further complicate this relationship.

The best way to resolve our own issues with race is to work through them *before* entering the therapy room. Regardless of our ability to do so, however, we will need to work to engage our clients and to convince them that we can hear them and work with them successfully. Their concerns about themselves as racial beings and their fears of interacting with others who judge them based upon their group membership may often be the grist for therapy. Can people who look like me offer me anything of value? Am I acceptable and valuable? Can I trust people who look different than me? Can I act freely in my world? Will my actions always be limited by my race?

In order to raise and answer these questions, we will use some of the same listening techniques that are useful for Euro-American clients. However, in some cases we will need different strategies. These listening-intensive strategies are discussed in the next two chapters.

ENGAGING CLIENTS IN A MULTICULTURAL CONTEXT

"Who are *You?*" said the Caterpillar.

This was not an encouraging opening for a conversation. Alice replied, rather shyly, "I-I hardly know, sir, just at present—at least I know who I *was* when I got up this morning, but I think I must have been changed several times since then."

"What do you mean by that?" said the Caterpillar, sternly. "Explain yourself!"

"I can't explain *myself,* I'm afraid, Sir," said Alice, "because I'm not myself, you see."

"I don't see," said the Caterpillar.

"I'm afraid I can't put it more clearly," Alice replied very politely, "for I can't understand it myself, to begin with; and being so many different sizes in a day is very confusing."

"It isn't," said the Caterpillar.

"Well, perhaps you haven't found it so yet," said Alice; "but when you have to turn into a chrysalis—you will some day, you know—and then after that into a butterfly, I should think you'll feel it a little queer, won't you?"

"Not a bit," said the Caterpillar.

"Well, perhaps *your* feelings may be different," said Alice: "All I know is, it would feel very queer to *me.*"

"You!" said the Caterpillar contemptuously. "Who are *you?*" (L. Carroll, 1865/1960, pp. 67–68).

As both the Caterpillar and Alice surely discovered, *being* understood and *feeling* understood are often immensely difficult tasks—two that are supported by the basic therapeutic and listening strategies foundational to all clinical work (Rogers, 1957)—but surely not used well by the Caterpillar. In the Euro-American culture, these strategies include using strong eye contact, smiling, keeping a relatively small and informal personal space, and using active verbal and nonverbal ways to communicate understanding, including nods, encouragers, paraphrases, reflections of feeling, and summarizations (Ivey et al., 1997). These strategies are clearly necessary for therapeutic change, but they may also be sufficient when used with people in power and with those who have a history of being listened to. This is particularly true for those in acute crisis rather than those facing chronic, long-term problems (K. I. Howard, Lueger, Maling, & Martinovich, 1993).

However, special considerations must be remembered when working with clients outside of one's own cultural group. As Vontress and his colleagues (1999) note, these clients

> . . . often feel uncomfortable in a cross-cultural relationship because they feel that they are being judged by someone who is affluent, more edu-

Before beginning this discussion, think about two times when you tried to talk to someone about something unpleasant. One should be a difficult time; the other easy. What made the first situation difficult for you? What made the second easy?

TABLE 8.1	A MODEL OF MULTICULTURAL ENGAGEMENT

Am I distressed? Greater levels of distress are necessary when negative responses are given to the following questions:

- Can I expect benefits from disclosing?
- Does the listener seem to listen to me?
- Can the listener understand me and my worldview and why I might have chosen to act as I did?
- Do I believe that I can help the listener understand me and my situation, even if it is initially difficult?
- Can the listener understand the contextual factors of cultural restrictions, oppression, poverty, and the like that impact me and prevent me from acting freely?
- Does the listener respect me, my culture, and my strengths?
- Does the listener see hope in me and my situation?
- Does the listener communicate these understandings to me?

Note: The more affirmative responses that a client can give, the greater the probability of engagement.

cated, and perhaps unfamiliar with the moral compromises and complexities of a less privileged existence. (p. 41)

This chapter proposes a general model designed to help therapists engage their clients and explore some of the unique considerations for working with culturally diverse clients.

A MODEL OF ENGAGEMENT IN THERAPY

Often, clients will test their therapists to determine whether disclosing in therapy will be safe. Because therapy entails risk, clients must be distressed, have a history where the client expects benefits from disclosing, and recognize that they have been understood. The therapist must be able to see the context for the problem, identify the client's strengths, and communicate hopefulness about the future. Finally, effective therapy requires significant assertiveness: the therapist's hopefulness and understanding must be communicated to the client (see table 8.1).

THE IMPORTANCE OF DISTRESS

Therapy is often difficult, and clients may experience more distress as they begin to address issues that they have avoided in the past. This distress, however, can provide the motivation and energy to work in therapy (Hanna & Ritchie, 1995; Kopta, Howard, Lowry, & Beutler, 1994; Frank, 1961). Clients who are not currently distressed may leave prematurely when asked to do the personally challenging things that are important parts of therapy, including accepting some part of the responsibility for their dilemma and taking control in order to change it. Change and the "unknown" can be so frightening that many people will avoid it unless their current situation is overwhelming enough or the future shows some potential for success.

Some clients are distressed and in enough pain that they are willing to try anything that promises a possibility of relief, *if* they foresee improvement. When the distress decreases, they often will become more hopeful and will develop a greater degree of self-efficacy (Bandura, 1982). This hopefulness in and of itself can give them the resources to cope effectively with stressors. At the very least, the relative decrease in distress will strengthen the therapeutic alliance and cause clients to see their therapists as more credible and competent (K. I. Howard et al., 1993). People in acute distress generally respond more rapidly to therapy than those with chronic levels of stress and anxiety (Kopta et al., 1994). People who are chronically stressed *and* distressed often feel profound hopeless about their future.

EXPECTED BENEFITS FROM DISCLOSING

Return to the two times when you needed to tell someone something: one easy, the other difficult. What were the perceived benefits of talking in each example? What were the expected costs of talking?

This afternoon, I watched the Cialdinias family (mom and her two sons) being interviewed shortly after a crisis. The youngest son Matthew had been at the center of a major brawl at his school. He agreed to come in for a therapy session only grudgingly ("You're going to tell me it was my fault. You can't make me say anything!"), while the rest of the therapeutic team stayed behind the mirror. His brother Jared thought therapy was a waste of time ("Why do I have to be there?"). His mother, a young and impoverished single parent, had gone through a series of bad experiences with other therapists and agencies and was forthright in saying that she didn't trust anyone ("Why should I?"). As long as none of these family members could identify any advantages to talking in session, they were silent and sullen. The frustrated therapy team devolved into asking a series of closed questions, which only created additional problems.

The team took an early break, and we talked about what we saw and decided to try to do three things in the rest of the session: (1) Use paraphrases and reflections of feeling almost exclusively; rather than attempt to discover "what happened," (2) listen for and identify family strengths that we observed during the session, and (3) offer the family homework before they left the session.

Although the first half of the session had been painful to watch, the tone quickly changed in the second half and, in fact, became almost playful. Matthew, without prompting, described the fight at school and how he thought his teacher and the principal had been unfair. We listened as he described the problem in a way that accepted more responsibility. Ms. Cialdinias began smiling at her son and even allied with the therapeutic team on several occasions.

What made the difference? Matthew and his mother found allies where they hadn't expected them. They were listened to respectfully, their requests for help in stabilizing the situation were understood and accepted, and realistic alternatives were offered and accepted. Matthew wasn't just a diagnosis, Ms. Cialdinias wasn't treated as "trash," and the situation wasn't hopeless, all of which were things they had expected and feared. Even Jared, who liked his younger brother, found something: His opinion was requested and valued, and he discovered things that he could do to help his brother (Both had been on the playground at the same time). Until this meeting, the three were unwilling therapy clients. The team and the family had had rough times, but all knew they were working together for a reason.

Costs of Change

Therapy is often a painful process, and the emotional costs of therapy and change sometimes can seem more prominent than the benefits of any possible change. For many people, change means loss, and while it is theoretically easy to imagine positive consequences of therapy, many people find it difficult to *believe* that it will actually happen. Unfortunately, *not* deciding to change is also a decision. Therapists can help clients recognize clear benefits from the beginning—just being open to the idea that Matthew was not "bad" was important to the Cialdinias family. Oz (1995) also recommends that therapists make the costs of *not* changing clear and salient and that clients incur some costs regardless of their decision.

Some decisions occur in the context of real value conflicts and are not a matter of choosing among neutral alternatives. A young man who is coming to terms with his homosexuality may choose to be open about his sexual and affectional decisions, but he may struggle with how to be open without hurting his conservative, religious parents (Oz, 1995). Both decisions—whether to be open or hidden—have significant costs. Becoming aware of each set of costs and the numerous possible solutions, including when, with whom, and how to be open, can destabilize the "stuck" situation and allow him to make a decision with which he can be comfortable.

THE VALUE OF LISTENING AND BEING LISTENED TO

When the Cialdinias family were being questioned by the therapists about the brawl at school, they shut down. They seemed to assume that their therapists would adopt the same blaming response that everyone else had taken with them. When the therapists took the time to listen actively and use encouragers, restatements, paraphrases, reflections of feelings, and

Most people within a culture appreciate certain listening styles, but there are very real individual and cultural differences. Think about the people you know who listen well. What do you like about the way they listen? What kinds of interpersonal listening styles do you find off-putting or offensive?

Talk to other people. How do their preferences differ from yours? Do you (or they) prefer different kinds of listening depending on the situation? What patterns are you discovering?

TABLE 8.2   CLASS-RELATED FACTORS THAT AFFECT THE THERAPEUTIC PROCESS

Relationship-related Values and Beliefs	Effects of Cultural Values on Therapy
Middle class • Expect and want to achieve further upward economic and social mobility. • Believe that being angry is culturally inappropriate for girls. Feel more controlled and restrained by social norms. • Are "appropriate," indirect, tactful, and respectful rather than direct and honest. Nonetheless, success is associated with speaking out appropriately. • Perfection, defined as achievement and interpersonal smoothness, is a goal. • Have boundaried discussions and tend to keep "dirty linen" under cover.	• May influence the nature of therapeutic goals and often will expect success at least in some realms. • May have greater difficulty expressing anger in or out of therapy. May choose to do what is "expected" rather than right for the person. • May underreport or dismiss own anger. Success in external spheres may be compromised by inability to be appropriately assertive. • May be out of touch with feelings that interfere with goals of perfection, beauty, and interpersonal smoothness. • May have difficulty disclosing problems, especially to parties who may judge them.
Lower class and working poor • May feel hopeless about the future and about their ability to meet material and vocational ideals of dominant culture. • Are often angry, cynical, and frustrated with authority figures. Believe authorities won't listen to them and are unwilling or unable to meet their needs. Anger serves a protective function. • Beauty and perfection are less important than strength, perseverance, and outspokenness. These qualities may get them labeled as "bad." • Are more direct in their verbal and physical expression of negative feelings. Believe girls' anger is inappropriate when it undermines close relationships. • May hide fear and pain under layers of toughness and invulnerability. May engage in dangerous behaviors as a way of self-medicating or demonstrating "toughness."	• May feel hopelessness that bleeds over into expectations about therapy. • Expect adversarial relationships with therapists and do not expect to be heard or have their anger validated and seen as "good." • The positive sides of these behaviors have often been overlooked. Recognizing and validating these positive aspects is often useful. • Accept anger and find ways to express it in adaptive ways. Be flexible in recognizing cultural limitations of previous definitions of appropriately expressed anger. • May need to hear fear and pain and keep client safe, while also acknowledging client's real strengths. May need to help client express strength in healthy and adaptive ways.

Note: These factors have largely been identified in Euro-American populations. From L. Brown, 1998; Liu, 2002; Pickett, 2002.

summarizations, the mother and sons became less defensive and began discussing their concerns in an active and open manner.

As this example shows, active listening is often a prerequisite for work with clients who feel excluded by those in power. Susan, a white, working-class 13-year-old said, "I don't talk to the teachers about [my opinions] because I don't think they would listen to somebody that disagrees . . . they don't find out our opinions about it." Rachel, also 13 years of age, attended the same working-class school and added, "It's like they're too busy to listen when we need to know something" (L. Brown, 1998, p. 181).

For many culturally different people, including the working poor, the world feels unfair. They feel they will be unable to succeed by following white, middle-class rules (see table 8.2). Adults and older children may attempt to equalize perceived inequities by not talking or by being verbally aggressive (Meichenbaum, 2000a). Toddlers throw tantrums instead. These examples of anger are difficult for many authority figures to address for two reasons. The first is that angry feelings may be followed by angry actions; the second is that more than one way to look at things exists, and in fact, the culturally different viewpoint might be right. When therapists think dichotomously and face other viewpoints that may be right (suggesting that theirs is wrong), they often feel threatened.

Especially when a client's history suggests that others will not listen, the therapist must develop a warm, sincere, and respectful relationship with the client. In these situations, the quality of the relationship can be more important than the tasks themselves (Diller, 1999; Hanna & Ritchie, 1995; McClure, 1999). Therapists may need to spend extra time listening to clients and validating their viewpoints. As we do this, we may remove the need for maladaptive ways of expressing anger. These recommendations are well within the mainstream of therapeutic research and grounded in the work of Carl Rogers (1957).

Listening occurs in an individual and cultural context (see table 8.3) that influences what its members see as good listening (Paniagua, 1998; Zhang, 2003a). African Americans, in particular, tend to be very active listeners even in formal public settings (e.g., church and public lectures). Unsolicited verbal feedback is the norm, and speakers often leave space for it. Many Native Americans tend to fall at the other end of the spectrum and perceive interruptions of a speaker as rude and immodest (Modesty is an important cultural value). Euro-Americans tend to be between these two and often interrupt one another. In fact, this kind of conversation is sometimes described by other Euro-Americans as "vibrant." Despite this, Euro-Americans can become irritated when they are interrupted too frequently, especially when interruptions introduce a topic change or otherwise invalidate or don't expand on the speaker's message.

Some aspects of nonverbal communication, especially facial expressions associated with happiness, sadness, anger, fear, disgust, and surprise are easily recognized, but others (e.g., embarrassment and amusement) are sometimes difficult to recognize and distinguish between (Keltner, 1995). Cultural differences seem to increase the difficulties, especially when low-intensity emotions are involved and when therapists have less experience with the speaker's culture (Bailey, Nowicki, & Cole, 1998). Problems increase when the emotions of people in crisis, our most common customers, are rapidly shifting and poorly identified. Francis, for example, was bewildered and thinking he was going crazy because he felt sad, relieved, angry, and guilty all within a short period following his grandfather's death. Knowledge of culture and context may be especially important in decoding these confusing and apparently conflicting emotions—emotions that

TABLE 8.3 **CULTURAL PATTERNS IN LISTENING AND DISCLOSING**

African Americans
- Are nonverbally expressive.
- See nonverbal communication as a more reliable barometer of truth, especially with Euro-Americans or people in authority.
- Do not use eye contact as a normal part of conversation because conversations often occur during other tasks. Eye contact is, however, generally greater when speaking than when listening.
- Do not regularly use head nods and minimal encouragers to maintain a conversation.

Arab Americans
- Use indirect eye contact often, especially with people of the opposite sex.
- Need little same-sex personal space.
- Use indirect, yet effective, challenges to elders and authorities.
- Communicate often in indirect ways, using metaphors, euphemisms, and extended introductions.
- Rarely share emotional issues with anyone outside of family. Issues of this nature are saved for trusting, deeper relationships.

Asian Americans
- Often view smiling as a sign of weakness and not as an indication of happiness. Smiling may be a response to embarrassment, shyness, or discomfort.
- Value silence and see it as respectful, especially with people of greater power, authority, or wisdom.
- See eye contact as disrespectful, especially with people of greater power, authority, or wisdom.
- Do not show affection, even handholding, toward a spouse in public.
- Speak in relatively quiet and reserved tones.
- Touching occurs about half as often as among Euro-Americans. Japanese, in particular, have strong taboos against touching strangers.
- Communicate indirectly to avoid shaming self or others or cause a loss of "face." Nonverbal expressions are often suppressed, except in extreme situations.

Euro-Americans
- Respond in relatively emotionally restrained and nonverbal, nonexpressive ways.
- Consider eye contact to be a normal and expected part of conversations. Absence of eye contact is assumed to imply shame, guilt, dishonesty, or poor self-esteem. Eye contact tends to be greater when listening than when speaking.
- Often consider pauses and stretches of silence in a conversation to be uncomfortable. Euro-Americans often will attempt to "fill up" these moments. Interruptions occur frequently.
- Expect others, including young children, to enter conversations freely, state their opinions clearly, and ask questions frequently.
- Often speak in relatively loud and frequently boisterous ways.
- Expect handshakes to be firm. Firm handshakes are seen as a sign of power, strength, and interest.
- Touch less frequently in formal than in informal situations, although when it occurs, it is indicative of greater amounts of power or status. The person with more power or status does the touching.

Latin Americans
- Will frequently engage in long and vigorous handshaking.
- Have personal space that is relatively smaller. Latinos frequently touch each other when talking.
- Speak in relatively rapid and often boisterous ways.

Native Americans
- Expect good listening to involve careful and silent observation of the listener. A large amount of the "information" in a conversation is assumed to be communicated nonverbally.
- See eye contact as disrespectful, especially with elders or people with more power.
- Speak in relatively slower and quieter tones. Long pauses may occur between speakers.
- Expect handshakes to be light. Firm handshakes are seen as "aggressive."
- May view asking direct questions or challenging the course of therapy as disrespectful.

Note: From Amer, 2002; Erickson & Al-Timimi, 2001; Halonen & Santrock, 1997; Keltner, 1995; Paniagua, 1998; D. W. Sue & Sue, 1999; Tafoya, 1990; Zhang, 2003a, 2003d.

Francis did not have the skills to understand and therefore was less able to help his therapist.

Potential Benefits of Warm and Empathic Listening

Empathic listening skills can be set aside or sacrificed when therapeutic power and prestige are strong (see table 6.1). Some of the psychotherapeutic "greats," for example, are rude, brusque, and even superficially insensitive in their work (cf. Ellis, 1971, in Ivey et al, 1997, or Whitaker & Bumberry, 1987). My Euro-American students from rural areas tend to respond much more positively to Ellis and Whitaker than to tapes of contemporary client-centered therapists. While my students *say* they believe that warmth is very important to the client-therapist relationship, they seem to prefer a brusque, genuine, active, and directive therapist.

Perhaps more than warm and empathic paraphrases and reflections of feelings, clients with a personal or cultural history of oppression prefer active, open, and expressive communications (D. W. Sue & Sue, 1999). For example, Asian Americans generally prefer a logical, rational, and structured style over an affective, reflective, and ambiguous one (Atkinson et al., 1978). African American therapy trainees often have a natural affinity for the use of active styles—advice, directives, paraphrases, and interpretations, in particular—while Euro-American trainees use more attending skills (Berman, 1979). Similarly, an open, active, and direct style is appropriate for the fast-paced, crisis-oriented work of hospital settings and with people who have acute or chronic physical illnesses (Belar & Deardorff, 1995).

Clients often enter therapy hesitant and unsure about the process, the person helping them, or both. Cultural values may also make therapeutic disclosures difficult initially (see table 8.4). Asian Americans and Native Americans, in particular, believe it is foolhardy to disclose to strangers (Paniagua, 1998). Many clients' early communications, regardless of cultural background, include the implied request, "Before I open up to you, tell me who you are and why you are safe to talk to" (D. W. Sue & Sue, 1999).

Active modes of intervening, including self-disclosures, advice, directives, sharing information, and interpretations, are a kind of therapist self-disclosure and they help clients understand the personal and professional values and stance of their therapists. Being active and open creates a safe therapeutic environment and thus increases a client's ability to disclose safely. Disclosures beget more disclosures, and an active style of intervention is often appreciated and particularly important for people with personal or cultural histories that may interfere with trust (Zhang, 2003g).

TABLE 8.4 **RELATIONSHIP-RELATED VALUES AND BELIEFS FOR DIFFERENT GROUPS**

Relationship-related Values and Beliefs	Effects of Cultural Values
African Americans	
• Race is often a barrier to developing relationships.	• Therapy may be stilted and ineffective until therapist discusses the impact of race with client.
• Many have external loci of responsibility and control.	• Medication may be seen as a racist attempt to ignore the client. Environmental influences on problem must be discussed and addressed.
• The church institution is often an important influence. Going to a therapist instead of church may be viewed as a lack of trust in God.	• Spiritual needs should be addressed, and the church and therapist should work together as allies.
• The culture values the wisdom and contributions of elders.	• Clients, especially elder ones, must be treated respectfully and generally be addressed by title, such as "Mrs. Johnson."
• Many have frequently experienced being "put off" or "put down" by agencies and may expect the same from therapists.	• Therapists must be sensitive to this fact and be respectful of the client's autonomy and opinions.
Arab Americans	
• Many have a strong familial network and often depend heavily on family for support and help with stressors.	• As they generally turn to family first for support, many have a difficult time disclosing issues to people outside of their family network. They may initially appear reserved.
• Individual happiness and individual goals are often less important than familial goals and family honor.	• They may become confused or feel guilty if individual goals are stressed in therapy.
• Years of political instability in their home country have often led to cautious attitudes and apprehensive worldview, especially toward Westerners. They expect their religious or political views to be misunderstood.	• Many find disclosing social or political views difficult, at least initially. Often, they expect to be misunderstood. Therapists must be willing to consider nonWestern perspectives of Arab life. Families may expect therapists to ally with more "Americanized" members of the family.
• Disclosure of psychiatric or behavioral problems is often seen as bringing shame to the family or Arab community, thus clients may fear being branded *majnun* (crazy).	• May have difficulty disclosing "problems" outside of familial network. Clients will need to be reassured about their mental stability and the confidentiality of therapy
• Communications are often hierarchical in nature, with fathers being the "head of the household." Mothers often have considerable power, but they express it indirectly.	• Therapists should acknowledge relative strengths and assets and be willing to see other patterns of communication and gender interactions as functional.
• They tend to express emotional pain in terms of physical symptoms.	• Therapists should consider this approach to communication a culturally-different style rather than "wrong."
• Insight is less important than action.	• Psychoeducational and action-oriented therapies will probably be preferred over insight therapies.
• Giving advice, especially within a hierarchical relationship, is normal and expected.	• They will expect to receive advice and may treat the therapist as an "expert." When the therapist does not use this style of interaction, this should be clearly explained.
• Time orientation is focused more on the present.	• Clients may be late without it being an indication of resistance. This should not be interpreted as such without evidence. Clients may not be interested in considering consequences for future events.
Asian Americans	
• Helping relationships are often formal, benevolent, and hierarchical, generally with the helper being older and more expert.	• Therapists may want to take special steps to demonstrate their expertness. Therapists may adopt formal, but benevolent, relationships and should not push early disclosures.
• Disclosure to strangers is seen as foolish and immature. Problems are "shameful."	• Disclosures will be limited until the therapist is no longer a "stranger." Some therapeutic self-disclosure may be necessary early in therapy.

(continued)

TABLE 8.4 *(continued)*

Relationship-related Values and Beliefs	Effects of Cultural Values
• The mind and body are seen as indivisible.	• Mental illness and other issues may be expressed as somatic symptoms.
• Interpersonal harmony is extremely important. Personal sacrifice may be necessary to maintain it. Wishes are often communicated indirectly.	• Being assertive and setting contradictory goals may be difficult, especially when doing so threatens a sense of interpersonal harmony.
Euro-Americans	
• Although disclosure generally occurs in a relationship, appropriate disclosures can occur in a "business setting."	• To the degree that therapy is seen as professional and as a "business," disclosures may be rapid and not relationship based, especially when confidentiality is guaranteed.
• Separation between church and state or other systemic influences is seen as normal.	• Systemic influences are not expected to be automatically engaged. Why other family members should be involved in therapy is often not understood.
• Insight, especially for middle class and educated Euro-Americans, is seen as an important goal.	• Clients may become irritated when therapy moves too rapidly without insight. Example: "But, what does it mean? Why do I do it?"
• Punctuality is often seen as a sign of respect.	• Clients may become irritated when sessions start late and become uncomfortable when they run long.
Latin Americans	
• Disclosure occurs within a relationship.	• Therapy may start very formally, but become less formal.
• *Respeto* (respect for authority figures and their wisdom) and *machismo* (manliness) are important values.	• The father may need special regard, and special attempts to join him should be made early in family therapy.
• Insight is seen as less important than action.	• Action and homework may be indicated even in the first session. Medication may be seen as an important part of therapy.
• The church is an important influence. Spirituality sometimes includes beliefs in evil spirits.	• Spiritual needs should be addressed. The church, folk healers, and therapist should work together as allies when indicated.
Native Americans	
• Silent listening is seen as respectful.	• The therapist will be expected to be a good listener and should allow some silence at the end of each statement.
• Disclosure to strangers is "foolish."	• Disclosures may be limited until the therapist is no longer a "stranger."
• Respect is due to one's elders.	• Clients, especially elder clients, must be treated respectfully and generally called by titles. They may ask about the therapist's age as a way to determine competence.
• Problems may be seen as interruptions in the harmony of spirit, body, and mind.	• Medications are often viewed with suspicion as a side-step of the problem. Spiritual harmony (a state of being that comes from within) must often be addressed, sometimes with traditional healers.
• Healing is often expected to be done in public, surrounded by one's family and friends.	• Change may need to occur in the community, often with a kind of "public confession."
• Action is seen as more important than insight into one's problems.	• It may be important for therapist to be relatively active and directive, such as giving homework. Use of ritual may be more important than insight.
• Being-in-time is more important than punctuality.	• Clients may often be late to appointments and may not see their tardiness as necessary or appropriate to apologize for. Lateness may not indicate resistance.

Note: These generalizations are also influenced by gender, class, and level of acculturation. From Amer, 2002; Erickson & Al-Timimi, 2001; Helms & Cook, 1999; Hines & Boyd-Franklin, 1996; Lee, 1990; Minuchin, 1974; Paniagua, 1998; D. W. Sue & Sue, 1999; Tafoya, 1990; Yi, 1995, 1998; Zayas & Solari, 1994; Zhang, 2003e. See also tables 3.3 and 8.2.

THE IMPORTANCE OF UNDERSTANDING CLIENTS AND THEIR WORLDVIEW

Having a good, empathic understanding of clients includes a willingness to set aside one's own worldview and values and to accept (at least initially) clients' understanding of their problems and their world. This is especially important for clients with personal or cultural histories of feeling misunderstood and devalued. The Cialdinias family needed to know whether or not their therapists would step out of their authority roles and move away from the (expected) natural alliances with the school and be willing to really listen to their concerns and perspective on the problems. As a result, one of the turning points in the session came when Mrs. Cialdinias apparently nonchalantly asked her therapist:

> MRS. CIALDINIAS: *What did you hear happened?*
> CATHRYN: *(nondefensively) By the time I called the school, [Matthew's] teacher had already left for the day. What the principal said was that another child called Matthew a name and Matthew hit him. The other kids got involved at that point. (She turns to Matthew) Did we get it right? (Information, checkout)*

Because Cathryn introduced some uncertainty about the nature of the interaction ("*What the principal said . . . .*") and checked out the principal's statement with Matthew, she communicated that she was willing to be objective and was not going to choose sides before getting all of the information. This simple, honest, and open response from Cathryn made it easier for both parties to work together.

Developing a Therapeutic Alliance

A number of writers have identified the therapeutic alliance as one of the most important tasks in therapy and one of the best predictors of therapy outcome (Asay & Lambert, 1999; Lambert, 1992; Meichenbaum, 2000a). Greif (1990) describes several things that therapists can do that can help us join with clients and families and can help them feel understood (see table 8.5). Sometimes, just finding similarities in therapist and client experience can begin to build the bridge that creates the therapeutic alliance. Whitaker, for example, included this joining exchange:

> DAD: *We're used to that on the farm.*
> WHITAKER: *You're used to that on the farm? I was born and brought up on a dairy farm. I should have brought my cow! I did a workshop and someone gave me a little toy cow with udders, in case I was*

What do you do to join with your clients or develop the therapeutic alliance? What things do you see others do?

TABLE **8.5**   **TECHNIQUES FOR JOINING WITH CLIENTS AND THEIR FAMILIES**

Structuring sessions
- Shake hands with family members when they arrive.
- Let everyone choose their seating arrangements, which shows respect of their autonomy and allows you to observe their usual way of interacting.
- Be aware of the personal space that is appropriate to their family style and culture and, if possible, stay within this range.
- Reassure clients and families, especially if this is their first time in treatment, that therapy often makes people uncomfortable. Frame dealing with problems and uncomfortable issues as a sign of courage, rather than as a sign of weakness.

Respecting individual and cultural differences
- Learn about each client's cultural and religious background. Respect this background and cultural differences.
- Respect each client's individual and cultural patterns and rates of problem disclosure. Moving too rapidly may scare some away from therapy. Others may need to begin work immediately and may become impatient when prevented from doing so.
- Honor family elders, especially in age-revering cultures and families. Be appreciative and playful with children without undermining family rules or authority.

Listening
- Learn about and use culturally-appropriate listening patterns.
- Especially initially, match your breathing, physical posture, language, and paralanguage to that of the family member you are most interested in reaching.
- Use your language—especially vocabulary, paralanguage, volume, and pace—to heighten clients' responses to you.
- Recognize individual differences in personal and family style and, while being genuine, match your style to theirs.
- Listen to and acknowledge the validity of your clients' pain. Track your clients' concerns by referring to their previous statements.

Recognizing and respecting clients' humanity
- Recognize and share common interests such as science fiction, computers, and backgrounds (e.g., "I grew up around there.").
- Recognize and acknowledge your clients' strengths, in addition to their weaknesses.
- Remember and comment on important dates and events, such as birthdays and anniversaries, including those mentioned in any previous sessions.
- Remember the names of family members and, when possible, those of girlfriends, teachers, friends, and after-school activities.

Creating respectful boundaries
- Some self-disclosure can create an atmosphere of safety and trust, especially early in therapy, and may be necessary with clients of some cultural backgrounds.
- Find ways to take notes when necessary, but do not let this create barriers to therapy.
- Send children out of the room when the discussion turns to issues that do not concern them, such as sexual problems. Be willing to see children alone when appropriate. While drawing appropriate boundaries, it can increase their comfort with disclosing in the future.
- Keep the length of the first session flexible whenever possible. More time may be needed to meet the family's goals because of family or cultural styles.
- While large gifts are often problematic, small ones are often culturally appropriate. Accepting small gifts can be respectful, if therapeutic goals and ethical issues are also considered.

Note: From Greif, 1990; Hahn, 1998; Lazarus 1993; Sue, 2000; Zhang, 2003g.

feeling lonely and wanted to cuddle up to a cow again (Whitaker & Bumberry, 1987, p. 8).

One outcome of feeling understood is a stronger therapeutic alliance. Clients' assessment of the quality of the therapeutic alliance predicts therapeutic outcome better than the therapist's or external observer's assessment (Bourgeois, Sabourin, & Wright, 1990; Safran & Wallner, 1991). As long as clients believe their therapists understand them and their problems, change can occur, even if the alliance is flimsy and ineffectual from the therapist's point of view. This "weak alliance" could, in fact, be stronger than any other relationship in the client's life.

OVERCOMING INITIAL BARRIERS TO UNDERSTANDING

Some clients have such a difficult time trusting other people that the therapeutic alliance needs to be renewed at every session. This can be seen in the following exchange that begins with Charley having just handed his journal to Derika and sitting quietly until she finishes reading):

CHARLEY: *Do you understand what I mean? I mean, do you* really *understand?*

DERIKA: *It sounds like it's very important to you right now that I understand your concerns and that you also don't believe that I or anyone can. While you're asking this here, I also heard some of those same ideas in your journal [when you wrote] "Can anyone hear me? Can you understand me? Will you work with me? Will you leave me?"* (Paraphrase)

CHARLEY: *Yeah, you're right . . . I always worry that you won't understand me. (Long pause) You know, my mom never really understood me or took care of me. Why should you be any different?*

DERIKA: *You're right to be careful, especially given your history. I'm wondering though, are there times when you do feel heard here?* (Sharing information, closed question)

CHARLEY: *(nodding) Yeah, most of the time I think you understand me. Like now . . . but, it's hard for me to believe you'll understand when I tell you something new.*

DERIKA: *I'm glad that most of the time it feels like I understand you. But when you think I'm not understanding, I want you to tell me as soon as you can. I want to know you, and I would appreciate it if you would tell me when I'm offtrack. (Self-disclosure, directive, self-disclosure)*

Because of his tendency to mistrust others, especially authority figures, Charley had difficulty feeling heard in therapy. In fact, what kept him there was that he felt very distressed, wanted to do something about it, and *sometimes* felt heard. Derika, in turn, accepted his perception of his world (that others do not understand and will take advantage of him), but she also helped him recognize the grays that existed between his dichotomous extremes. By emphasizing the *experience* of being heard and understood, instead of whether or not he *was* understood, she was able to circumvent a struggle that might otherwise have occurred. Nonetheless, this was the first issue they needed to address every week for several months.

Derika, an upper middle-class Euro-American, was at an initial disadvantage in her work with Charley. Nevertheless, she did several things that made it more likely for Charley to feel understood. First, she validated rather than dismissed Charley's feelings. Instead of pretending that she was perfect and never made mistakes, she readily admitted her own humanity (that she doesn't always understand) and requested his help in becoming a better therapist for him. She admitted that his concerns may have a reality basis. Second, she understood the impact of the history of emotional neglect upon his ability to feel understood and accepted his perceptions rather than demanding that he recognize her empathic understanding immediately. Finally, she treated him respectfully instead of condescendingly. Rather than relating to him as though he were "broken" and unable to work things out with someone else, she engaged him as a real partner in the therapy process.

THE VALUE OF UNDERSTANDING IMPORTANT CONTEXTUAL FACTORS

Throughout this book, we have been talking about the role of contextual factors that make important contributions to the ways in which clients perceive and respond to stressors. These factors include the

- Nature of family and community supports and stressors (Mervyn, chapter 1)
- Confluence of losses (Jackson, chapter 3)
- Familial and systemic prejudices about young African American males (Jackson, chapter 3)
- Cultural pride (Rashelle, chapter 4)
- Cultural and religious expectations (Manuela, chapter 6)
- Class conflicts (Manuela, chapter 6)

While these are important issues, the range of influences and moderating factors is limitless. It is impossible for any one person to have personal experience with all groups. One would have to be a gay; Black *and* White *and*

Hispanic; HIV-positive; upper-class; middle-aged; drug abusing; abstinent; sexually abused; depressed; female quadriplegic who's also a single parent. Because people believe that they are more likely to be understood by someone similar, I take it as a compliment of the highest degree when clients assume that I am a Christian or have a history of sexual abuse. They are saying, "You really understand me!"

Group similarities do not guarantee understanding, however, and are not always desired. Some people will look for a culturally similar therapist, while others will choose to go outside their reference community in order to maintain privacy and confidentiality (Paniagua, 1998). Some will be uncomfortable if members of their reference group even work in the waiting room. Others will feel that having members of their group or culture working at a site increases the probability that culturally relevant and appropriate services will be provided.

Because of the real limits imposed upon therapists' personal experience, we must find other ways to improve our ability to counsel diverse clients. These ways can include developing a diverse set of friends, volunteering, and becoming active in other communities, but they can also involve watching movies, reading novels and works of nonfiction, listening to clients, friends (and even strangers), traveling, and going to lectures. Understanding others requires that we as therapists step outside our "safety zone" into communities that are sometimes very different from our own (Diller, 1999).

D. W. Sue and Sue (1999) suggest that by simply admitting our limitations of knowledge and experience, respecting these differences, and demonstrating a willingness to listen and learn, we can break down these barriers and help clients become comfortable.

Building a Cognitive Understanding

When first working with someone from a different group, we should ask ourselves a series of questions: How has the dominant society affected members of this group? How does being a member of this group make life easy? How does it make things difficult? How might it cause the problems seen in therapy? Are symptoms normative or even adaptive for the culture and context (Hays 1995; Knight & McCallum, 1998)? For example, depending on one's values and whether or not one sees depression following retirement as normal, we may make very different treatment recommendations for two 65-year-olds facing retirement. We may choose to normalize reactions and symptoms, refer to a peer support group, challenge maladaptive thoughts, refer for medication, or hospitalize. If we think it may sometimes be problematic, how would we recognize those times? As we do these things, however, we also need to broaden the context and consider

TABLE 8.6   INDIVIDUAL AND CULTURAL FACTORS IMPACTING WILLARD'S AND MARSHA'S REACTIONS TO RETIREMENT

Willard
- African American culture is generally respectful of its older members, yet he equates retirement with "growing old," "falling apart," or "being useless."
- He was born at the end of the Depression, and his family never completely regained their previous quality of living. He is concerned about whether he and his wife will have enough money to live on.
- His best friends are five to ten years younger than he is and have not yet begun talking about retirement.
- Work has been his hobby. He wonders what he would do instead.
- His relationship with his wife is rocky, and he is unsure about whether he wants to spend much time with her.
- His father and older brother died in the first year of their retirements.
- His health has been failing, and he believes that this is the first indication of an inevitable decline, as was the case with his father.
- His daughter and two young grandchildren recently moved home after his daughter's divorce. The daughter is not working and is receiving only small child-support payments.

Marsha
- The larger culture is youth-oriented, but she is well-respected in her community and holds an elder position in her tribe and church. She looks on her gray hair and wrinkles as badges of wisdom.
- She was a young child during the Depression, but survived well. She knows that her community will help her if she needs it because she has helped other tribal members.
- Several friends have made good transitions to retirement. They meet several times weekly for breakfast, something she is looking forward to being able to do with them.
- She is an avid traveler and looks forward to being able to travel abroad more frequently.
- She divorced her husband 15 years ago, but has developed a strong and stable group of friends.
- Most relatives, except her mother, lived long and healthy lives during their retirements. One aunt (now 99), lives independently and is not taking medication of any sort.
- While she has been having a few mild health problems, her illnesses generally have been short-lived and transient, and she expects current concerns to easily be resolved.
- Her three children also live on the reservation and keep in close touch with her.

the impact of cohort differences and political history and learn relevant folkways, life experiences, and different word uses.

Willard and Marsha, each retiring in the near future, raise these issues (see table 8.6). Although both are facing the same stressor, they experienced it differently because of their context and the meanings that they drew from it. Marsha, a Native American, created a supportive community, while Willard, an African American, anticipated further defeat. Their unique contexts help us identify issues for treatment.

Rather than facilitating listening, thinking about cultural differences can prevent it. To prevent this, we must listen to the individuality within each context. Both Willard and Marsha struggled with losing their health and looks, with redefining life's purpose and goals, and with the changing relationships with family and friends, but they experienced these potential crises differently because of the unique meanings that aging and retirement held for them. Similarly, people with a history of abuse often struggle with questions of control, responsibility, safety, trust, and self-esteem, as well as whether they are and how they could be lovable. Some survivors, however, become promiscuous risk-takers, while others become cautious and celibate (Gil, 1999). We will return to these questions in chapter 11, when we specifically discuss the importance of created meanings and their relationship to behavioral outcomes.

Ignoring Differences

Working with people from other contexts or cultures can be very different or very similar to working with people from one's own culture and context. Fewer problems can be expected when the therapist is familiar with the concerns raised and the therapist or client is either bicultural or lives in a relatively integrated community (Knight & McCallum, 1998). However, these factors may also serve as stumbling blocks if the therapist *assumes* understanding without recognizing the importance and impact of those differences that do exist. Furthermore, the therapist might easily assume that some variables, especially racial similarities, are especially important, while ignoring the contributions of other variables such as gender, class, or history of sexual abuse—which may actually be more salient obstacles (Paniagua, 1998). For example, Levinson (2000) said that, in many ways, his heritage as a Russian Jew was more important than his affectional orientation. On the other hand, fathering a child was a singularly important and often isolating decision which would perhaps be better understood in the context of his identity as a young gay man.

On the first day of class, I often ask my students to introduce themselves to the person sitting next to them and identify similarities and differences between them. Generally, they find it easier to identify the similarities rather than the differences and will sometimes identify a series of trivial similarities in background and interests, while denying the impact of their differences in race, gender, and physical ability. This selective inattention may be because both parties see identifying differences in a public setting as threatening to their new and tenuous relationship ("Differences may blow us apart").

Therapists may emphasize similarities in order to create a therapeutic alliance, although clients may see differences that can assume huge importance later. Acknowledging the differences in worldview is acceptable. However, many people who are visibly "different" and may be a minority in a group have had to educate people outside of their group about their culture and worldview, more often than they would like. It is the therapist's responsibility to educate himself or herself about this group *and* to hear and understand how each client is unique (Paniagua, 1998).

Handling Contextual Differences

There are several ways to respond to potential differences in worldview, but it is important to first acknowledge their existence, as Derika did with Charley. With African American clients, it is often important for therapists of other cultural groups to acknowledge race and racial differences and to discuss their implications from the very first session. When race is ignored, the therapeutic relationship gets compromised. Clients may close down the discussion, avoid concerns, or talk in frustrated and anxious manners with multiple interruptions in the conversation (C. E. Thompson & Jenal, 1994). In the following discussion, Joe hears Darnel's concerns without dismissing the role of race:

> JOE: *I sense some major hesitations . . . it's difficult for you to discuss your concerns with me. (Feedback, interpretation)*
>
> DARNEL: *You're damn right! If I really told you how I felt about my coach, what's to prevent you from telling him? You Whities are all of the same mind.*
>
> JOE: *(angry) Look, it would be a lie for me to say I don't know your coach. He's an acquaintance, but not a personal friend. Don't put me in the same bag with all Whites! Anyways, even if he was, I hold our discussion in strictest confidence. Let me ask you this question, what would I need to do that would make it easier for you to trust me? (Self-disclosure, directive, self-disclosure, open question)*
>
> DARNEL: *You're on your way, man!* (D. W. Sue & Sue, 1999, p. 47, names and types of therapeutic leads added for clarity and consistency).

In this example, Joe, a Euro-American therapist, did two things to counter the concerns of Darnel, his African American client. First, he addressed Darnel's concerns openly, honestly, and genuinely. Imagine if he had calmly responded to Darnel's first statement with "What would telling your coach mean to you?" or responded angrily with "What do you mean, we're all of the same mind?" These are questions that at least partially dismiss Darnel's concerns by ignoring the role of context. Second, Joe's language became less formal and more direct in his second lead, as his verbal style mirrored Darnel's. This response, in addition to being more genuine, also joined with Darnel: "We both should be angry about the barriers that prevent Blacks and Whites from connecting and understanding each other." After the first session, continuing to raise race as an issue may create the perception that racial differences are uncomfortable for the therapist or that the therapist is attempting to play Savior (Paniagua, 1998).

Clearly, Euro-American therapists should address racial mismatches in therapy, but culturally different therapists should also be prepared to discuss these issues with their clients, even when they are members of the same racial or cultural group (Paniagua, 1998). Many African Americans, for example, find it difficult to disclose personal problems to other African Americans. We could expect that racial identity would interact with this process, such that people at either immersion or emersion racial identity statuses would have special problems working with Euro-American therapists, while people at the conformity or dissonance statuses would have fewer problems and may even prefer a Euro-American therapist (see table 7.3, p. 149).

These problems may be exacerbated when class is also a barrier between therapist and client. In this case, African American clients (and others) may fear that their African American therapists have "sold out" or bought into majority group values and norms (Helms & Cook, 1999; Paniagua, 1998). Paniagua recommends dealing with this potential problem in the here and now:

> LATICIA: *Blacks sometimes feel uncomfortable discussing problems with other Blacks. I'm wondering how you feel about working with me. (Information, question in the form of a self-disclosure)*

Being sensitive to issues of oppression and the adaptive nature of failing to disclose begins to build our clients' trust in us and in the therapy process. Respecting the person and context allows us to build a more open and genuine relationship and brings contextual issues into the ongoing therapeutic conversation (Helms & Cook, 1999).

Bridging the Gap

The gap between people of two different cultures can be more inferred than real, but both therapist and client can attempt to bridge this gap. This is seen in the work of Polster (2000), a European-born male working with Gloria, a Latina. Polster took generally very appropriate approaches to helping Gloria become comfortable enough that they could work together. First, he asked where she had been born and then tentatively shared his own experience of being different, with the apparent hope that she would respond to his self-disclosure with one of her own. Second, he attempted to transfer her strengths and admittedly supportive system to her school environment, which apparently was mostly young Euro-Americans. Gloria also attempted to bridge this gap, mostly by suppressing her voice. Unfortunately, by acquiescing and being "nice," she blocked a real connection.

Gloria said, "I want to know why I'm sad," while Polster worked in the here and now about her connection with him (Polster, 2000). Their miscommunication may be partially attributable to cultural preferences about the helping relationship, with Latin Americans generally preferring a hierarchical and action-oriented therapy. In this case, her words ask for insight, but she seems to be asking for immediate change. His approach, while action-oriented and set in the present, was relatively indirect. She did not immediately understand why he chose to talk about her interactional style rather than her depression.

Polster's (2000) work might have been more successful if he and the client had discussed his goals for their work and reached an agreement. For example, he might have said:

> POLSTER: *Gloria, I think you're sad because you see walls between people and cultures when they don't exist, and it leaves you feeling lonely. Can we try a little experiment?* . . . . *(Interpretation, directive in the form of a closed question)*

This interpretation makes his rationale for future work explicit; "irrelevant" work becomes more relevant. It also sets up a more cooperative relationship, rather than one where *respeto* is immediately pulled—a value that created even greater distance between the two. Of course, the problems in their interview were probably equally attributable to the fact that the interview was completed in front of an audience of about 2000, something Gloria readily admitted.

THE BENEFITS OF RESPECTING CLIENTS AND SEEING THEIR STRENGTHS

When our strengths are recognized, we often feel more powerful. Explore this by listening for someone's strengths. Observe him or her while you listen and notice shifts in body posture, tension, and language across the course of your conversation. How do these things shift as you jointly identify strengths?

How do you get people to recognize strengths? The next time you're listening to a problem, paraphrase the concerns then ask about how they are handling it. What is working, even a little bit? When they have a difficult time identifying their strengths or the coping skills they use with this problem, ask whether they have dealt with similar problems in the past. If so, how did they get through those periods? Are there parts of that experience that may be useful in dealing with the current problem? Pay attention to the things they do well and let them know that you heard these in an honest and open way.

Some people may react negatively when you attempt to find strengths in these periods. If so, consider whether the people are feeling heard. Before you can give a different perspective, they will need to feel heard in their current one. If they need to have you spend extra time listening to the "problem," be careful not to get caught by the weaknesses and the problems. Remember to pay attention to the strengths that they are overlooking.

With some people who feel very stuck and resist finding strengths relative to the stressor, I change the subject and ask them to tell me about another time, one when things were going well. What strengths do you hear? How can these be transferred to the current problem? How can these be built into their life at this point or expanded?

People who smile frequently are generally judged to be warmer than those who do not (Ivey et al., 1997). Without warmth, positive messages are lost or negated. Imagine hearing "You did a nice job," from one person whose voice was animated and who smiled warmly and from another person whose voice and face were expressionless. Who would you think was more sincere?

Warmth, positive regard, and respect are important and perhaps even essential to treatment (Ivey et al., 1997; Rogers, 1957), but they are not afforded all consumers of mental health treatment (see, for example, Michener, 1998; Shimrat, 1997). Vontress says:

> I have come to despise the professional games and bureaucracy that we dispense as our means of helping others. No wonder clients often come to hate counseling centers; these organizations often reflect the insensitivity of the client's world instead of offering a place of refuge and healing. (in Epp, 1998, p. 12)

The problems Vontress identifies may be related to therapists' and caseworkers' poor skills, high stress levels, alliance with some family members against others, or lack of awareness of how their behavior is not being respectful (or even knowing that respect is due). Each of these is a problem resulting from therapists' poor or insufficient training and socialization for a stressful and demanding position. When therapists and workers are disrespectful, they may simply be passing the indignities they've received down the proverbial food chain. Conversely, their objectification of consumers of mental health services may be a way of convincing themselves that they are different (and safe) and that they will never suffer the same kinds of depression, anxiety or paranoia as their clients.

Anna Michener's autobiography (1998) was often disdainful of the treatment offered within the mental health system, but she also described a variety of things that mental health professionals did that seemed either "respectful" or "disrespectful" (see table 8.7). While it was easy to make her feel disparaged by denying basic privileges, simple things could make her feel respected or special. Note, however, that these things were not generally basic and expected things like food, water, and a bed, but were things out of the ordinary, at least for that context, for example, her teacher offering to bend the rules somewhat to bring her hamster to the hospital classroom. For a child who was so deprived of what many of us see as "basic needs," having a teacher smile and listen to her felt "respectful" and was fondly remembered.

To engage clients, therapists generally need to treat them in a respectful manner. Ivey and his colleagues (1997) describe how respect, warmth, and positive regard are interrelated ideas. Respect involves recognizing

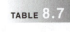

TABLE 8.7 **MENTAL HEALTH PROFESSIONALS' BEHAVIORS THAT MICHENER (1998) DESCRIBED AS EITHER NOTABLY RESPECTFUL OR DISRESPECTFUL**

Disrespectful	Respectful
Listening	
Not being listened to.	Just being listened to and taken seriously.
Being diagnosed or having decisions made for her without allowing her to contribute to the process.	Being allowed to have an independent opinion about her problems and treatment.
Not having history of abuse taken seriously or investigated.	Having history of abuse taken seriously.
Being criticized for behaviors that are normal for a teenager, such as talking to a boyfriend.	Smiling, looking at client kindly, and touching client softly.
	Having her opinions about problems and treatment listened to and respected.
Basic rights and privileges	
Being denied basic privacies and confidentiality.	Being given basic privacy and privileges.
Being made to wait for privileges or information without being told why.	Being given privileges in a kind or timely fashion.
Being given an age-inappropriate and poorly maintained waiting room.	Being given age-appropriate, well-maintained services.
Having inaccurate and poorly written reports written about client.	Having reports be accurate, insightful, and well-written.
Being forced to take medications against wishes, even though the medications made her ill.	
Being punished for doing something "right," such as comforting someone who was upset.	
Being given punishments that were "illegal," such as being put in solitary confinement for violating rules instead of keeping self or others safe.	
Extra privileges	
Not being given a blanket when room was cold.	Being carried when ill (when no one had done that before).
Being denied things essential to normal life such as hobbies, exercise, and fresh air.	Having arrangements made to have a favorite pet brought to the hospital classroom.
Being taught by people who did not care about teaching or about their students.	Being allowed to take makeup, stuffed animals, and comforter to hospital.
Being given outdated textbooks and being denied age-appropriate reading materials.	Being given noncontingent reinforcement.

strengths and communicating these to the listener in a warm, empowering manner. Note the difference that this makes in Shostak's (1981) interactions with Nisa, a !Kung tribal woman:

> Every day Nisa visited our camp, and every day she reminded me how much Nancy and Richard [the previous team of anthropologists] had done for her. She arrived in the morning, sat around, watched the confusion our presence always generated, and talked to the people who waited for medicine or tobacco . . . . After the first day, I started to dread these times. Her voice was loud, sharp, somewhat frantic, and [she was] constantly seeking attention, and it seemed never to stop. . . . Her voice persisted. I couldn't ignore it, with its barrage of thinly veiled criticisms. I felt I needed a place to go where I could close my ears and eyes, where I could stop hearing and stop responding. I had to do something.
>
> Finally I decided that since I had to listen to her anyway, I might as well get her to talk about something I wanted to hear. I had asked other women at Gausha about the drug properties of various roots and plants, but these interviews had not been very satisfying . . . . At last I approached [Nisa] "I have some questions I want to ask you. Would you like to work with me?" She broke from her conversation and smiled broadly. Catching my eye, she said "Aiye!" which means, literally, "Mother!"—but this time it also meant "Of course I will, I'd love to."
>
> It now seems a strange way to have begun a relationship that was to become so important to me, but it was only after I had approached her in this way that her attitude toward me changed. She had been trying to talk to me all along, but it was only on the subject of Nancy and Richard that she felt we had common ground. Now I had asked her to start something new. It was as though she had been waiting for me to see that she had something to offer. (pp. 29–30)

Of course, both Nisa's *and* Shostak's behavior changed at this point. When Shostak could see Nisa as someone with something to offer, she behaved differently. The change in Nisa's behavior supported and enlarged the changes in Shostak's behavior.

Although we want to acknowledge our clients' individual strengths, recognizing their culture-specific strengths and coping strategies is equally important (Stevenson & Renard, 1993). See table 8.8. This is especially important for QUOID clients—quiet, ugly, old, indigent, and dissimilar culturally. For example, many older adults are unable to bring youthful speed to problem solving, but their greater life experiences and expertise may allow them to hold and work with apparently contradictory emotions and experiences simultaneously. This is an important strength to recognize and acknowledge (Knight & McCallum, 1998; Steele, 1997). Similarly, accessing the strengths our clients bring to therapy, even when they are in crisis, often increases our credibility and may be particularly necessary with

---

Think about a problem that you currently feel stuck in. What options do you see? How likely is it that you will find a solution? How do you feel about that?

Now, try to brainstorm other solutions. If you feel too stuck to do this on your own, ask someone to help you. When brainstorming, remember that your goal is not to identify the "correct" solution, but to identify as many options as possible. Don't exclude the ridiculous or the absurd at this point, although you may do so when you choose one or more solutions on which to follow up. How likely do you feel it is that you will find a solution now? How do you feel physically and emotionally? Try putting one small piece of this plan into place. How do you feel now?

TABLE 8.8	THEREPEUTICALLY IMPORTANT CULTURAL STRENGTHS OF AFRICAN AMERICAN FAMILIES

Community and Cultural Patterns
- Community is both an important support system *and* the center of interactions.
- Spiritual orientation is important, and the church is often a hub of the community.
- Emotional expressiveness—especially novelty, liveliness, and spontaneity—are valued for its own sake rather than seen only as problems with impulse control.
- Understanding others' emotional expressions is seen both as an important part of the communication process and as a way of coping with outsiders.
- Oral traditions such as stories, preaching, interactive music, talking, and listening are important modes of communication.
- Negative social forces may knock one down, but resilience is believed to be an important part of African American nature.
- Having a healthy cultural paranoia is seen as normal and adaptive. African Americans' trust of Whites must be earned. Hiding one's true feelings may be an important coping mechanism in the face of racism and oppression.
- Hard work is valued and expected.

Family
- Extended kinship networks and nonblood social supports are viewed as essential. The family is not defined by nuclear boundaries.
- Children are taught to respect themselves and to be happy.
- Parents are expected to be active disciplinarians and guides to their children.
- Children born out of wedlock are generally accepted.
- Family roles are flexible and adaptable.
- Family cooperation is emphasized.

Note: From Paniagua, 1998; Stevenson & Renard, 1993.

people who are mistrustful about whether they can be or will be understood (Stevenson & Renard, 1993).

THE VALUE OF SEEING HOPE IN CLIENTS AND IN THEIR SITUATION

Hope is widely believed to be a necessary aspect of successful therapy (Asay & Lambert, 1999; Lambert, 1992; Frank, 1961; Meichenbaum, 2000a). Students and athletes with high levels of hope have the best outcomes in their courses and athletic events (Curry et al., 1997). While greater amounts of hope were associated with better outcomes in these settings, the relationship between hope and outcome may be curvilinear for addictions and habits. For example, Haaga and Stewart (1992) suggest that moderate levels of hope, as opposed to high or low, predict the best outcomes from a smoking cessation program. This is perhaps because hope is moderated by skepticism and, thus, risky behavior is avoided. Self-efficacy is an important predictor of change, but it should be realistic.

Hope alone, however, is not enough, but must be matched by knowing how to circumvent a problem and having an ability to actualize the plan. Because many clients enter therapy depressed, think dichotomously, and are unable to identify other solutions ("I must go on like this forever and ever unless I kill myself"), it is often a task of therapy to identify potential solutions. This responsibility, while initially the therapists' becomes the clients' as they feel stronger and have a greater sense of self-efficacy. Failing to help clients identify their own solutions fosters dependency in our clients, rather than an active and creative hopefulness. How can clients generate solutions even when stressed? How can they put these plans into practice?

Actively Demonstrating Hope

Although therapeutic change depends upon listening and empowering, the therapist is *not* a passive or nondirective change agent—far from it! In fact, therapy seems to be especially successful when the client perceives the therapist to be effective and to be expecting positive change (Kirsch & Lynn, 1999). This can happen in a number of ways:

- By being competent and knowledgeable about people, cultures and change.
- By informing them of the inevitability of change.
- By setting up situations in which change is very probable.

Shaundra, a client with a number of vague and serious somatic symptoms, had gone from physician to physician to find relief. After having everything from a brain tumor to thyroid problems ruled out, she was referred to me. With other things ruled out, it became pretty clear that she was severely depressed with a set of mixed anxiety symptoms. It was clear to me why she should be depressed—having had significant, severe, and chronic stressors in her life—but she couldn't see this context for the first three months that we worked together. To her, the stressors she had in life were normal. At discharge, however, she said that one of the most important things I had said to her was a flippant response (that I'd made and forgotten) at the end of our first session: "I've helped people much worse off than you."

Shaundra was a fighter, but she had never been offered hope before. I really listened to her and told her that things could be different, and because I was "an expert," she believed me even though others had been unable to help and even though she couldn't see the path that I was offering her. As with most of my clients, I gave her a very simple intervention at the beginning of therapy, one that I thought would be helpful and that would give her a measure of success. In this case, it was to practice simple breathing techniques to help her relax at various points throughout the day. This simple intervention was enough to prime her expectation that she could change successfully and that she was able to work consistently toward this goal.

This technique was the first in a number of steps to increase her self-efficacy (Bandura, 1997), a standard element in therapy's repertoire. Over the course of Shaundra's therapy, we discussed the significant strengths that she already possessed, the ways that she was already partially meeting her goals, and the ways to identify other steps that would move her farther along the path to change.

Concretely Demonstrating Hope

Furthermore, this type of therapy is often concrete and goal-oriented. While *understanding* the role of context is important, it is also vital for clients to *do* something different. Helpful ways of making this change involve helping clients identify their superordinate goals and specific and concrete steps toward the goal and helping them learn ways to handle the problems that will inevitably crop up (Gollwitzer, 1999; Marlatt, 1996). Gollwitzer reported that potential changers who identified specific plans regarding their desired behavior ("I'll spend 30 minutes exercising first thing after getting dressed in the morning") and what they were going to do when they hit a problem ("*If I go to a party where people are drinking, I will get a glass of tonic water with a twist so no one will ask if I want a drink*") were much more successful. Vague goals ("*I'm not going to drink*") are considerably less effective in helping clients meet their goals.

Being empowering and being directive or goal-oriented are not contradictory ideas. When I am working with a client, I try to be no more directive than is necessary at that point in time. Obviously, this can be different for highly motivated and self-directed clients than for clients who are in crisis and significantly ambivalent about change. There are various ways to approach this. With some clients, I will ask them what *they* think about an issue. With others, I will ask what homework they should have. Because my clients often give themselves much more difficult homework than I would, I may accept their homework or simplify it as needed, while also giving them homework with which they could easily expect to be successful:

> HARMONI: *We've had a very difficult but, I think, very productive session today. Have you thought about what your homework should be?* (Feedback, open question)
> ALEX: *I think Margrete and I should sit down and talk at least once this week. Maybe try to work things out on our own some.*
> MARGRETE: *I could do that.*

HARMONI: *That sounds like a good goal. Perhaps you could choose a single problem to talk about and use some of the listening skills that we discussed today . . . (Smiling) I'd also like to see you do something else hard. Are you ready for it? (Feedback, directive, directive, closed question)*

MARGRETE: *(Laughing) Oh no! What do you want us to do this time?*

HARMONI: *I want you to have at least one date this week. (Directive)*

ALEX: *That sounds good, we never go anywhere. But we don't have any money, and we can't get a sitter with kids like ours.*

HARMONI: *(Smiling) Can you make it to the grocery store? (Yes.) Well, I told you this was going to be hard. Can you make going to the grocery a romantic date? (. . .uh). It doesn't have to be the grocery store, but my point is that you can make anything a date—even if you're only buying potatoes. I'd like you to find some way to have a date next week, even if it has to be going to the grocery store. (Laughing) I want to hear about this! (Closed question, information, closed question, information, directive, self-disclosure)*

ALEX: *(Laughing) That does sound hard! I bet we could try!*

My goal, particularly after a difficult session like the one between Alex and Margrete, is to help clients be successful. The assignment used here was designed for this purpose. It also served other goals. It introduced a sense of humor into our work together, and it strengthened our therapeutic alliance. It also suggested that life was more than just the problems that weighed them down and that they needed to have fun together. A severely distressed couple that had a very difficult time getting out for dates took the elevator to my office alone—while sending their sons up the stairs! This working-class, Euro-American couple defined their life around work and parenting and took a Calvinistic approach to life, which seemed to say that life shouldn't be *fun.* Their dates, then, served as a touchstone as we talked about the more difficult parts of their lives.

Being hopeful is not the same as being naïve or overlooking problems and obstacles. Becoming aware of strengths, having a hopeful view of the future, accepting weaknesses, and planning for potential obstacles all have their place in therapy (Marlatt, 1996). Even critical feedback can be motivating when it is perceived as do-able and coupled with optimism about the client's potential for solving the "problem" (Steele, Spencer, & Lynch, 1993; Steele, 1997). Note this in the following example:

DREW: *You're right. You have a rough row to hoe. You've made some major mistakes with your children, but I believe you can get back on track and be a good father to your children if you keep these things in mind and take it one day at a time. You can't turn back the clock, but you can create your own future. (Feedback, self-disclosure, information)*

THE IMPORTANCE OF COMMUNICATING UNDERSTANDING TO CLIENTS

Understanding our clients is important, but it is fruitless when the understanding is not *communicated* to them. If Derika understands Charley, but he believes that she doesn't understand him and she does nothing to change his viewpoint, then her empathic understanding is in vain. With some people, nonverbal correlates of listening, including head nods, eye contact, facial expressions, and minimal encouragers, will be enough to communicate understanding. But with others, active listening such as paraphrases, reflections of feelings, and summarizations with frequent checkouts will be necessary to accomplish the same task. Notice that Derika needed to communicate her understanding explicitly ("It sounds like it's very important to you right now that I understand your concerns and that you also don't believe that I or anyone can").

CONCLUSIONS

We have thus far discussed a general model of engagement that is similar to models described elsewhere, but there are significant individual *and* cultural differences that influence it. We should know and be able to use culturally appropriate forms of listening, but also be aware of individual differences. What does a client want in a relationship? How does she know that she is being understood? What can *we* do to create a relationship whereby she feels readily understood? Table 8.9 summarizes many of the barriers to therapy from the client's point of view that have been discussed in the last two chapters, as well as ways in which therapists can challenge these barriers.

Lazarus (1993) refers to therapists who are able to change their presentation styles to match the needs of their clients as genuine chameleons. The word "chameleon" suggests the flexibility in presentation style necessary within a single workday: the shy child, the aggressive adolescent, the paranoid adult, and the overwhelmed and depressed elder. Each of these clients may require a different interpersonal style and skills, and we need to be alternately playful, direct and down to earth, open and honest, or serious but soothing. Although we need to shift how we present ourselves in

TABLE 8.9	COMMON BARRIERS TO THERAPY AND WAYS OF ADDRESSING THEM

Barriers	Guidelines for Resolving Problems
• Clients feel "broken" or hopeless.	• Identify individual and cultural strengths and partial solutions to problems from the very beginning. Offer realistic hope.
• Clients feel ashamed or guilty.	• Accept clients as they are. Challenge clients' beliefs that they are shameful. Normalize their experiences and reactions when appropriate.
	• Do not push clients to disclose more rapidly than they are comfortable about doing so, but at the same time give them opportunities to disclose.
• Clients do not feel understood or valued by therapists.	• Determine where clients feel misunderstood and clarify misunderstanding. Accept clients' belief system and worldview except when maladaptive. Choose interventions that are consistent with clients' worldviews.
• Clients expect that their therapists will hide feelings, will deceive, or will abandon them.	• Be open, honest, respectful, and genuine in all interactions. When clients believe that you are hiding, deceiving, or leaving (or may do these things), respond honestly and openly rather than defensively.
	• Report contacts with third parties in an open and honest fashion.
	• Relate issues to real familial or cultural factors that may cause these expectations.
• Clients see therapists as condescending or disrespectful.	• Address condescension and disrespectfulness honestly and cordially when they arise in the course of therapy.
• Clients take a "one down" stance relative to their therapists, and they expect advice.	• Engage clients in therapy in an active, egalitarian, and empowering fashion.
	• Accept this "one down" tendency while gently challenging clients to think for themselves.
• Clients have an individual or cultural history of being discriminated against or of not being respected.	• Be respectful. Address individual and cultural barriers to building a relationship honestly and respectfully in the first session and as needed in therapy. Acknowledge issues of privilege and discrimination in an honest fashion and when appropriate.
• Clients expect that their privacy will be violated.	• Receive explicit releases to get information from external sources. If telephone contacts cannot be made with client in the room, report the nature and content of contact at next session.
	• Identify other potential sources of losses of confidentiality such as a very public entrance or a coworker who is a friend or relative of the client. Resolve these in collaboration with the client when these issues are unique to the client.

(continued)

TABLE 8.9 *(continued)*	
Barriers	**Guidelines for Resolving Problems**
• Clients do not find what they are looking for in therapy.	• Assess clients' worldview and attitudes about therapy at first session and give something they see as valuable from the very beginning. This may be homework or a partial solution for many people, although Native Americans often prefer just feeling heard.
• Therapeutic interventions are different than clients' expectations about the therapeutic process.	• Explain interventions in a straightforward and respectful manner, especially when they violate client's expectations. Negotiate therapeutic goals and process.
• Clients perceive therapists as dismissing them when they give "less valuable" interventions.	• Clearly describe the rationale for interventions that may be perceived as less preferred such as group therapy, brief therapy, medications, or use of paraprofessionals.
• Clients' culture, folk traditions, and traditional healing patterns are ignored or treated disrespectfully.	• Consider whether more culturally acceptable interventions are appropriate and find ways to meld traditional healing strategies with psychotherapy. Consult traditional healers as appropriate.

Note: Based on Paniagua, 1998, Vontress et al., 1999.

the course of a single day, the word "genuine" suggests that the therapist must remain honest and authentic while doing so.

These processes will be easier for some people than others. Some therapists are more flexible and have a broader range of authentic presentations. Thus, they can work successfully with a wider range of people. Regardless of our clients' specific needs over the course of the day, we must be "active, engaging, open, direct, assertive, and energetic" to greater or lesser degrees (Belar & Deardorff, 1995, p. 33).

THE TELLING AND THE LISTENING: HEARING CONTEXT

I am a medical student currently doing a rotation in toxicology at the Poison Control center. Today, a woman called in because she caught her young daughter eating ants.

I quickly reassured her that ants are not harmful and that there would be no need to bring her daughter into the hospital. She calmed down, and at the end of the conversation happened to mention that she fed her daughter poison to kill the ants. I told her that she had better bring her daughter into the emergency room right away. (Source unknown)

Think about something that was or is difficult for you to disclose. What was or is difficult about telling? If you were finally able to disclose it, what was it about the situation or the person that made this possible?

THE TELLING

This story is purportedly true, but it reminds us that sometimes the "problem" isn't what it first seems to be and that often people fail to disclose their real concerns early on. We may believe that people should prioritize and identify those things that are of significant concern, but for many reasons, they often can't.

Being Able to See the "Problem"

Why don't people share their concerns? Sometimes people don't share relevant information because they have little insight into the factors impacting their behavior. Shaundra (see chapter 8, p. 191) asked me over and over again why should she be depressed. Over several months, she told me of the significant poverty she lived in, her son's diagnosis with a progressive and degenerative muscular disorder, the emotional and medical neglect that she incurred as a child, and the physical abuse she received. Why should she tell me these spontaneously? These were "normal." Bones that were never set when she was a child were not described as neglect. She did not refer to her father's whippings as abuse. She had learned to expect that no one—not her parents or anyone else—would be there for her or would attempt to meet her needs.

It was hard for me to understand how she could *not* be depressed given her life history. But, the fact is that we often perceive our own experiences as normal. As long as Shaundra overlooked class issues, her history of abuse and neglect, and her son's illness, she was not able to acknowledge problems and label them in a way that would be helpful in therapy.

An important therapeutic goal is to help our clients see the problem, to pathologize what they have mistakenly accepted as normal and, in the case of abuse, to transfer the realm of responsibility from our clients to the adults who have hurt them. I wanted Shaundra to begin to identify those things in her life that could be causing her depression. The poverty, anticipated loss of a child, history of abuse and neglect had to be thought about differently. Rather than saying, "I'm a bad person because bad things happen to me," I wanted her to learn to say, "These are unfortunate events, but I'm not bad because of them." Other important questions for her to consider were: How can I live more effectively in spite of them? How can I recognize the difference between those people who will hurt me and those who will support me?

How do culture and context come into play here? The therapist who cannot recognize the impact of Shaundra's history of abuse, or the various anniversary dates that Mervyn faced (see chapter 2), or the impact for Rashelle's being one of a few African Americans in her high school and community (see chapter 4), or the difficulties Manuela faced in considering divorce (see chapters 6 and 7), would likely fail to build a strong therapeutic relationship (cf. C. E. Thompson et al., 1994).

Stages of Change

Telling anyone about the most shameful parts of one's life takes trust. Most people have had to swallow their pride at some point in their lives to tell someone they know and trust about something they were ashamed of ("Mom, I'm failing English" or "Dad, I'm pregnant"). This process is even scarier when we can reasonably expect a negative reaction. Most people can only disclose shameful parts of themselves to people they know and trust and from whom they expect—at least with their head, if not their heart— a positive reaction.

Imagine a client's ambivalence about telling these scary parts of herself to a therapist, especially early in therapy. While the client may want to get better, taking the first step may seem insurmountable ("What if she doesn't hear and understand? What if she hears, but judges? What if she hears and understands, but can't help? What if she can help, but the pain of trying will be overwhelming?"). Imagine a starving dog eyeing a juicy steak on the other side of a huge electrified fence and wanting to get it, but being afraid of the anticipated shock. A client who is ambivalent about therapy and change is in this same kind of approach/avoidance conflict.

Prochaska's (Prochaska & DiClemente, 1982; Prochaska, 1999) work on stages of change is important to keep in mind at this juncture (see table 9.1). Not everyone is ready to change when entering the therapy office. People in Precontemplation do not even recognize that there is a problem. Arrested for a fourth DUI and sent to court-referred treatment people will say, "I don't have a problem." But, of course, they do. When her husband says they have problems in their marriage ("We have to fix them or I'm leaving"), the wife is baffled. These clients are rarely self-referred and are often frustrating to work with because, before the problem can be addressed, it must first be seen.

Few clients, however, enter therapy unaware of the problem (Precontemplation) or ready to attack it immediately (Action). Most are in Contemplation and deeply ambivalent about change. They may see a problem such as a bad marriage, tobacco addiction, or abusive parenting, but they are afraid of what will happen if they try to change things ("What if I leave my marriage and never find anyone else?). For some clients, simply telling the whole problem requires more trust than they have.

TABLE 9.1	STAGES OF CHANGE
Precontemplation	There is no intention to change in the foreseeable future. Many people are unaware or under-aware of their problems. Often, they feel forced into changing by a family member who is bothered by the problem.
Contemplation	Although they are aware that a problem exists and are seriously considering change, they haven't yet made a commitment to do so. They often are evaluating options and may be significantly ambivalent about changing.
Preparation	People in this stage intend to change and are taking small steps in preparation for continued change, such as delaying the next ciga-rette or decreasing the number of cigarettes they smoke each day. They intend to take action in the near future.
Action	People begin to modify their behaviors, beliefs, experiences, or situa-tions in order to overcome the problem.
Maintenance	People become aware of and then address the pitfalls that undermine continued change. They work to prevent relapse, and they consoli-date changes made in the action stage.

Note: From Prochaska & DiClemente, 1982; Prochaska, 1999.

Loss   Liev worked with me for several months before he was able to disclose that he'd had a severe history of physical, emotional, and sexual abuse. He was able to tell me that he'd been raped on multiple occasions by his beloved older brother; that he'd been beaten by his father; and that he'd watched helplessly as his mother had been attacked on numerous occasions. It took another year to tell me of his fears that he had multiple personalities. A month later, he shared his fears that his severe and dis-abling headaches were related to brain injuries from a car accident when he was a young child. Each time, he reacted as though I would think he was a terrible, awful person and that I would tell him I could no longer work with him.

Liev's problems can be conceptualized in many ways. Perhaps he was testing me to see whether I would stay with him regardless of what he told me. Perhaps he was inventing new and more spectacular stories to engage me with and keep my attention. Perhaps his disclosures were related to class differences—as a man raised in an upper middle-class family, he was expected to keep his mouth shut and not complain about his family's dirty laundry in public. Perhaps he had begun to see these new stories as rele-vant to the therapeutic process and trusted me enough to share them.

One of the most common statements I hear in therapy is "You're the only one I've ever told this to." As Rogers (1957) said, experiencing uncon-ditional acceptance is fundamental to the changes clients see in therapy. The experience that one is acceptable to another regardless of circumstances enables people to develop the trust to disclose in and out of therapy. And, of course, successful disclosures increase the experience of trust.

Fear What will we hear if we disclose this scary part of ourselves? Recently, Dan went to see his psychiatrist. His previous antidepressant had been unsuccessful, and he had made a very serious suicide attempt the night before. His psychiatrist, a warm and friendly man, was someone he had met only once before. The doctor, in a hurry, assumed that his bright and capable client would outline the problems clearly. He did not directly ask about suicidal ideation. Dan did not tell him about it, because he was afraid he'd be hospitalized (since the office was in the hospital and Dan had had a terrible experience in another psychiatric hospital). Clients' fears and ambivalence about disclosing problems are often grounded in a context and, thus, makes sense. It is not our clients' jobs to disclose information, but ours to make disclosure easier.

This experience, as Beckman and Frankel (1984) initially reported, is a common one. Many people bring several concerns to a doctor's office. However, they may fail to report their most important one until the doctor asks, "Is there anything else?" Frequently, the first complaint to a physician is used as an icebreaker. Later complaints are made once it feels safe to make them. Unfortunately, as Marvel, Epstein, Flowers, and Beckman (1999) later replicated, physicians allow patients fewer than 25 seconds to state their concerns before redirecting the discussion and beginning a series of closed questions to follow up on the initial complaint. Even when the ambivalence of many clients is remembered, identifying and following up on a problem may mean overlooking others that may be more important.

Should we as therapists assume that this complexity is irrelevant to therapy? People have the same concerns about their mental health as they do about their physical health, and they often have greater levels of fear and shame about these concerns. Especially with severely ambivalent clients, the therapist should assume that initial complaints need to be followed up on, *even if it takes 25 sessions!* Using open questions ("What else would you like to talk about today?" or "What other concerns have we not yet discussed?") can be a very helpful approach to eliciting greater disclosures (Ivey & Ivey, 2003).

Responses in Therapy

Clients *and* therapists contribute to these problems. When we give advice, judge, try to one-up, criticize, or plan ahead for our next response, it can interfere with our clients' willingness to disclose. When they are in an immediate crisis such as getting a diagnosis of diabetes, having someone close commit suicide, or being discriminated against, clients will want to hear a solution to their problems. But hearing someone jump immediately to conclusions to "solve all my problems" can make them feel helpless and even a bit resentful. When we try too hard to rescue them prematurely, they will tend to avoid disclosing problems, or they may repeat the "problem" over and over again until they feel heard and understood. A reflection of feeling ("It sounds like you're scared about being told that you have diabetes . . . ") and some encouragement to think about similar situations that they handled well can help people identify strategies and resources in other aspects of their lives that could be very helpful.

Even when clients know that they can't readily identify a way out on their own, it is helpful when others help them solve the problem rather than doing it for them. When I am working with someone with chronic physical pain, I generally have some ideas about the kinds of things that can increase and decrease the pain. For example, pain is generally worse in the evening, when people are stressed or when they have physically overextended themselves. Having someone chart correlates of the pain and pain levels may provide redundant information. But, just having a chart of their pain can be very useful for at least two reasons: First, a pain chart may throw in a few monkey wrenches, like when Nick, a 19-year-old man with spina bifida, enjoyed dancing at a local under-21 club. Although doctors had not believed he could ever learn to walk, he still wanted to dance and meet women his own age. Of course, the dancing also caused him severe pain the next day! Second, when people can identify the patterns for themselves, they are more invested in the change process and they feel empowered to discover and identify successful strategies for change themselves.

THE LISTENING

Finding a balance that *supports* without *doing for* can be difficult. Often, any intervention requires first understanding the client's frame of reference. What does the client see as happening? How bad does it feel? Where does it hurt most? Only when clients recognize that their therapist understands and accepts them will they allow interventions to begin that could change the crisis they face.

Listening to the Client First

The importance of listening is illustrated in the following sets of dialogue between Andor and Jalyse, a caseworker and client respectively. They are from different classes and different genders, and they have different parenting histories. Jalyse is a young, privileged Euro-American caseworker without children. She uses words like *yeah, and,* and *also,* as well as *no* and

TABLE 9.2   WORDS OR BEHAVIORS SIGNALING HIDDEN CONFLICT OR COLLABORATION

Conflict	Collaboration
Key words "But," "not," "no," "instead," "although," "however," "on the other hand," and "you don't understand."	**Key words** "And," "too," "also," "yeah," "MmHmm" Some cultural groups rarely use minimal encouragers (the Chinese, for example) and view them as "disrespectful" under some circumstances (e.g., African Americans).
Dichotomous language "Terrible," "awful," "never," "always," and "failure" especially when used to describe the therapeutic process.	**Gray language** "Sometimes," "occasionally," and "a problem."
Inconsistent language Words and ideas of the speaker and listener do not match or are inconsistent. For example, the speaker's "black" is followed by the listener's "white."	**Consistent language** Words and ideas of the speaker and listener match or are consistent.
Nonverbals Poor or glaring eye contact, a backward lean, closed posture, body tension, and a lack of synchronicity between speaker's and listener's movements.	**Nonverbals** Good eye contact, a forward lean, open body posture, and synchronicity between speaker's and listener's movements. Members of various cultures may not display each of these. For example, eye contact is seen as "disrespectful" by many Native Americans.
Paralanguage Increased hesitations, disruptions, staccato speech, and stutters. Periods of awkward silence may end only when the therapist intervenes to end it. These problems may also be due to shame, embarrassment, discomfort, and the like. Members of some cultural groups may become more quiet or passive and may otherwise follow cultural rules about hierarchical relationships. Others may become more verbally direct in their disagreement.	**Paralanguage** Paralanguage is relatively smooth. Few hesitations, disruptions, stutters, or awkward silences occur.
Follow-through Homework is completed inconsistently or forgotten. The subject within or across sessions is changed. Self-disclosures are minimal or shallow and, rather than increasing over time, they decrease in frequency.	**Follow-through** Therapeutic ideas are followed up, expanded within therapy with additional examples, and even extended outside of therapy.

Note: From Helms & Cook, 1999; C. E. Thompson & Jenal, 1994.

but (see table 9.2). Afterward, we'll consider how these words signal whether Andor feels listened to and whether Jalyse and Andor are working together (using the former words) or at odds with one another (using the latter words).

> ANDOR: *Last week I had one of the hardest days of my life. I thought I'd never get through it. First, school was canceled, and I had to find something to do with the kids. Then, the kids just began bouncing off the walls. I wanted to kill them!*
>
> JALYSE: *It sounds like you might have been doing some things here that made your day more frustrating than it had to be. You should ask*

your mother to babysit for you on snow days, but more importantly, I would be finding some ways to change your self-talk. (Feedback, advice. Jalyse assumes that Andor needs help solving this problem.)

ANDOR: *But it just seemed to keep going like there was no end in sight.*

JALYSE: *Do you notice how you're using catastrophizing and stabilizing language here? (Closed question)*

ANDOR: *I don't care what kind of language I'm using. I was trapped at home with kids who wanted to be outside running, and instead, they had to do it inside with me. I was afraid I was going to lose my job because I had to call off work three days in a row while school was canceled. I just felt overwhelmed.*

Notice that Jalyse's interventions make sense, but she used poor timing. Watch how this conversation changes once Andor feels listened to.

ANDOR: *Last week I had one of the hardest days of my life. I thought I'd never get through it. First, school was canceled, and I had to find something to do with the kids. Then, the kids just began bouncing off the walls. I wanted to kill them!*

JALYSE: *That sounds like an overwhelming and frustrating week! (Reflection of feeling)*

ANDOR: *Yeah, it was. I felt completely helpless in the face of everything going on around me.*

JALYSE: *How did you handle it? (Open question. Jalyse assumes that Andor did handle it and asks about the solution.)*

ANDOR: *Oh, this is embarrassing . . . First, I sat down and cried. Then, I called my mother and asked her to sit for me. Then, I realized I was making a mountain out of a molehill. I know that I've done a good job at work, and it's unlikely that I'm going to be fired just like that. I know that I can do something to handle this. I always have. And I guess I've listened to the stuff you've said about how the way I think about things makes things worse. I just decided I wasn't going to do this anymore!*

JALYSE: *Wow! I'm impressed that you were able to put our ideas into practice like that! Perhaps now would be a good time to review the specific kinds of thought errors you were making initially and think about what you did that worked, so that it will be easier next time your world comes crashing down around you. (Self-disclosure, directive)*

ANDOR: *And I also want to find ways to get to the point that I don't have to think that way in the first place.*

In the second dialogue, Jalyse listened to and respected Andor. Her simple reflection of feeling ("That sounds overwhelming and frustrating") enabled him to calm down and think more divergently. As Jalyse asked about his successes, Andor was able to review his actions and recognize that his approach was much more successful than he had initially believed and that he was on the right track. Furthermore, perhaps because of the context for this conversation, he was able to relate his own actions to the therapeutic interventions and goals. This style of intervention—using listening, empathizing, empowering; asking about natural solutions; and creating a natural reframe—characterizes the contextual approach and often prevents apparent barriers from being real ones.

Just Listening

Although Rogers (1957) identified empathic listening as a necessary and sufficient part of the therapeutic process, unfortunately, many clients do not feel heard by their therapists. This may be due to the clients' own problems in feeling heard, but as F. Shaw (1998) described, it may also be because we have become complacent and unwilling to challenge our therapeutic preconceptions:

> [My psychiatrist] always seemed to me less interested in finding out what I thought or felt than in having confirmed some assessment she had already made. And in that environment, organized around her own style of communications, all her statements were self-confirming. (p. 74)

Just witnessing a person's story respectfully can be helpful. A 53-year-old survivor of a Croatian concentration camp describes his experience like this:

> You were nobody, nothing, because they can step on you, kill you, humiliate you at any moment of the day or night. . . . When you have no self-confidence, you feel hopeless and helpless. You can do nothing, you cannot contribute to anyone, not even to yourself. (Weine, Kulenovic, Pavkovic, & Gibbons, 1998, p. 1723)

However, being able to describe his camp experience and having it listened to made a difference.

> When I speak to someone who listens to me, and who respects me, and when I can tell my story to such a person, then I feel good. I don't feel like a zero, and I have felt that way in concentration camp, or even coming to this country. (Weine, Kulenovic, et al., 1998, p. 1723)

Emotional healing can happen outside the therapy room—this process can be a useful adjunct to or substitute for therapy. For example, most Bosnians view the notion of disclosing their stories for individual catharsis to be self-indulgent. Telling stories of their concentration experiences to make a public record *for familial and societal purposes,* however, has been appropriate and healing, and it dramatically decreased the incidence of post-traumatic stress disorder (Weine, Kulenovic et al., 1998). Really listening to clients in helpful ways may require us, as therapists, to access culturally acceptable forms of healing.

Listening for the Bigger Picture

It is certainly important to listen to what a person *says*, but it is also important to help them look beyond what they see and are currently aware of and perceive the context for the stories they disclose. Context may include temporal setting—our reaction to bickering children is different when on vacation and well-rested than when stressed and overwhelmed—as well as situational factors such as being in a church as opposed to an open park. People can be influenced by these factors without being aware of them.

Think about context in terms of the Gestalt idea of figure and ground. The ground—the context, including race, culture, time, situation, and the like—influences the figure, which is whatever people focus on or think is important. A child who fidgets during a dinner of hot dogs and fries at home will get a different reaction than the same child who squirms around at a fancy restaurant. Parents are likely to be more understanding of a two-year-old playing with her food at the dinner table than with a fourteen-year-old playing with her food.

Some contexts are easy to see and appreciate. Others are readily overlooked. Josef Alber's painting *Homage to the Square* makes this point well. His simple painting has two squares, one on a red background and another on a blue one. The painting's apparent simplicity is misleading, however. Most people conclude that the two "identical" internal squares are different shades of purple, but this is not quite the case.

Alber's painting is unimpressive to anyone unaware of the contrast effect being taken advantage of in the painting, which causes each purple to look different. Similarly, it is easy to overlook the role of context on our own behavior or in the behavior of our friends and clients. Once we are aware of the role of context, either on the painting or in our lives, we may attempt to screen it out. We can look at Alber's painting, trying to screen off the surrounding colors to see it for what it really is. This is possible to some extent, but in doing so we change our perception by providing yet a different context. We cannot see the square without a context.

Being Unaware of Context

Sometimes, we can be aware of the context for our observations and compensate for it, but at other times, we can be unaware of it and ignore its effects. In these cases, a better metaphor is of a painting displayed under unusual light. When we are unaware of the light and its influence, we misinterpret the stimulus.

Can you have a circle without its surround? Try cutting a circle out of a sheet of paper. What do you see? Try covering up the edge of the circle. What do you see?

What is the context for a behavior or problem? How do time of year, your age, culture, family, ethnicity, strengths, and weaknesses influence your perception of this issue or problem? Can these be removed?

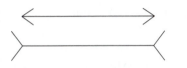

FIGURE **9.1**

The Müller-Lyer illusion. the arrows' middle lines are the same length.

In Duncan's classic study (1976), people either observed a Euro-American or an African American bump another person. The Euro-American's behavior was attributed to being accidental more often than the African American's behavior, which was more often seen as intentional. Similarly, S. Hoyt (1998/1999) showed people "job tapes" of an "upper-class" or "lower-class" applicant. The upper-class applicant was consistently judged more favorably than the lower-class applicant, despite both giving identical responses in their interviews—and being the same woman.

What happens when we try to observe behavior without paying attention to context? What happens when someone believes that she *can* be fair and *can* compensate for context? Illusions like the one seen in Alber's painting are very powerful and difficult to compensate for, even when people know they exist. Although we may know about the Müller-Lyer illusion (see figure 9.1), it is difficult to compensate completely. Duncan (1976) and S. Hoyt (1998) suggest that the same may be true for behavioral illusions.

Alternative Explanations

One problem we therapists face in listening to clients is the ease of accepting the simple, straightforward explanation and failing to look for alternative explanations. However, truly empathic listening requires thinking divergently, approaching the person and the problem in different ways than has been done in the past, and looking to see which is the best and least-pathogenic explanation.

This willingness to shift conceptual frames and think critically is seen in the following story. Jakob came to therapy very depressed and had a difficult time understanding why. He was a deacon in his conservative Christian church. He had a good, well-paying job and had recently expanded his business. He described his wife and children as attractive, kind, generous, and successful. They were widely regarded as "the perfect family." However, when he would describe his family as "perfect," his face would pucker, as though this notion was distasteful.

When asked about this, Jakob admitted that there were some problems, but that he knew he had it much better than most ("I shouldn't feel this way"). Although his marriage had been violent in the past, it no longer was. His wife was faithful and had kept a good home. Nonetheless, he described her as "very critical" toward him, and his children thought he was the "good parent" and wondered why he stayed with her.

How does becoming aware of context aid our understanding of this situation? Several issues are important. First, Jakob lived on the cusp of two worlds—the spiritual and the worldly. On one hand, his worldview emphasized many traditional biblical views of family, especially one where women were to be submissive to their husbands. His family failed to conform to this picture. On the other hand, his friends from work thought he should divorce his wife. His religious beliefs prohibited divorce except for grounds of infidelity, ongoing violence, or spiritual schisms within the family. (Notice that the traditional and normative frames are generally identified with "shoulds," which can be challenged or enlarged in therapy.) Second, his family did not match his religious ideals—he believed that they should read, study, and live the Bible on a daily basis—yet the family was widely seen as "perfect." This made him feel like a hypocrite at church. Thus, he began avoiding the very things that kept him happy and healthy in his daily life (prayer, reading the Bible, and going to church). Third, his family of origin was calm and cooperative. While he wanted to say that his wishes were "unreasonable," he found this difficult because his childhood had been, by his own description, ideal.

Helping Jakob to become aware of his expectations and to reframe his experience did not immediately remove his depression, but helping him become aware of the cultural context for, and the reasonableness of his concerns, was productive. Helping him see his experience in a way that neither his worldly friends nor his spiritual family and church could allowed him to feel listened to, understood, and safe in a way that he had not felt lately.

Choosing Stories

The process of reframing may be an art, but it's also grounded in basic scientific skepticism (see table 9.3). Therapist and client can be collaborating scientists, with each challenging the other about the validity of assumptions determining the problem. Together, they need to ask, "What is the source

---

TABLE 9.3   **SKEPTICAL AND OPEN-MINDED "SCIENTIFIC" STYLE OF THINKING THAT IS CONSISTENT WITH A CONTEXTUAL VIEWPOINT**

- What kind of evidence is offered to support the claim?
- Can hidden motives and assumptions explain the claim?
- Can other explanations of the phenomenon be observed?
- Do mitigating factors exist?
- Is the person who is making a negative claim feeling threatened?
- Is the person making the claim really an expert?
- Is the claim extreme and thus unreasonable?
- Is the reasoning fallacious?

of this viewpoint?" What assumptions underlie Jakob's thinking that may blind him to other ways of seeing the problem and the world? Jakob believed that he "should" be able to work in a worldly setting and achieve worldly successes without sacrificing spiritual goals. He attempted to meld two cultural worldviews that did not readily accommodate one another. To what extent is such an attempt reasonable and possible? And, if possible, how can he do so?

Throughout our lives, without being aware of it, we absorb stereotypes about both our own cultural group and others ("African American men are irresponsible parents and can't hold a good job!" or "Women are emotional and nurturing," or "Homosexuality is an abomination against nature"). Both client and therapist need to ask, "What evidence, if any, is offered for this position?" We must work with our clients to examine these messages and then challenge them when they are harmful.

Painter (1999) argued that being a White or a light-skinned Black has been seen as beautiful throughout the history of the United States. For evidence of this, she argued, just look at the skin color and hair texture of African American television actresses and popular musicians, especially when compared to their male counterparts. This value, White is good, also seemed to influence modifications of Sacagawea's portrait on the new dollar coin, which progressively became younger-looking across drafts and gained more "White" features (Reiter, 1999). The definition of beautiful, however, has fluctuated to match the group's status, whenever groups have come into or have gone out of favor. For example, when Irish immigrants were poor and oppressed they were seen as "ugly" (Painter, 1999). But as their fortunes improved, Irish American women became increasingly "beautiful." Painter's work challenges us to ask, "What hidden motives and assumptions influence our conclusions? How do these conclusions protect groups in power?"

We have already talked about assumptions that keep people from being objective about groups, but we must also challenge our assumptions about individuals. Vicki was scapegoated by members of her family, especially by those who assumed that she always followed the way of least resistance to find the easiest way out of things. As a result, even when she was successful in business, her family often found ways to dismiss her. Because her own successes were very different than those of her six older brothers and sisters, they had a difficult time seeing her work as valuable. Vicki internalized their view of what she was and minimized her successes. In effect, her family's view became a self-fulfilling prophecy. Therapeutic change required that she challenge the family's assumptions and develop her own picture of who she was and what she wanted to be. Therapy helped her find a picture that would work for her.

When we draw inferences about a person or group's behavior, we also need to be aware of factors that argue against otherwise pejorative conclusions. In chapter 1, we discussed how people often judge strangers and members of out-groups more negatively than themselves. In therapy, we must challenge this tendency and probe other explanations for the behavior of individuals or groups. Are some of these explanations less blaming?

For example, anonymous sex in bathhouses, especially in this age of AIDS, is maladaptive and even deadly, but are there some explanations for this behavior that make sense? One hypothesis, of course, is that when a group is marginalized by society and its members face a deadly plague, they may self-medicate with sex to affirm who they are by engaging in the very behavior that defines them to outsiders. Counterintuitively, sex can help them deny or avoid thinking about the disease. These coping strategies are maladaptive, but understandable in the context. This reframe may make a gay man's behavior more understandable to him and his therapist and may enable them to identify treatment goals that would be both acceptable and positively affirming.

Humans take pride in being rational beings and thus different than other animals, but they are rarely as rational and objective as they think they are. Human emotion often colors human thinking. As we review events with clients, it's important to consider whether a group or individual is being threatened. Discussions of "floods" of immigrants and why we should restrict immigration frequently have economic justifications behind them ("There won't be jobs for us!"). Feminists have suggested that sexual harassment is an attempt to maintain the status quo in the workplace. Painter (1999) pointed out that evaluations of beauty are related to the group's status. When the group is accepted and thus less of a threat, its members are rated more beautiful.

The feminist manifesto The Personal Is Political reminds us to challenge the status quo. In effect, as our clients tell us a story about discrimination or a firmly accepted reaction within their family, we need to challenge their conclusions that *they* are the problem rather than something they symbolize or fears they raise in the group or person in power. Our job is to question the reasoning leading to a conclusion. What is the evidence supporting it? Is the claim extreme, and thus, untenable? Is the person making the claim knowledgeable? For example, Vicki must challenge her family's assumptions about her worth and potential by questioning why some but not all parts of her life seem to inform their decisions. She must ask why her family has identified her as a "screwup," rather than also seeing her strengths. A man who is denigrated for his affectional orientation, but also for the anonymous sex of other gays, must question the common explanations for his behavior and wonder whether these are used to maintain the status quo. How else can he view himself and his behavior? Which will free and empower him? Which will enchain him?

CONCLUSIONS

All ideas should be examined and thoughtfully challenged in the therapeutic process. In this chapter, we have assumed that clients often cannot tell us why they feel the way they do. But, by listening sensitively and empathically, we can hear the shame, fear, and ambivalence that often serve as barriers to disclosure. Moreover, we must break the conceptual frames that blind the client *and* the therapist. A person's behavior may not make sense to us, but it will generally make sense to him or her. To understand this "senseless" behavior, we must become aware of context and think critically about it. This requires that we become aware of the context for the problem and of the client's (or group's) assumptions and challenge the reasoning that leads to a conclusion. Doing this will often lead us to less-pathologizing assumptions and more helpful interventions for clients. Looking for other explanations for behavior and exploring the relationship between these and the knowledge base we have will enable us to be more successful.

EGALITARIAN AND EMPOWERING RELATIONSHIPS

A small child was crying, frustrated because she couldn't tie her shoes. Her grandmother, choosing not to tie the girl's shoes herself, sat down to teach her granddaughter the steps. The girl's father asked impatiently, "Why don't you just do it?" to which the grandmother replied, "I can't afford to. I'm too busy."

When a client comes to us with a problem, as the grandmother in this story demonstrates, we have three options:

- We can leave the client floundering.
- We can solve the problem for the client.
- We can teach the client how to solve it for himself or herself or help them get to the solution on their own.

Often, it can feel more efficient to be directive and just give the advice that will solve the "problem." Chapter 9 touched on some of the problems caused by "just giving" advice. In chapter 10, we'll enlarge this theme and discuss some of the problems caused by "doing for." At the same time, we'll examine some of the advantages of "doing with."

WHAT EMPOWERMENT *Is*

Support can take any of three forms: emotional, informational, or instrumental (Helgeson & Cohen, 1996). Emotional support includes both verbal and nonverbal indications of concern and understanding. Informational support educates, guides, or advises. Instrumental support includes provision of services, goods, or money that help to meet a person's needs. Each of these three kinds of support is often necessary, but our goal as therapists is to choose support that empowers rather than to create dependency, which can undermine self-efficacy. In their review of the cancer literature, Helgeson and Cohen reported that emotional support was preferred by people with cancer and was positively correlated with adjustment, while instrumental support was least helpful. This seems to be especially true when the support is from loved ones rather than from strangers.

Empowering interventions leave people feeling stronger and more powerful, and with greater self-efficacy. Rather than expecting others to identify and resolve their problems, they will feel capable of looking inside and deciding what they want, when they want to ask for help, and when they do not need it. Eva Oliver clearly describes the kind of helping that empowers:

> I think the answer is it's better to help a person some and let him help himself some. And then, as he helps himself, then give him less until it balances out. In other words it's like raising a child. Once you have it, you have to keep nurturing it until it grows to stand on its two feet. So, just saying, "In two years we're going to cut them off"—no. Because you created this system and kept them babies all this time. And now, all of a sudden, you're going to cut the cord? Uh-uh. That won't work. (Roberts, 1998, p. 82)

Empowering interventions should give no more help than is needed. They should generally start from "more helping," especially when the person is distressed or in crisis, and move to "less helping" as the person becomes stronger and more capable.

Some interventions are clearly empowering. When describing what made her job training program successful, Eva Oliver (Roberts, 1998) clearly articulates empowering interventions:

> They gave us a lot of love. They made you believe in yourself. It was a hug, a pat on the hand. It was a time of healing. It was a time of learning. They taught you how to dress for an interview, how to talk, what to say, what not to say. And they gave you that extra pat on the back: "Girl, you can do it. This is the greatest class that ever came through here." And then they sent you out the door . . . "I'm going to conquer the world." If the first job didn't come through, they'd send you to another, giving the sense all the time that they cared, that they believed. (Roberts, p. 83)

These same ideas apply equally well to therapy. We can listen deeply to our clients, be open about our thoughts and plans, ask clients what they want as goals, discuss treatment options, and ask what they want as homework between sessions. We can believe that our clients can *and will* make it. This sense of hopefulness seems to be one of the most essential aspects of empowerment. Consider the following scenarios:

> COURTLAND: *I've had a terrible week. My neighbor turned me in for using again and . . . they took my kids!*
>
> AMADO: *What do you want to do?* (Open question)
>
> COURTLAND: *I don't know. It's all so overwhelming. What do you think I should do?*
>
> AMADO: *How about if I call Child Protective Services to find out what you need to do?* (Makes phone call.) *They want you to get off drugs, finish your diploma, and move to a larger apartment where each of your kids can have their own room . . . What do you want to do?* (Sharing information, open question)
>
> COURTLAND: *I just don't know. What do you think I should do?*
>
> AMADO: *I think you should start at the easiest place, by getting a job. What you can do is go down the hall and . . .* (Courtland's eyes glaze over) *Courtland, I feel like I'm doing this all by myself. Don't you want this?* (Advice, directive, self-disclosure, closed question)

Amado attempts to have Courtland resolve these issues for herself by consistently turning to her with open questions at each fork in the road. However, every time Courtland indicates that she is helpless, Amado responds by *saving* her. Each rescue attempt seems to leave Courtland more passive and helpless than the last. Contrast the hopelessness of that scenario with this one.

> COURTLAND: *I've had a terrible week. My neighbor turned me in for using again and . . . they took my kids!*
>
> AMADO: *That's terrible! What do you want to do?* (Reflection of feeling and open question)

COURTLAND: *I don't know. It's all so overwhelming. What do you think I should do?*

AMADO: *This is a difficult situation, and it sounds like you're having a hard time making a decision here. What are your thoughts? Where would you like to begin? (Feedback, open questions. Asks for her opinion a second time without beginning to solve the problem.)*

COURTLAND: *Well, I want my kids back, and I'll do whatever it takes. But I don't know what they want me to do and . . . and I don't feel like they'll listen to me when I call. Could you call for me?*

AMADO: *That has to be frustrating for you. I could call, but it might be more to your advantage to call and find a way to get them to listen. Perhaps you could call, and I could coach you if you get stuck. What problems do you usually have? (Reflection of feeling. Logical consequences. Directive. Open question.)*

COURTLAND: *Yeah, that makes sense. Sometimes I find myself yelling or even shutting down when they tell me what to do. It's like they treat me like I'm stupid or something. I want to do it better.*

AMADO: *I can let you know if I hear you doing those things. (Self-disclosure)*

Both conversations start out the same way, but they diverge in the second scenario when Amado asks Courtland (for the second of three times) what she wants to do in this situation to resolve the problem. Because of his continued questioning ("What do you want to do?"), they agree on a second goal beyond the superficial one (get her children back). They also agree that it would be helpful to find ways to get Courtland's caseworkers to listen to her. In the latter exchange, Amado initially identifies this goal, but Courtland accepts it and expands on it. In doing so, Courtland, who had been passive and helpless previously, becomes Amado's active and collaborative partner in treatment.

Furthermore, although Courtland assumes that she *will* get stuck ("I don't feel like they'll listen to me when I call."), Amado assumes she can call and introduces optimism about the outcome of the call ("I could coach you *if* you get stuck."). In this case, Amado introduces uncertainty about negative outcomes by taking Courtland's view of the situation and shifting it in a more optimistic direction by using the word "if" as opposed to "when." If Courtland had assumed an optimistic situation was uncertain ("*If* I get my children back . . .), Amado could have shifted her view in a more hopeful direction ("*When* you get your children back . . . "). See table 10.1.

Clearly, Amado's second set of interventions is empowering, but the *possibility* for empowerment comes through Amado's empathizing with Courtland's frustration and her feelings of being overwhelmed. Without this empathy, Courtland probably would have felt that Amado was moving

TABLE **10.1**	**WORDS THAT NURTURE HOPE**
Introducing certainty, especially about positive outcomes:	
When	"When you get into school you'll need to spend a lot of time thinking about your future, and I expect that you'll begin to re-think yourself on all fronts."
Is/are/will be	"It will be much easier once you begin recognizing self-defeating thought habits."
Yet	"You haven't turned the corner yet, but I'm confident that we'll see changes soon."
Introducing uncertainty, especially about negative outcomes:	
If	"If you flunk out of school, we'll have to think about where you want to go next.
Seems/looks like/ feels like	"It feels like it would be overwhelming if you lost your job, but you have always coped well before, and I am confident you can do it again."
May/might	"It may look like there's no way out, but I'm confident that you will be able to find a way of resolving this soon."
Possible	"It's possible that you'll have another panic attack when we go to the mall, but we've learned ways to cope with anxiety before it becomes overwhelming, so I expect this time will be different."
But (to accept the client's view, then shift it):	"It sounds like a very overwhelming week, but you've learned something about when you're in pain and how to change it."

Note: Based on ideas from O'Hanlon & Weiner-Davis, 1989.

Reread the second dialogue, omitting the reflections of feeling—the first statements in the first three of Amado's four leads. How do you react to these changes? Do they make a difference? If so, why?

her too quickly. Table 10.1 shows this as well: the therapist empathizes with the client's feelings ("It feels like it would be overwhelming if you lost your job . . . "), but introduces some uncertainty by saying that it would "feel" overwhelming rather than agreeing that it would "be" overwhelming. Furthermore, the second exchange ends on a more hopeful and realistic note with the comment about the client's good coping skills and how they would be helpful in the situation.

Empathic listening is foundational to our ability to help our clients shift their points of view. Most people need to feel safe before they can take the steps toward change. Being listened to empathically gives them the safety to accept the reframe and the ability to hear the confrontation, follow the directive, take the risks, and express opinions.

Voices: Lost and Found

One of the most apparent changes that occurs when we act in an empowering fashion is that clients begin to regain their "voices." As a result of Amado's patient questioning and his assumption that Courtland had useful

TABLE 10.2 WAYS IN WHICH PEOPLE INDICATE THAT THEY RECOGNIZE AND ACKNOWLEDGE THEIR "VOICE"

Without a "Voice"
- Have difficulty expressing an opinion.
- Frequently say "I don't know," even when they have an opinion. They may express an opinion if given more time and opportunity.
- Will accept others' opinions even when decisions go against their own interests or values.
- May switch decisions easily, based upon what they believe will please others.
- Frequently believe that they cannot disagree with someone *and* maintain that relationship.

With a "Pseudovoice"
- Will express a strong opinion about issues even without having a strong opinion.
- Opinions often seem uninformed or have little data to support them.
- Have difficulty listening to or accepting others' opinions unless they agree with their own.
- May switch decisions suddenly based on external factors, including the popularity of a stand or others' opinions.
- Often believe that they must look out for their own needs first.

With a "Voice"
- Will express strong opinions when they have strongly formed beliefs, but may reply "I don't care" when they don't.
- Opinions generally seem informed. If they say they like or don't like Chinese food, it's reasonable to assume that they have tried Chinese food in the past.
- Even when they have an opinion, they will listen to others' arguments.
- They may change their decisions, but only after considering any new information received.
- Believe that they can disagree with someone *and* maintain the relationship.

opinions, his client's stance changed significantly. She went from "What do you think I should do?" to "Could you call for me?" to identifying a specific problem and finally to understanding where she needed help. In the process, she became an active partner with Amado. Her sense of what she wanted to do and where she wanted to go was now clear.

Table 10.2 shows a number of clues about how people recognize their voice and how they feel when giving it away. In general, people who have a voice in their own lives tend to move freely in their actions, rather than allow themselves to be buffeted by fate or by the decisions of others. They are able to recognize their own goals, values, and wishes, give voice to them, and act on them when it seems to make sense. However, they can also listen to others and consider the merits of their arguments. When Courtland allows Amado to make decisions for her or when she makes decisions blindly based upon what Amado or her caseworkers want, she has given up her voice. This is true even when her decision is diametrically opposed to that of Amado or her caseworkers.

If Courtland decides that she is a good mother *only* because her caseworker believes she's *not* and even if she screams her conclusions from the tallest buildings, she remains without a voice. Her ability to act powerfully, freely, and responsibly depends upon how she considers others' opinions before acting either to validate or to reject them. Having a voice does not mean taking a dependent or a rigidly autonomous stance, but rather an interdependent one that assertively listens to the opinions of others yet develops them for oneself.

Cultural Values That Influence Decisions to Empower

Although healthy and autonomous stances generally make sense in Euro-American society, the approach is not accepted across cultures. Asian cultures, for example, value the opinions of elders more than Euro-American society does. Making a decision in such a "free" fashion can seem disrespectful to Asians and can violate their value system. However, within the two cultures, valuing an elder's opinion and choosing to accept or reject it will often remain a possibility. These cultures do not value all elders' opinions equally, but both value those whom they perceive as "wise."

> On one particular evening, the teacher invited one of his brightest students to walk with him. This boy was troubled by the contradictions in Buddhist doctrine.
>
> "You must understand," said the teacher, "that words are only guideposts. Never let the words or symbols get in the way of truth. Watch."
>
> With that the teacher called his dog. "Fetch me the moon," he said and pointed to it.
>
> "Where is my dog looking?" asked the teacher of the student.
>
> "He's looking at your finger."
>
> "Exactly. Don't be like my dog. Don't confuse the pointing finger with the thing being pointed at. Words are only guideposts. Every man finds his way through other words to find his own truth." (modified from McLean, 1998)

Traditional Asian cultures may be thought of as protecting against "pseudo-voices." To them, these are strongly expressed but poorly considered opinions. Children and young adults are expected to consider and use the values of their elders as guides to the development of values and to the decision-making process. As Asian children mature, these guideposts may be refined or rejected.

However, autonomy and self-respect are important values in Euro-American cultures. Interventions that foster these values also foster self-esteem and vice versa. This is a central theme of Schlink's (1995/1998) book *The Reader*, a story in which the narrator struggles over whether to share information that, on one hand, could reduce the culpability of a woman prison guard on trial for her crimes following World War II, but on the other hand, would be costly to her self-esteem. The narrator's father argues that sharing the information would be disempowering:

"... [W]ith adults I see absolutely no justification for setting other people's views of what is good for them above their own ideas of what is good for themselves."

"Not even if they are happy about it later?"

He shook his head. "We're not talking about happiness, we're talking about dignity and freedom. Even as a little boy, you knew the difference. It was no comfort to you that your mother was always right." (pp. 141–142)

As the narrator's father observes, that which people believe will make others happy, and even what they believe will make themselves happy, often does not. In effect, the narrator and his father conclude that allowing another to knowingly make a decision for herself is better for her in the long run. This is not an easy process for Schlink's narrator or for therapists. The narrator, at least partially, struggles with his decision and wonders whether he took the easy way out or helped foster the woman's autonomy.

Schlink's (1995/1998) book raises an important distinction. Empowerment is not the same as a laissez-faire strategy. When many of our clients enter therapy stressed and overwhelmed, they may not have the resources to make good decisions for themselves. We need to help them explore their options, but true empowerment neither tells a person what to do nor allows them to do it on their own, but encourages a thoughtful decision with all options available. Some empowering interventions are described in table 10.3.

Finding a Voice

In *The Wizard of Oz,* the Scarecrow, Tin Man, Cowardly Lion, and Dorothy search for brains, a heart, courage, and the ability to go home, respectively. After they "melted" the Wicked Witch of the West, the Wizard gives them symbols of the gifts they had possessed already, but hadn't recognized. They had brought back the Wicked Witch's broom and hat successfully, a task that had seemed impossible to them before, and they were finally able to recognize that they already had the very skills they were seeking. The dilemma faced by Dorothy and her friends is similar to the difficult tasks Milton Erickson gave his clients—ones that taught them that they *could* meet their goals (J. Haley, 1993).

As discussed earlier, we as therapists have three primary options when a client is in crisis: (1) ignore their plight, (2) solve the problem for them, or (2) teach them how to solve it. Therapeutic interventions can empower clients to discover or develop what they already have but don't yet recognize. Most clients would not believe a therapist who glibly tells them that they already possess the skills they need. Solving the problem or telling them to do so without helping them to identify the necessary skills would be frustrating and even disempowering.

TABLE 10.3 WAYS IN WHICH THERAPISTS CAN EMPOWER THEIR CLIENTS

Therapeutic Relationship
- Set up egalitarian relationships. Treat your clients as collaborators. Brainstorm together.
- Let your clients see you as a real person, as someone who sometimes makes mistakes. Exposing weaknesses to someone who's "perfect" can be difficult.

Seeing the Person
- Recognize clients' strengths and validate them.
- Recognize the influence of context on their behavior and help them to see it rather than blame them inappropriately for problems.
- Listen to and learn from their views on the world.
- Problematic behavior may make sense to them and may be attempts to solve a problem.
- Challenge stereotypes and view your clients as people rather than as labels.
- Recognize when clients are members of oppressed groups. Be open to talking about prejudice, oppression, and privilege.

Problem Definition and Goal Setting
- Listen to your clients' perceptions of problems and treatment goals.
- Help them to recognize behavior patterns rather than only identifying patterns for them.
- Ask about the periods of time when the problem is absent.
- Ask about points of light in their life rather than assume that there are problems everywhere.
- Listen to their "solutions." Even when they offer an incomplete solution, the germ of a complete one may be present.

Treatment Process
- Ask whether they want or need therapy services. Choose the least restrictive, most appropriate service available.
- Discuss your rationale for decisions. Obtain informed consent on all interventions.
- Rather than solving their problems, teach them how to do so themselves.
- Consider the impact of your interventions on other aspects of their system. Do the interventions strengthen or diminish other aspects of the system and the client's support? Should a member of their natural system offer this service?

Many clients deny having the skills to solve their problems successfully. Oftentimes, they think dichotomously when they are depressed, stressed, or anxious ("I can *never* make her listen to me. We fight *all* the time!"). Being empowering means challenging the artificial and unrealistic black-and-white notions and discovering the grays ("Tell me about the good times. *When* are you a good parent? What's different?"). Although the good times may not happen as often or be as successful as clients would like, their successes can be acknowledged and enlarged in therapy.

These ideas are consistent with Berg's (1994) and de Shazer's (1988) work. Both Berg and de Shazer assume that the kernel of a solution exists in the client's current successes and that these successes should be nurtured and developed. Therefore, they would ask a family, "When *isn't* it a problem? What are you doing when you do get along?" They assume that no problem exists 100% of the time or to the same degree. Their questions are both hopeful and empowering.

In the dialogues between Andor and Jalyse in chapter 9, Jalyse is superficially helpful by telling Andor how to solve his dilemma (see first dialogue, p. 203). In the second dialogue, however, Jalyse assumes that he is already solving his problems successfully (or she would have read about the deaths of his children in their newspaper!). Because she makes this assumption, Jalyse asks about his successes. Although Andor left the first dialogue still frustrated and overwhelmed, he recognizes his successes in the second and is able to identify places he wants to continue to explore in the future. A strong and empowering assessment of a problem will include an examination of current successes as well as the failures.

Hearing Their Voices

Clients may deny having opinions, values, and goals. Being empowering means believing that our quiet, passive clients have opinions that have been silenced. This silence robs them of both voice and power. As the last exercise can reveal, believing that clients have been silenced is not a naïve or baseless belief, but rather one that can be demonstrated in many people.

Even people who deny having an opinion ("I don't know") will have one when given sufficient time. This is an important point. The voice that they are denying is often one that they see as dangerous to themselves or to others (Gilligan, 1991; Lorde, 1984b). However, their assessment may be habitual and grossly inaccurate ("I must be quiet. Whatever I say will be hurtful, or alienating, or dangerous"). If clients truly don't have opinions, therapy should help them recognize and make decisions. However, if they have opinions but because of uncertainty, lack of practice in recognizing their opinions, believing their opinions are unimportant or hurtful (or any number of other reasons) are unable to express them, the therapeutic goal has to become helping our clients recognize and express their views.

> TAMMI: *What would you like to get out of therapy? (Open question)*
> JOCELIND: *(Voice rising and becoming more shrill) I don't know what I want anymore. I just don't know!*
> TAMMI: *Take your time. We don't have to identify all of our goals right now. Perhaps you could start by describing some of the times when you run into problems and the times when things seem okay . . . (Directive, sharing information, directive)*

WHAT EMPOWERMENT *ISN'T*

It is certainly empowering to have someone listen deeply to you, believe in you, see hope that you can find a path through your troubles, and work with you toward a solution, but it is often difficult to identify whether or not other kinds of interventions are also empowering. Consider the following examples drawn from an in-home family therapy agency:

Throughout the next week, pay attention when people (or you) say, "I don't know." Give them a minute to explore or expand on their ideas. Ask them to make a guess or say, "What do you think?" What do you find when you give them a little more time? Is this different for some people or some situations?

- The therapeutic team went to the de la Cruz house for a regularly scheduled appointment. Mrs. de la Cruz met them at the door, informed them of her father's suicide, and said that now wasn't a good time to meet. What would be the most empowering response from the therapeutic team? Would it matter how the de la Cruz family had responded to grief in the past?
- Aphrodite was running into problems at school and was in serious danger of being kicked out. School administrators requested a meeting, but asked that her parents not be invited. What would be an empowering response to this request? Would your response depend upon the parents' relationship with the administrators? Would it make a difference if you were meeting to develop a game plan to ensure that future meetings went more smoothly?
- The Johansens entered an agency with a series of significant stressors. These included head lice, thousands of dollars in unpaid bills, the 7-year-old identified patient acting out in school, and an older sibling diagnosed with leukemia. If the team offered to take the 7-year-old to the park after school, would this be empowering? Would it be empowering if family members asked the team to do this? Would it make a difference if their request came early in therapy, when both parents were spending considerable time at the hospital with the sick sibling, rather than later in therapy when the family had been stabilized to some degree?

The answer to these difficult questions is "It depends." Interventions that include clients in the decision-making process are often more empowering than those that exclude them. Therapists are less empowering when they make decisions *for* the family, than when their relationship is relatively egalitarian and they make decisions *with* the family. These options are less empowering than when clients make decisions independently. The point at which this process gets muddied, however, is when clients make decisions reflexively without thinking about them. Often, the therapist's task in therapy is to slow the process down and assist thoughtful and divergent decision making. If we simply tell clients what to do, we are not being empowering. If we encourage clients to thoughtfully consider their options, our intervention becomes empowering.

If the de la Cruz family had been handling grief well in the past (and a therapeutic goal was not to learn to handle grief better), leaving the house when Mrs. de la Cruz indicated that it wasn't a good time to talk would be an appropriate response. However, if the family tended to avoid strong, negative emotions and that this generally caused the family greater problems, it might be more therapeutic (and empowering) to remind Mrs. de la Cruz of their decision to deal with painful emotions in a direct and honest way and to ask whether the family was approaching this crisis differently than in the past. If she were to say that they were talking about the suicide and doing a good job, a good response would be to respectfully bow out. If, however, she were to say that they were not handling it well but that the time to talk was still wrong, a good reply would be to ask about another time to meet. If she were to say they were handling it poorly, but that she was scared to talk, a good response would be to ask if now might be a good time to meet. The question should be motivated by real curiosity, rather than being rhetorical in nature.

For Aphrodite, having a meeting with the school alone might be considered, but only if a therapeutic goal was to develop a game plan to work together more effectively. However, work on a plan with the school should not happen without the family's input. Developing a plan *for* Aphrodite would shift the balance of power away from her family and would suggest that we (the therapists) did not believe that they (the family) could assist in developing a healthy and productive treatment plan. It's always a good idea for therapists to share the nature and content of any external communications with clients, even when there is material they will not like hearing and even if the information is routine.

Work with families can help them find ways to stabilize and to develop healthier interpersonal interactions and sounder relationships with others. Having a therapeutic aide take the Johansens' son to the park may be therapeutic and even empowering early in treatment while the family tries to identify ways to cope with overwhelming stressors, and hopefully find stability. However, later in therapy this same action becomes less productive, especially if the family has ways of meeting this need on its own. It is important to remember to ask, "What will you do when we end therapy? How will you get your children to the park then?" If they don't see any ways of doing this, perhaps their treatment goals should include finding ways to increase the breadth and strength of their support network.

Note that these and other interventions can be therapeutic *and* empowering. Therapists always have a range of options at their disposal. Some of these may be empowering, others therapeutic, but only some are both. Because we always have multiple options for solving the problems a client or family faces, we should always choose the most efficacious *and* empowering path (see table 10.4).

EMPOWERING THE INDIVIDUAL *AND* THE SYSTEM

Nicola saw Tamia, a shy 8-year-old, and offered her a small piece of candy. Tamia's face lit up, but Tamia's mother became quiet. Elena, who saw this exchange, took Nicola aside and asked her what she thought had happened.

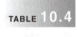

TABLE 10.4 EVALUATING INTERVENTIONS FOR THERAPEUTIC EFFICACY AND ABILITY TO EMPOWER

Problem

Josef (age 15) has been acting out in the home and at school for the past year. He has been truant, is failing three subjects, and is often gone for days. His father is frustrated and has asked for help with school issues.

Interventions

- The therapist suggests that she meet with the school to discuss school issues. *This is therapeutic, but not empowering.*
- The therapist suggests to the frustrated and overwhelmed father that he go to the school and talk to Josef's teachers about school issues. *This may be empowering if he is able to do this meeting successfully on his own, but it is of questionable therapeutic efficacy otherwise.*
- The therapist and the family discuss the situation and brainstorm alternatives. Together, they decide to request a joint meeting with appropriate members of the school. During the meeting, they work to make sure that the family's viewpoints are expressed well and that the school's suggestions are heard. *This is therapeutic and empowering to all members of the team.*
- The therapist and family discuss the problem and decide that, over the next week, the family will identify several ways to handle these problems and will choose from among the options. The family identifies a number of ways to approach this issue. Some are useful, some are not, but the family is able to identify a good strategy with the therapist. *This is therapeutic, and potentially even more empowering.*

Nicola was puzzled. She had been nice, and Tamia had appreciated the small gesture. But, as Elena pointed out, although Nicola's innocent act may have created a relationship with Tamia and even encouraged her to think of herself as someone who deserved to be treated well, it also served to undermine Mrs. Brown's parenting. She had stolen Mrs. Brown's ability to decide what and when her daughter should eat. Since it was late afternoon and Tamia was a finicky eater, a piece of candy was a bigger deal than it seemed at first glance.

Later that same week, Sanjay offered to go with Mrs. Brown to a multidisciplinary team meeting. He was not the primary therapist working with the Browns, but because he had worked with them previously, he believed that his action would empower Mrs. Brown and give her voice greater strength, especially at a meeting that everyone expected to be very difficult. While Mrs. Brown appreciated his act, it undercut the treatment team by sending Mrs. Brown the message that the team would not be able to understand or support her as well as he could.

Both of these acts defined the impact of a therapeutic intervention narrowly. While these interventions affected the identified patient, they also affected the greater system of people. Although empowering Tamia and her mother were desirable consequences, the goals could be accomplished in many different ways. The goal should be to intervene in a way that will support and empower the *entire* system. Nicola and Sanjay, however, approached this question dichotomously and did not consider the entire range of possible solutions.

Because Nicola and Sanjay worked at a family therapy agency, these considerations were especially important. Their goals included engaging Tamia and improving her self-esteem, but also empowering Mrs. Brown as a parent. Because they anticipated continuing to work with the Brown family after the multidisciplinary meeting, the treatment team needed to be left in a position with enough power to be able to intervene successfully, yet the other agencies needed to be listened to and engaged in the treatment plan.

How could they meet these goals? Nicola's dilemma was relatively simple. She could ask Mrs. Brown whether Tamia was allowed to have candy and then respect her decision. Sanjay's situation was somewhat more difficult, but only because it required him to pay attention to the greater system. He can, however, be empowering if he talks to the treatment team and shares anything that could help them engage the Brown family in treatment. As part of the larger treatment team, he could also ask the therapists for their insights about working with the Brown family. The therapists could enter the multidisciplinary team meeting maintaining a respectful attitude toward the other agencies and share the treatment team's insights, while still listening to the input of other members of the multidisciplinary team. In this way, the family, Sanjay, the therapists, and other agency representatives are left in a powerful position believing that they have something to offer (see also table 10.4c).

OBSTACLES TO BEING EMPOWERING

Few of us have seriously thought about the relevance or importance of being empowering. In fact, most of us have perceived stepping back and failing to offer help as a problem. This section discusses some of these obstacles to being empowering and reframes potential "advantages" of unempowering interventions as problematic.

Being Helpful

Being empowering is difficult. It also flies in the face of many motives we have for entering this field. Students often say they are coming into this field because, "I've always wanted to help people, and my friends say I give good advice." Our own assessment of our success as helpers often includes some measure of how helpful we are. In addition, many people feel helpless and powerless, but they expect advice and even ask for it, even though they may ignore the advice or become resentful when they get it.

Can we be useful even if we aren't "helping"? Certainly. The grand-mother who taught her granddaughter how to tie her shoes was more use-ful than her son would have been had he jumped in and tied the child's shoes himself. Similarly, it is possible to be very useful in the course of ther-apy, even as the client performs the bulk of the work of identifying goals and going down the path of meeting those goals.

Clients in Crisis

Does this mean that we, as therapists, should be nondirective and should simply facilitate client work? First of all, listening and facilitating client progress is by no means "simple." It requires significant work and training. Second, the question underestimates the importance of strong listening and facilitation, both of which are fundamental to any therapeutic work. Fi-nally, our decision to be directive needs to be a thoughtful one rather than a reflexive one. Generally, clients only need significant directiveness when they are in crisis, but even then, we should provide as little as needed to sta-bilize the client.

> MARTY: *If I am hearing you correctly, the last week has been pretty rough and you're thinking about killing yourself after you find a place for your children to stay. We've talked about this before, and you know that I think this is a permanent solution to a temporary prob-lem. What can we do to get you over this bump—big bump—in the road? (Summarization followed by open question)*
>
> RAFIQ: *I don't know what to do. I DON'T KNOW WHAT TO DO! That's why I'm here!*
>
> MARTY: *You're right. That is why you're here, and I'm happy you're able to see that one part of you does want to live. It must be frus-trating to want to stay alive, and yet be unable to find any way to stay safe. Do you remember what worked in the past? (Feedback, interpretation, self-disclosure, reflection of feeling, and closed question)*
>
> RAFIQ: *No! (Long pause) Well . . . I remember that we agreed we were going to meet every week until things were okay and that I could call you if I needed to. (Pause) I also told my sister how I was feeling, so she would know where I was coming from.*
>
> MARTY: *That's a good start. Anything else? (Feedback and open question)*
>
> RAFIQ: *Well, I still carry around that list of things to do when I get stressed, but I don't look at it as much anymore. It's right here in my wallet.*
>
> MARTY: *Ah! Did it work before? (Closed question)*

RAFIQ: *Yeah. I guess it did. Maybe I could look at it again.*
MARTY: *Would this be enough to keep you safe? (Closed question)*

Marty has a clear agenda during this conversation and approaches it in a structured manner. However, she takes a respectful and collaborative stance and does not jump in to be more directive than necessary. If she had simply reminded Rafiq of his past successes and suggested that he use the same strategies, she would have met the same immediate treatment goals—without approaching her larger goals for therapy. She would have failed to empower Rafiq, failed to help him develop a strategy for making healthy decisions, and failed to identify skills that he could use independently when in crisis. Because Rafiq eventually was able to describe what worked and identify treatment choices, he became more committed to staying alive and more invested in the strategies they identified together (G. C. Williams, Rodin, Ryan, Grolnick, & Deci, 1998). Because he was treated in a respectful manner even when he was "falling apart," he will be more likely to see himself as competent, capable, and someone deserving of respect.

Being patient with clients who are angry and frustrated can be very difficult, as it was with Rafiq, and giving them time to calm down and identify solutions can be difficult as well. Being able to do this successfully requires *believing* that clients have the resources to be significant partners in their own therapy. They are no more and no less important to the course of therapy than the therapist. Patience with them requires the therapist to challenge their beliefs about the clients' resources and whether or not they can solve their own problems and access those resources now.

Rafiq's saying, "I don't know what to do. I DON'T KNOW WHAT TO DO! That's why I'm here!" is an example of how Marty needs to identify Rafiq's cognitive, emotional, and social resources in order to assess his current ability to weather this crisis (refer to table 10.5). She needs to appraise his self-efficacy regarding this and other issues and determine how his available resources can be brought to bear in this situation. If she believes that he is a very capable person who underestimates his own abilities, she may simply remind him of his successes. If he thinks dichotomously and can only identify two extreme alternatives without assistance ("I'm going to go on like this forever unless I kill myself!"), Marty may need to focus on helping Rafiq brainstorm other options. But, if he has few cognitive and emotional resources and only sees himself as helpless, she may have to be considerably more directive.

Her assessment of his ability to handle frustration and to ride out crises will also influence her decision. If Marty believes that Rafiq is volatile and unpredictable, and has a history of potentially lethal suicide attempts, she may do more to help him stabilize than if she were to know that he gets upset easily but uses these feelings to make adaptive changes. Her perception

TABLE **10.5** **QUESTIONS FOR IDENTIFYING INTERVENTIONS THAT EMPOWER**

Resources
- Would the client be able to solve this problem under other conditions?
- Has the client solved this problem in the past?
- How capable does the client feel about solving the problem this time? Is the client's assessment of self-efficacy reasonable?
- What preexisting resources or resources developed in the course of therapy does the client have that would be useful in solving this problem?
- What makes the problem difficult to solve this time?

Accessibility of Resources
- Is the client able to access these resources? If not, what prevents this?
- What level or type of prompting will be needed to access and to use available resources?

Response to Mild Frustration During Crisis
- How frustrated is the client?
- How has the client responded in the past when asked to continue working on a problem while frustrated?
- How does the client usually respond to frustration?
- Are both the therapist and client willing to accept the consequences of this frustration?
- If a safety plan is necessary, will the client likely follow through with it?

that he is significantly at risk would make her less patient and more directive in this crisis. If neither Rafiq nor anyone else is at significant risk, Marty can afford to move more slowly and be more empowering, even as Rafiq views himself as helpless and incapable.

Directiveness: When and Why

The importance of being empowering cannot be overemphasized, but the interventions discussed so far have been fairly directive and often action-oriented rather than insight-oriented. Why?

We may often think that directive approaches are action-oriented and unempowering, but these three dimensions have no necessary relationship. An insight-oriented approach, for example, can be directive and unempowering in the same way that stereotypical psychoanalytic approaches can be, and an action-oriented approach can be nondirective and empowering in the same way as a few of the experiential movement therapies.

Nondirective, insight-oriented stances can be very powerful and empowering interventions (as with person-centered therapy). However, even when used well, they are not well-accepted by all clients. The importance of being directive when a client is in crisis has been established, but some clients, particularly among Hispanic and Asian American cultures, tend to expect their therapists to take an active and authoritarian approach to the problems that they face (D. W. Sue & Sue, 1999). In particular, being active and open provides clients with clear information about the therapist's viewpoint, which seems to be especially important to them. Second, active approaches often focus more on external or societal factors that are causing the problems, such as poverty and discrimination, and less on internal and intrapsychic factors, such as low self-esteem and passivity. Such clients may respond very well to therapy that is structured, clear, and explicit.

Furthermore, being open when responding to clients' questions, as opposed to hiding behind therapeutic neutrality, can help foster the trust necessary for successful therapeutic change. This is especially important when working with clients who have significant problems with trust, either as a result of abuse histories or oppression (Ivey et al., 1997). Often, as with the following example, clients can lay a series of tests for therapists throughout the course of therapy. These are best responded to in open, nondefensive ways.

> ELYSE: *This is all so overwhelming! I don't know how I'm going to get through this.*
>
> FAITH: *This is hard stuff, but we can do it together. Because of the problems you've come with—the flashbacks, nightmares, and dissociation—we may need to spend some time talking about your history of abuse. You're going to need to be open in describing your memories about the rapes and your thoughts and feelings about them. (Feedback, sharing information)*
>
> ELYSE: *That's all going to be hard . . . .*
>
> FAITH: *I'm also going to ask you to check your expectations about how I'm going to respond by reading my face. Check to see if I understand you. See if I find you as shameful as you seem to think I will. (Directives)*
>
> ELYSE: *How can you understand me? You were never raped by your brother.*
>
> FAITH: *You're right. I don't have a history of child abuse. I had a very serious boyfriend who was abusive, however, and I remember my feelings and thoughts from that period. It helps me understand some of the stories I've heard from other clients . . . (Pause) But, I'd like you to stop me if you think I'm not understanding you. Sometimes I can be so dense. (Self-disclosure, directive, self-disclosure)*
>
> ELYSE: *This is going to be hard . . . .*

In this example, Faith is very directive about the nature of therapeutic interventions for dealing with post-traumatic symptoms. However, her stance is also empowering in that she validates Elyse's feelings and concerns, responds openly to her requests, indicates her own fallibility, and communicates that there is a place for each of them in the therapeutic exchange (Saba & Rodgers, 1990). Although this is probably not the last time Elyse will assume that Faith cannot understand her, particularly since she has a history of people not understanding her or appreciating her concerns,

Pay attention to your inter-actions in and out of for-mal helping settings over the next week. Think about times when you are being directive. Why do you choose this approach? How do you feel doing so? Spend some time thinking about your reactions to your client (or anybody else) and yourself.

Now identify a time when you were less direc-tive. Consider your reac-tions under these circum-stances. What differences do you notice?

it does begin to address her concerns in a therapeutic fashion. The success of her intervention can be seen in Elyse's shift of subject form and verb tense, from "That's all going to be hard . . . " to "This is going to be hard . . ." which suggests greater commitment.

While everyone walks into novel situations with expectations about how others will respond to them based on their worldview, clients with a history of abuse or oppression may especially assume that others will mistreat them or be unable to understand them. This is a valid assumption, especially for those who were often mistreated or misunderstood by the important people in their lives. These clients in particular seem to need more struc-ture and less ambiguity in therapy, but they also need an open and respect-ful stance from their therapists.

Needs: Met and Unmet

The interventions discussed so far can be helpful and even useful, but they can also be unempowering. When this happens, the reasons are more telling about us than about the person we are supposed to be helping. Marty could have chosen to be directive with Rafiq because of the sense of power it gave her. Faith could have described her own history of abuse as an attempt to resolve her own survivor guilt rather than to help Elyse (Helms & Cook, 1999). These motivations can undermine, rather than sup-port, therapeutic goals.

It feels good to be needed. Being able to help a person resolve a prob-lem can be wonderful, and it can make one feel all-knowing and powerful. These grandiose feelings can be compounded when significant apprecia-tion or praise is received ("I've never been able to tell anyone this before. No one has ever been able to help me with this in the past. How did you know to do that?"). In addition, being able to identify a strategy for solving a problem can make us feel competent, successful, and good at our jobs. These are powerful reinforcements.

It can also feel awful to allow someone to "take the long way" in solving a problem. Watching someone struggle painfully to solve an issue that you know can be resolved readily can be very difficult. Some clients react with criticism, "Can't you see I'm floundering here? Just tell me what to do." Even if our clients don't react in this way, we may make the same criticisms of ourselves ("How do I know if she isn't too fragile and helpless to be able to find her way out? This may have worked in the past, but how do I know it will work now?"). Our beliefs and self-talk can make choosing interven-tions that empower easier or more difficult.

These criticisms from others and ourselves can expose our basest fears. Because therapy is an art and a science, a general path toward addressing our client's concerns may be apparent, but a specific path is almost never identified clearly. As soon as a new client presents issues that seem easy to work through, a monkey wrench invariably appears in the system, perhaps because we stopped listening.

USING LONG-TERM GOALS TO IDENTIFY EMPOWERING INTERVENTIONS

As competent therapists and "nice" people, we want to give our clients good service for their money. Good service is generally defined in terms of how well we meet our clients' immediate treatment goals. Being relatively nondirective and having the product-oriented and time-focused approach of managed health care that so strongly influences contemporary psychotherapy, can seem incompatible with the goals. However, *less* may be *more* when we enlarge the picture and look at both the short-term and long-term treatment goals.

- Courtland's immediate "problem" was that she wanted to get her children back. However, she also wants to *keep* her children. To do this she may need to identify ways to make decisions when in crisis and learn to work more effectively with her caseworkers, as opposed to being alternately passive or aggressive.
- The de la Cruz family wanted to get through the crisis caused by the suicide, but their long-term goal was to learn to grieve in a positive way that worked for and strengthened the entire family.
- Aphrodite's family wanted to set up an effective plan with the school, but they also wanted to learn to work more effectively with other agencies as well.
- The Johansen family may have wanted someone to spend time with their son during his sibling's illness, but theirs was a stop-gap approach. In the long run, they needed to identify strategies for giving him positive attention, either through their own immediate efforts or by engaging extended family and friends.
- Rafiq's immediate goal was to find ways to cope with stressors and not attempt suicide. He had been successful doing this in the past, and now he needed to prevent relapses. This meant identifying and using sound coping strategies more rapidly.
- Elyse wanted to have her flashbacks and nightmares stop. This goal depends upon her ability to exercise healthy control over her life and memories. Giving away her control is not a good strategy for meeting this goal.

In each of these situations, less was more. Jumping in and solving their problems may stabilize them during a crisis, but would not address any of the long-term goals (When clients are truly in over their heads, stabilization in and of itself can be a useful goal). Assisting them to identify strategies to meet their goals is effective both in the short term *and* in the long term to the degree that we can prevent future relapses with the same problems (Helms & Cook, 1999).

Although the work described here is less directive than some approaches, it provides a structure that meets therapeutic goals in a timely, yet empowering fashion. Outcome work at one in-home family therapy program demonstrated that the work had been successful at immediately stabilizing the family *and* in preventing out-of-home placements following termination (Motter, Slattery, & Bean, 1999; Pfendler, Slattery, Hollis, & Bean, 1996).

THERAPY AS MENTORING

An empowering stance in therapy is very similar to a mentoring type of relationship. When people are given a voice in the decision-making process and when they are listened to and given real treatment options, they experience greater opportunity for growth in the long run. Furthermore, because many clients have the tools already within them to solve their problems (or they have these tools readily obtainable), therapy should remind them of the healthy solutions they've used in the past and should help them use these tools to solve similar problems in the future. Clients should never be prompted to become dependent on the therapist to meet their goals. Dependency does not foster long-term needs. As the saying goes,

> Give her a fish, and she will be hungry the next day. Teach her to fish, and she will never be hungry again.

When we mentor, we recognize and nurture a person's strengths. Similarly, when we are doing therapy, we can recognize strengths even though our clients are overwhelmed and doing poorly. F. Shaw (1998), for example, includes this note written by her physician, shortly before she was admitted to the hospital:

> Fiona began being weepy on Monday after discharge [from the maternity ward] and has gradually deteriorated over the last few days. She last ate 2 slices of bread at noon yesterday and is still drinking. She seems to be caring for her baby very well and continues to breast-feed.
>
> She is a very articulate, intelligent lady and is well aware that there is a problem. She had previous eating and depressive problems in the past. Depression and weight loss while in hospital with an orthopedic back problem as a teenager and then [eating problems] as a student. She felt these problems were cured after her first pregnancy.

> She cried the whole time I was with her and blames herself for all the problems! (p. 30)

Clearly, this doctor saw Shaw as a competent person and did not ignore the seriousness of her depression. Shaw described interactions with people who were like himself as being calming and even helpful, while those people who treated Fiona as a number were less calming and helpful.

The belief that our clients can be successful in meeting their goals is an important one. Our belief in their ability to reach their goals seems to become a self-fulfilling prophecy. Rogers (1983) described his evolution as a teacher in response to incorporating his theoretical ideals,

> I ceased to be a teacher. It wasn't easy. It happened rather gradually, but as I began to trust students, I found they did incredible things. (p. 26)

Think about a time when someone mentored you. How did it feel? What made it work? What short-term and long-term advantages and disadvantages did you draw from this relationship?

If there were disadvantages, were these peculiar to this relationship or would you expect to see them across mentoring relationships? Why?

Similarly, our clients can do incredible things when we believe in them.

Identifying the people who our clients see as mentors in our early assessments identifies who they can turn to when they are struggling when the person is a contemporary figure in their current support system. We can help clients enlist the real or imagined support of these mentors. When clients, as with Mervyn (see chapter 2), see historical figures, such as JFK and Job, as mentors, we can begin to wonder with them whether these figures experienced any similar problems and what they did to resolve them. These experiences can be a touchstone for the balance of therapy ("Job survived when he was tested, so can I. Moreover, I can be active and strong, even when I'm afraid, just as JFK was").

CONCLUSIONS

In addition to our short-term goals with our clients (stabilizing their current symptoms), we have long-term goals (empowering them and preventing relapses). Although we can meet short-term goals by providing a crisis phone number, it is to our clients' advantage if we give them the skills to solve their own problems now and in the future. Unfortunately, being empowering is often difficult, because there are numerous barriers to doing so. Should we take care of our clients, which is part of being the "nice" helpers that motivated many of us to enter the field, or if not, when and how should we attempt to move beyond this unempowering stance?

An especially important barrier to being empowering is our inability to identify empowering interventions or to challenge those that are not empowering. Being empowering is difficult to do consistently, particularly because two clients in superficially similar situations may require different strategies of intervention. Particularly early in one's career, it will be difficult to distinguish between empowering and distancing interventions, between caring, enabling and "doing for." Distinguishing among these is best handled through a process of personal reflection and consultation with peers and supervisors. This is an ongoing process; even seasoned therapists should challenge themselves on these issues and continue to identify ways in which they steal their clients' power.

The residents and interns I teach believe that their medical schools have told them, in the case of a dispute, that their patients are always right and that they are, conversely, always wrong. If so, it's a perverse misinterpretation of the importance of the client in the change process, generally, and of empowerment, specifically. Although clients contribute significantly to change, and their opinions are important (see, for example, Asay & Lambert, 1999; Lambert, 1992), the therapist (or doctor) is equally central to the change process. We should not put one ahead of the other or forget either's contribution. All parties profit from a powerful therapist *and* an equally powerful and empowered client.

MAKING MEANING

'A long time ago, there lived a child named Ling-ling who was a good artist. After her mother's death, her father's favourite concubine began to maltreat her by showing preference towards her own children. Ling-ling had no one to play with and spent her time painting. Her pictures became famous and were sold for many taels of silver. Her stepmother now grew jealous. One night, she crept up to Ling-ling's bed and stuck a dirty nail into the child's hand, spreading faeces on the nail to cause an infection.

'In a few days, Ling-ling's hand became red and swollen. Though the nail was removed, pus poured from the wound. However, Ling-ling continued to paint.'

'Now, a strange thing happened. The wound never healed, but Ling-ling's paintings became better and better. The more the pus exuded, the greater the beauty of her work. In the whole of China, there was nothing like it. The pain in her hand seemed to imbue Ling-ling with an essence of invincibility, enabling her to *zhan er bi sheng, dou er bi ke* (prevail in every battle, overcome every adversity) (Mah, 1997, p. 273).

Nietzsche said, "That which does not kill me makes me stronger." Certainly, one way of looking at Ling-ling's successes after being wounded is that she was able to transform her pain and sorrow into personal and artistic beauty. While this process occurs easily and naturally for some people—sometimes within days of a trauma (Park, 1999)—it doesn't for everyone.

Finding meaning *is* a normal and natural part of life. People impose meaning and order upon their lives even when it does not otherwise make sense—they wear lucky socks, rub a lucky coin, or eat a special meal before a big event. However, people don't always find *positive* meanings. In the best of all possible worlds, the ways we think should give us the strength to deal with difficult times and places. Unfortunately, when some people leave difficult experiences, they believe that they are bad and are being punished for real or imagined sins. They may also come away believing that other people are bad in this dog-eat-dog world or that life is random and pointless. Each of these beliefs is a kind of meaning making.

Meaning-related Health Outcomes

The search for meaning is associated with a variety of psychological and physiological impacts. For example, women undergoing surgery for breast cancer have lower levels of distress when they have higher levels of acceptance and more positive ways of looking at the world (Carver et al., 1993). People with perceived benefits following a heart attack, such as closer family relationships or stronger personal values, reported less depression and more life satisfaction (Affleck et al., 1987). Caregiving partners of men with AIDS who looked at their experiences in a positive light also reported more positive moods during the caregiving process and even after their partners' deaths (Moskowitz, Folkman, Collette & Vittinghoff, 1996).

Positive health-related outcomes have also been widely reported after disclosing a trauma, writing about it, or somehow finding meaning in it. These changes were reported by "normal" populations having no significant diagnosed health problems. Changes were also reported by populations with severe and debilitating illnesses. People who have more difficulty expressing their emotions have poorer immune system function than those who are more emotionally expressive (Esterling, Antoni, Fletcher, Margulies, & Schneiderman, 1994). After writing about a stressor, people make fewer visits to their health center and show improvements in autonomic activity and immune system function (Esterling et al., 1994; Pennebaker & Beall, 1986; Pennebaker, Colder, & Sharp, 1990; Pennebaker, Hughes, & O'Heeron, 1987; Pennebaker, Kiecolt-Glaser, & Glaser, 1988; Petrie, Booth, Pennebaker, Davison, & Thomas, 1995).

These outcomes can be quite dramatic. HIV-positive men who reported making changes in their life values and priorities following the death of a close friend or partner had a smaller decline in lymphocyte function than those who had not (Bower, Kemeny, Taylor, & Fahey, 1998). These changes translated into a lower rate of AIDS-related mortality over a 4–9-year follow-up period. People who perceived benefits like changes in life philosophy and in personal values after their first heart attack were less likely to have a subsequent attack and had lower death rates over an 8-year follow-up (Affleck et al., 1987). Children of mothers who saw benefits following their child's hospitalization in a neonatal intensive care unit had developed more optimally by their two-year follow-up (Affleck, Tennen, & Rowe, 1991).

POST-TRAUMATIC OUTCOMES

Frankl (1959) wrote about his attempts to make meaning during his imprisonment in Auschwitz, and he stirred the field's interest in meaning making under adversity. However, little research (as opposed to theoretical speculation) has been done on making meaning following cultural adversity. Most has centered on medical trauma. Some studies have examined natural disasters (e.g., earthquakes), while others have looked at personal traumas like sexual abuse and car accidents. Discrete and notable acts like sexual abuse and cultural genocide have been easier to study, however, than the more everyday acts of prejudice, harassment, or discrimination.

Negative Post-traumatic Outcomes

Most people agree that drops in functioning often follow traumas. Diagnoses of post-traumatic stress disorder (PTSD) increase after rape, sexual abuse, and cultural genocide. Survivors of the Bosnian civil war who now live in the United States have high rates of post-traumatic symptoms (Becker, Weine, Vojvoda, & McGlashan, 1999; Weine, Vojvoda et al., 1998). Cambodian survivors continue to experience post-traumatic symptoms years later (Kinzie, Sack, Angell, Clarke, & Ben, 1989). People with severe mental illnesses were considerably more likely to report lifetime histories of trauma (98%) and of co-morbid PTSD (43%) than do people in the general population, 8–9% of whom are diagnosable with PTSD (Mueser et al., 1998). Women with rape or sexual abuse histories have significantly higher rates of PTSD, major depression, substance abuse, and other psychiatric disorders (Rodriguez, Ryan, Vande Kemp, & Foy, 1997). As many as 20–25% report symptoms of PTSD as much as 30 years later (Rothbaum, Foa, Riggs, Murdock, & Walsh, 1992; Widom, 1999). United States prisoners of war were still significantly more depressed, had more post-traumatic symptoms, and were living with stomach ulcers 40 years after the end of World War II (Kluznik, Speed, Van Valkenberg, & Magraw, 1986; Tennant, Goulston, & Dent, 1986).

Relative to major acute stressors, oppression and discrimination are often difficult to study because they can occur frequently enough and in small enough doses that they feel "normal." Sometimes the observer may suspect its presence, while the person experiencing it denies its presence (Smaby, Slattery, Creany, & Motter, 2000; Steinpreis et al., 1999). Even when these daily traumas are acknowledged, identifying the place where they first occurred and tracking the course of healing can be very difficult. Nonetheless, discrimination and other racist incidents may possibly be both less severe than many of the previously described traumas and also more chronic in nature. Among African Americans, reports of discrimination and other racist events are correlated with poor psychological and physical health (Landrine & Klonoff, 1996).

Post-traumatic damage seems to develop as a result of the kinds of meanings that are drawn following a trauma. Nash, Hulsey, Sexton, Harralson and Lambert (1993) report that even when they controlled for family environment—a predictor of pathology—women who were "sexually abused in childhood must more often contend with a distressing sense that something about them is fundamentally damaged" (p. 282). Social and cognitive mediators of trauma, however, predict outcomes better than isolated and objectively defined events alone (Nash, Neimeyer, Hulsey, & Lambert, 1998). Social support and the way survivors later perceive themselves after trauma strongly predict outcomes (Brewin, Andrews & Valentine, 2000;

Nolen-Hoeksema & Davis, 1999). People often withdraw and lose previous sources of social support, which increase relapse rates in those with severe mental illness (S. L. Brown, 1991; Mueser et al., 1998). Children in chaotic or dysfunctional families, who are least likely to receive support, were more likely to report a history of PTSD symptoms (Widom, 1999). Substance abuse often increases after a trauma and worsens the course of other mental illnesses (Mueser et al., 1998).

Have you ever seen yourself as "broken" or "undeserving" because you are a member of a group or because something bad happened to you? Do you admire anyone who has been sexually abused or divorced or is gay or Latina (or a member of any other group)? If so, can you really be "broken" because of your membership in this group?

Herschel, for example, felt "dirty" when he was beaten after his neighbors discovered he was gay. Although he continued to go to work, he stopped answering his phone and stayed at home at night drinking. His friends were initially outraged by the attack, but they did not know how to help him. After being pushed away on numerous occasions, they eventually stopped visiting. Herschel did not receive help until after his second serious suicide attempt. As can be seen in his story, negative meanings, poor social support, substance abuse, and inadequate coping strategies are factors that contributed to his problems after the assault. But as one improves, others generally do also.

Post-traumatic Growth and Positive Outcomes

Understanding post-traumatic growth is often complicated by the fact that people will report growth even when they show no measurable improvements in adjustment (Park, 1998). Considerable disagreement exists about these non-findings, however. Does the need to have something positive come from trauma cause people to report growth, even when there is none? Are we overly rosy in our assessments of growth because returns to baseline functioning feel much better than previous despair? Are measures of growth and adjustment insensitive to real post-traumatic changes?

Despite these problems in interpretation, the anecdotal literature of growth following a trauma is often compelling. People have stopped smoking after being diagnosed with cancer, have stopped drinking after being arrested for driving under the influence, and have worked to get legislation passed to change medical procedures following poor treatment under traumatic circumstances (Bloom, 1998; Park, 1998; Rabasca, 2000). In fact, Park, in summarizing one view of this literature, suggests that perceiving growth may in and of itself be a positive aspect or an outcome of effective coping. When Herschel began to reach out to others and found that he was accepted, he felt able to overcome his hurdles. Despite the fact that he was no better off than before his beating, he felt better about things than he had felt for quite a while and believed that he could survive anything life could throw at him. His improved self-concept and self-efficacy were important changes.

Although post-traumatic growth is difficult to measure, it is clear that post-traumatic damage is not inevitable. Although 25% of women with histories of rape do not show recovery even 30 years after the event, the other 75% report few symptoms (Rothbaum et al., 1992; Widom, 1999). Kluznik and his colleagues (1986) reported that one-third of the POWs they studied 40 years after the end of the war had fully recovered. Weine, Kulenovic, and their colleagues (1998) report significant drops in post-traumatic symptoms over the course of study among a group of Bosnian survivors who were not receiving traditional psychotherapy. Survivors of the Holocaust were described as being remarkably resilient and well-ad-justed (Kahana, Harel, & Kahana, 1988). Women in mental-health profes-sions reported significantly greater histories of child abuse and trauma than did a comparable group of female professionals. But they reported having better outcomes (D. M. Elliott & Guy, 1993)!

THE MEANING OF FINDING MEANING

Members of the psychology field spent a considerable part of the 20th cen-tury emphasizing the importance of reinforcements, punishments, and pat-terns of reinforcement schedules in determining people's behavior. How-ever, Bergin and Garfield (1994), in summarizing Bandura (1986), conclude that

> [B]ehavior is not controlled by its consequences so much as it is by fore-thought and by personal constructions of its meaning or value in relation to internal cognitive assessments, self-reflections, and controls. (p. 823)

What and how people believe determines how they act. In the best of all possible worlds, meaning provides clients with a sense of purpose that directs their future actions (see table 11.1). A search for meaning can help in identifying life goals and in obtaining the energy and motivation to reach them or to get through bad times. The kind of meaning developed can in-crease or decrease clients' feelings of stress and sense of control. The ways that people, their culture, and their significant others interpret events

TABLE 11.1 **CONSEQUENCES OF FINDING POSITIVE MEANING IN DIFFICULT EVENTS AND TIMES**

- A sense of purpose and direction
- Goals and a sense of vision for the future
- Hope
- A sense of control
- Decreased stress
- Bridge gaps across difficult times
- Increased tolerance for pain

determines whether something is even identified as "traumatic" (Helms & Cook, 1999).

Having a sense of purpose is a powerful predictor of general life adjustment (Park & Folkman, 1997). Those who believe that life just happens and that there is no way to resolve or overcome stressors, often end up feeling defeated both by the event in particular and by life in general. They also have a difficult time addressing even those stressors that can be changed (Alloy & Seligman, 1979; Seligman, 1975). On the other hand, developing a sense of meaning and purpose ("I can learn from mistakes and avoid making them again") enables people to develop a sense of hope for the future, even if their hope is of an afterlife, and it can be a bridge between stressful periods.

Many authors attribute improvement to the meaning-making process (Kahana et al., 1988). It is important, as discussed earlier, to remember that meaning making, social support, and coping strategies tend to be confounded and tend to change together. Having good social support and using effective coping strategies, in addition to fostering hopeful meanings, can help most people survive and thrive despite being traumatized (S. L. Brown, 1991; D. M. Elliott & Guy, 1993).

Principle of Personal Deservedness

Think about something difficult in your life. It could be an illness, an accident, a death, an assault, or something similar. How do you think about it now? Who or what caused it? Who or what do you blame? Do you believe you could have or should have done something to prevent it?

Identifying why an event occurred and who or what was responsible for its occurrence can help people make sense of trauma (Park & Folkman, 1997). One of the common principles organizing a person's attributions about events is the principle of personal deservedness. People often expect that good things will happen to good people and that bad things may, should, or will happen to bad people (Park & Folkman, 1997). People tend to blame other people for the bad things in their lives (see chapter 1), while excusing themselves when in similar predicaments (Gilbert & Malone, 1995; J. Greenberg et al., 1982; Jones, 1979; Zuckerman, 1979). Unfortunately, people tend to use self-blame when they are depressed.

The type of stressor also seems to contribute to people's response style. While it's possible to find an "escape clause" for natural disasters and "acts of God," people find it more difficult to excuse themselves for a "personal" trauma or for their response to a natural disaster, such as failing to hold onto a child in the midst of a tornado (Nolen-Hoeksema & Morrow, 1991). Thus, we might expect that people who saw themselves as responsible for a trauma would be self-blaming and drawing more negative attributions (Delahanty et al., 1997). People who had been sexually abused or had experienced other interpersonal traumas often attributed the traumatic events to themselves rather than seeing the event as truly random (Catlin & Epstein, 1992). People who blamed themselves had significantly lower self-esteem, believed themselves to be less worthy of love, perceived the world as less meaningful (and more maleficent), and placed less value on interpersonal relationships than people not reporting these sorts of traumas (Catlin & Epstein, 1992). Their views of the world seemed to be mediated by the number of positive and negative events in their lives, which had a cumulative effect. Although these are correlational data and biased by self-report, people reporting more positive and fewer negative events had more positive global meanings (and vice versa).

A Sense of Control and Hope

Returning to the event from the last reflective writing, how did your sense of control change afterward? Did it increase, decrease, or remain the same? Can you do anything to stop the event from recurring or from having a lesser effect on a second occasion? If your sense of control changed, how did it affect your self-concept and view of the world?

People who see themselves as responsible for negative outcomes generally experience less depression than those who saw themselves as random targets (Delahanty et al., 1997; Shapiro, 1989). They also abstain from substance use more successfully (Bradley, Gossop, Brewin, Phillips, & Green, 1992). People who felt responsible for their car accidents were less likely to develop PTSD than people who believed others were to blame (Delahanty et al., 1997).

This relationship between depression and responsibility is counterintuitive, but it can be adaptive to blame ourselves for specific and controllable actions, while being maladaptive to blame ourselves for stable, unchangeable aspects of self (Bradley et al., 1992; Delahanty et al., 1997). The first scenario may leave a person feeling somewhat hopeful ("I can do things differently next time"), but the second may produce a profound sense of hopelessness ("This is the way I am, and I can't do anything to change it").

The importance of this sense of control and hopefulness has also been found with rats and dogs. Richter (1957) found that wild rats would drown within minutes whenever they were held tightly until they stopped struggling and then released into a vat of water where they were forced to keep swimming. Those rescued immediately before they drowned, and thus given a sense of hope, were able to swim for an additional 60 to 80 hours. Similarly, dogs that were given an insoluble task and then subjected to electrical shocks whenever they failed it, gave up and did not attempt a solvable task in the same setting, even when the task was otherwise easy (Alloy & Seligman, 1979). This result has been replicated in multiple settings and has been proposed as a model for depression (Seligman, 1975).

Schlenker and his colleagues (Schlenker, Britt, Pennington, Murphy, & Doherty, 1994), in summarizing the literature, describe the positive consequences of having a sense of control. People with greater perceptions of personal control tend to be more creative, have greater cognitive flexibility, and can learn better. They are more intrinsically motivated, they procrastinate less, and they expend more effort but persist longer when they encounter obstacles. Their problem-solving abilities are also stronger. They have more realistic levels of aspiration, higher outcome expectations, and greater motivation for challenging tasks. People with greater senses of personal control also experience less pressure and tension, evaluate themselves more positively and, while they may experience greater distress initially, they often have better psychological health.

Even negative meanings can give people a sense of control when the meanings can help them act differently in the future. Seeing possible behavioral changes rather than unchangeable attributes is generally much more successful (Janoff-Bulman, 1979, 1992; Tennen & Affleck, 1990). Herschel, for example, did better once he began to attribute his problems to being naïve about whom he could share his affectional orientation with, as opposed to attributing the problems with his being gay. He reconsidered when and how he wanted to disclose his affectional orientation and moved to a more GLBT-friendly neighborhood and job.

Disclosure or Isolation

Post-traumatic meanings may interfere with a person's ability to talk with others about the event. This is especially true when survivors blame themselves for the predicament that they now face (Nolen-Hoeksema & Morrow, 1991). Shame, embarrassment, and guilt are barriers to asking for and receiving much-needed social support.

It may be easier to get emotional support after certain types of trauma. For example, support comes easier after an earthquake than it does for a sexual assault. Nolen-Hoeksema and Morrow (1991) suggest that this may be because few people blame others for earthquakes, while many survivors of sexual assault, racial discrimination, and ethnic attacks are blamed or expect to receive negative reactions. In addition, earthquakes are often the primary conversation for weeks afterward. Anyone who wants to talk about it has many willing listeners. With assault, however, family and friends of the survivors may have a difficult time hearing about the event and often expect that it should be over, typically soon after the physical wounds heal. Consequently, survivors of personal traumas get hit with a triple whammy: (1) shame, (2) isolation, and (3) disillusionment about their support system, not to mention the physical injuries. They may become revictimized in the course of asking for help (see table 11.2).

As the meaning of these personal traumas shifts during therapy, so do shame and isolation. When survivors stop blaming themselves and begin to blame the system that allowed others to objectify, discriminate, or assault them, they also generally find it easier to share their experiences with others. In addition, as they successfully disclose their experiences without receiving negative responses, their own personal meanings often become more tolerant and forgiving. Therefore, one of the most important gifts

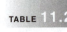

TABLE 11.2 FORMS OF SECONDARY VICTIMIZATION FOLLOWING ETHNIC VIOLENCE WITHIN AN IMMIGRANT'S NEW COUNTRY

External Consequences
- Time off work, associated loss of self-esteem incurred from loss of job, and income while recuperating
- Financial costs associated with counseling and court appearances
- Loss of insurance
- Loss of available income to send to family still in other countries
- Retaliation, both within and without the family, for reporting

Internal Consequences Stemming from Victimization
- Shame about their culture or their country of origin
- Feelings of being "second class" within their new country
- Perceived loss of masculinity or "head of household" status for male victims
- Loss of trust in their new country and in the hopes they had about their new life

Internal Consequences Related to Asking for Help
- Encountering prejudices of system caregivers regarding their ethnic group
- Difficulty understanding laws, systems, or services in new country
- Communication problems or language barriers

Note: Expanded from S. L. Brown, 1991.

therapists can give clients who present with a history of trauma is to simply listen and give free acceptance of them and their stories.

MEANING-RELATED COPING STRATEGIES

Choose a story in your life, especially one that is or was challenging for you in some way. Identify several ways you have thought about the problem, your role in it, and the relative involvement of environment, luck, and responsibility. If this is too difficult, choose a client who is stuck in thinking about a personal crisis or trauma.

Do some stories leave you feeling more hopeful and better about yourself, the people around you, and the nature of the world around you? Do some leave you feeling worse? What advantages do you see in telling each story? When or why might you choose to tell one rather than another?

Oftentimes, particular coping or defensive strategies follow the meanings people draw (see table 11.3). Allan, who was diagnosed with lung cancer, saw himself as "bad" and believed that the cancer was a "punishment" for unnamed and unidentifiable sins. He continued to punish himself. He withdrew from others, neglected his personal appearance, wore clothes that he did not like, and played music that depressed him. Eliza, who saw herself as "broken" after being molested by an uncle, gave up and became dependent upon others around her. Suzan believed that her attackers were acting out the misogynist attitudes of her culture, so she chose to distance herself from men, surround herself with supportive women, and become politically active in the local women's center. Because coping responses are directly related to beliefs, it is important to assess meanings carefully and shift them in more adaptive directions—directions that permit realistic coping and produce the ability to enjoy life (Park & Folkman, 1997). In addition to identifying cultural and diagnostic issues, assessments should examine broader belief systems that assist or complicate treatment (Belar & Deardorff, 1995).

In addition to assessing an individual person's belief system, it is also important to assess and intervene with the beliefs of the important people in

TABLE **11.3** ATTRIBUTIONS MADE AFTER A HEART ATTACK AND THEIR CONSEQUENCES

Attributions	Consequences
Negative	
No one can do anything to stop God's plan.	Hopelessness; no change in health behaviors.
Life is unfair. Bad things happen to good people.	Anger, especially toward God; may give up on "being good."
I'm out of shape, but there's nothing I can do to be healthier.	Hopelessness about prognosis; no change in health behaviors.
Joe was a marathoner, and he had a heart attack, too. It doesn't make a difference what I do.	Benign acceptance of fate; no change in lifestyle.
We all go sometime. My time may be soon. I can't face this.	Denial of health problems; may show increased avoidance and some use of negative coping behaviors such as substance use and irregular sleeping and eating habits, which increase risks to health.
Positive	
I can control the probability that I will have a second heart attack.	A change in lifestyle, especially an increase in health-promoting behaviors.
This is my wake-up call to live my life as I want to live it.	A shift in behaviors to align these with preexisting values and priorities or newly identified values and goals.
God gave me a second chance. How can I pay Him back?	Perhaps no change in health behaviors, although positive changes in attitude and reordering of priorities.

the person's system. These include family, friends, caseworkers, physicians, and therapists. A woman who cannot conceive and is blamed by her family and friends and is seen as less feminine as a result, will have a more complicated reaction to her diagnosis than one who receives a more positive and accepting response (Belar & Deardorff, 1995). Children whose nonoffending parent (usually the mother) is seen in therapy and is doing well there have much better outcomes than those children whose nonoffending parent is not seen (Meichenbaum, 2000b).

MODE OF ACTION

While findings about the physical and psychological consequences of our belief systems are provocative, the mode of action by which changed morbidity occurs is still poorly understood. Do people who have discovered a positive meaning after having a heart attack have lower rates of morbidity because they now think about their lives differently or because they have made adaptive lifestyle changes? Certainly both can lead to improvements in sympathetic nervous system activity, blood pressure, and heart rate. They could, in turn, lead to better morbidity outcomes. More research, like the kind conducted by Bower et al. (1998), is needed. This is research in which lifestyle, cognitive style, and morbidity are assessed by following and tracking the target population over a number of years.

Pennebaker and his colleagues (1990) suggest that disclosing a stressor serves two functions. First, it removes a stressor that increases the probability of disease processes. Second, writing or talking about a traumatic situation allows difficult events to be understood and assimilated. According to the hypothesis, those events that are not assimilated are more likely to remain as unwanted thoughts.

C. L. Park, in a personal communication dated October 6, 1999, suggests that successful outcomes may be predictable *before* the heart attack actually occurs. People who recognize a discrepancy between their worldview and their beliefs about the heart attack would be expected to attempt to close this gap. When someone is pessimistic and has external loci of control and responsibility, a heart attack may not initiate either a change in meaning making or in coping responses. Why should it? The heart attack makes sense and future heart attacks are out of their control. However, Park predicts that people who can develop benign or even positive ways of seeing their heart attacks would be more likely to make the kinds of lifestyle changes that could help them rehabilitate following a heart attack and prevent its recurrence. While they may retain an external locus of responsibility for their behavior, it is notable that they are also accepting more control over their future health.

The time orientation of positive attributions tends to be more future-oriented rather than past- or present-oriented. People who imagined experiencing a negative event tended to be more self-blaming, depressed, or angry when they focused on the present rather than when they thought about the future (Boninger, Gleicher, & Strathman, 1994). This was particularly true when it was clear that they could do things differently next time, such as planning for the next race.

Thinking about the future gives a person a greater sense of control than does ruminating about the past. People with serious health problems, especially those with irreversible illnesses such as HIV/AIDS, tend to have a difficult time perceiving control, but they can still find peaks and joy in the rest of their lives (Folkman, 2001).

Finally, Emmons and Colby (1995) suggest that positive changes associated with finding meaning could be at least partially attributable to building a social network that is perceived by the person as supportive. When they draw negative meanings from an event, people are more likely to withdraw

TABLE **11.4** **LU'S CONNECTEDNESS TO HER SUPPORT SYSTEM BEFORE AND AFTER DOMESTIC VIOLENCE AND SUBSEQUENT THERAPY**

Prior to Violence	Following the Violence	Following Therapy
Friendships Described self as "outgoing," with a large number of acquaintances and a few close friends.	Isolated in new community. Felt like people gossiped too much. Felt "exposed."	Renewed several friendships with people who had previously been important to her. Felt less "paranoid" about others' reactions toward her.
Family Was a pampered only child; received everything she wanted as a child; always felt special in this context; felt closer to her mother than to her father.	Withdrew from her family because she was living in a different town 150 miles away and because she was embarrassed about the abuse; parents confused about her distancing. Husband alternately angry, violent, and conciliatory, blaming her for abusive episodes. Had two daughters (ages 2 and 5) whom they both adored; both girls quiet and anxious.	Disclosed the violence to her parents who were initially angry at her husband. Her parents were later supportive of both of them and the changes they made. Both identified healthier ways to communicate about problems as they occurred rather than waiting until they blew up. Husband quit drinking. Oldest daughter became more independent and began sleeping through the night.
Work Described self as a hard worker who readily found work and was promoted quickly.	Productivity declined somewhat but remained within normal limits; took an increased number of sick days. During last performance review, her supervisor asked what was wrong. She replied, Nothing.	Described her work as easier to focus on. She took considerably fewer sick days.
Community Resources None identified.	A supportive sitter. Neighbors avoided family following overhearing shouting from their house.	Positive relationships with domestic violence agency, individual and family therapists, her daughter's school, her sitter, and one neighbor.
Community Contributions Was a cheerleader in high school and active in a number of service projects.	Identified none.	Became active in the domestic violence support group and organized fundraising projects for the agency. Read to her daughter's kindergarten class weekly.

from those who are important to them and will often stop making the interpersonal contacts that would otherwise be helpful. This pattern can be seen with Lu, a previously outgoing woman, who withdrew from her family and friends after becoming involved in a violent relationship (see table 11.4). During this period, she believed that she was both causing and deserving of the violence. She began to draw more positive meanings in therapy ("The violence wasn't something I deserved, although I can develop better ways of communicating with my family and friends, and cope with stressors better"). In addition to these changes, she renewed her relationships with family and friends and developed a stronger support system, principally by accepting the support offered by others.

MANY PATHS TO A SINGLE GOAL

While there are many ways of intervening after a trauma, most of these intentionally or unintentionally create new meanings about the event and person. Three less formal strategies are described below. Weine, Kulenovic, and their colleagues (1998), writing about testimony therapy, a "nontherapeutic" approach to collecting, listening to and believing stories of trauma, state that *testimony therapy*:

> offers the possibility of affirmatively addressing these aspects of the Bosnian experience, supporting strengths inherent in the survivors' struggles to recollect, to find meaning, to communicate, and to learn and teach what it means to survive political violence and to be Bosnian (p. 1721).

This process uses a culturally acceptable way of telling stories about a confusing period in the participants' lives, most of whom would not accept traditional individual therapy, and it affirms successes in the face of overwhelming disaster.

A similar, nontherapeutic process is used by African American fathers of academically high-achieving sons. Greif, Hrabowski, and Maton (1998) reported that these fathers acknowledged that prejudice and discrimination existed and that life was not fair, but nonetheless they maintained high expectations, taught their sons not to let stereotypes and bias keep them from achieving, and encouraged them to identify and use positive strategies to succeed. The fathers acknowledged their sons' perceptions of events and challenged them to make the events different.

In a segment of dialogue taken from an African American men's support group, Elligan and Utsey (1999) describe a similar pattern of acceptance of the person and experience, while encouraging more adaptive responses:

> CARROLL: *Man, every time I go around them they always have some fucked-up remark that's hostile in a subtle way. One day, my program director asked me what my research interests were and before I could say anything, he replied: "Oh, I forgot you're interested in that minority bullshit." Man, I almost lost it. I started to tell him what I really thought about him.*

LUTHER: *What do you think that would have gotten you? You need to get what you're there for and leave everything else alone. You're not going to be of any use as a psychologist if you don't complete your degree. When I was in school during the '50s, I had better not even look at them the wrong way or I might have been thrown out of school. So I kept silent, got my degree, and then joined the small team of psychologists devoted to helping our people heal the psychological scars inflicted by the White colonizers.*

DAMIEN: *I don't agree. I think you can address that kind of behavior without jeopardizing your status in the program.*

FARRELL: *What would you have done in that situation?*

DAMIEN: *I might have said something to the effect of, "Well, I'm sorry you feel that my interests are bullshit, but they're important to me and as the program director I would have expected you to be more supportive."*

GREGORY: *That might have worked.*

LAMAR: *I guess that's why I'm not in graduate school. I know for a fact that if that dumb-ass motherfucker said something like that to me, I would have given him an iron fist to the third vertebrae and paralyzed his colorless ass. (Laughter among the group members)*

ALHADJI: *When I was doing my graduate work in Florida, there were some [White] students from South Africa in the program. Keep in mind that this was during the early '70s when this was a hot issue. In those days, I was a noncompromising revolutionary and told the department chair that I was not going to attend classes with the racist South Africans. I stood my ground, and I still graduated. So I don't think there is a right or wrong way to handle a situation similar to this one, as long as you are comfortable with your decision or behavior and are prepared to deal with the consequences of your actions* (pp. 161–162, names added for clarity).

As the group members accepted Carroll's experience, they also challenged him to think about it differently and brainstorm ways to respond to this blatantly racist event (Elligan & Utsey, 1999). Lamar suggested physical or psychological violence, while Luther suggested silence within the system until gaining sufficient power to change it. Damien suggested polite assertiveness, and Alhadji proposed a noncompromising resistance. They powerfully helped Carroll brainstorm options for what seemed like an immovable obstacle and, in so doing, challenged him to draw new meanings about his experience ("I can succeed without sacrificing my sense of self as a powerful Black man"). In the process, they encouraged him to develop a positive self-image and sense of self in his culture.

In each case, despite their surface differences, participants are encouraged to share their experiences with a valued listener. The listener, much like a therapist would, accepts the feeling of outrage and, especially in the last two examples (Elligan & Utsey, 1999; Greif et al., 1998), helps them identify other ways of coping.

MULTIPLE STORIES FOR THE TELLING

Stories are a choice. Rarely do people have only one way of looking at the world. We can choose to see the glass as half empty or half full. We can see ourselves as lucky to have the little we have or focus on the places where we have been cheated in life.

Our stories are also generally internally consistent even when our lives are not. Even when stories are told with all of the contradictions of life, they are often *heard* as consistent themes. Ceballo (1999) describes this process in terms of her own interview research with Mary, an African American woman. At the initial set of interviews, both women saw Mary in a single, internally consistent manner, which was as a strong woman who was resilient in the face of adversity and as a person who was able to use relationships as a source of strength. At an interview two years later, Ceballo heard the contradictory themes. Mary was both angry with her father for his neglectful parenting, *and* she missed him when he was away. She appreciated the value of families, intimate connections, and therapeutic disclosures, while also maintaining her own privacy. She was ashamed of critical episodes in her life and had difficulty sharing these with the people around her.

Although Mary may have talked about only one set of themes initially, the contradictory themes were probably also present. However, Mary had difficulty accepting and staying with Ceballo's story of her life, perhaps because Ceballo (1999) had failed to "hear" both themes before supporting the "strong story." Ivey and his colleagues (1997) point out the importance of starting where the person is, really hearing that person, and having the understanding recognized, *then* attempting to do something to change the story. Mary needed to reach some closure about the confusing parts of herself before she could accept the "heroic" (and equally true) story that Ceballo saw for her.

Spend some time writing or thinking about a stressful event in your life. Perhaps it involved physical or mental abuse, health changes, a loss of someone important, or an anticipated relationship change. While acknowledging the ways you may have been hurt, think about what you gained from and how you dealt with the stressor itself. This process may be easier if you are not writing about a "hot" issue. How does this change in perspective affect how you feel?

CHOOSING STORIES THAT HEAL

Chodorow (1999) notes that our sense of meaning about our lives is not static; rather, it is continually created and recreated throughout our lives. A mother's closeness is comforting at the age of four, but can be suffocating at fourteen. The teenager may reject the closeness when things are going well ("She doesn't trust me"), but appreciate it when overwhelmed by external stressors ("She understands and comforts me"). Our stories, like any belief, support or undermine us and can cause anger, pain, sadness, joy, and fear.

Because the stories of our lives are not internally consistent and because we think differently about the same event at different points in time, there are several different stories we could tell. Perhaps some stories are more growth-promoting than others. Frankl (1959) described his own, often harrowing, experience in Auschwitz during World War II. Although it would have been easy for him to focus only on the meaninglessness of life or on how people are fundamentally bad, he drew different conclusions. During his imprisonment, he focused on his wife and family and attempted to make sense of his life and world. He even composed *Man's Search for Meaning* in his head. As he thought about himself and the people around him, he concluded that a sense of meaning was not sufficient to survive Auschwitz, but it certainly was necessary. Those people who felt they had nothing to live for had a difficult time putting one foot in front of another on the long enforced marches across country with little food. Those who had a sense of meaning and purpose could bridge the otherwise hopeless periods in their lives.

Some people are able to find positive reframes easily. When Mah (1997) was reunited with her aunt after the Cultural Revolution, she was appalled by the living conditions under which her aunt lived. Her aunt responded:

> I often think of life as a deposit of time. We are each allocated so many years, just like a fixed sum in a bank. When twenty-four hours have passed I have spent one more day. I read in the *People's Daily* that the average life expectancy for a Chinese woman is seventy-two. I am already seventy-four years old. I spent all my deposits two years ago and am on bonus time. Every day is already a gift. What is there to complain of? (p. 225)

Other people are not able to change their viewpoint as easily to find healing reframes. After the death of his son, Mervyn (in chapter 1) saw his life as over, or at best, as something to be endured. Jackson's family (in chapter 3) saw him as someone not worth caring about, and they actively rejected them. Rashelle, in chapter 4, saw herself as impotent and having nothing to offer. In the course of therapy, Mervyn began to see ways that he could honor his son *and* go on. Jackson's family saw how he *was* connected to them. As they acknowledged this, Jackson was able to stop pushing them away. Rashelle came to identify her real personal, familial, and cultural strengths and began using these more effectively.

Because multiple ways of looking at anything exist, one piece of the therapist's job is to help clients identify the hopeful stories about their lives.

This does not, however, mean changing reality (i.e., the glass is full), but acknowledging both the good and the bad. Jackson, for example, while caring about his mother and aunt, was also running into problems at school and using drugs heavily. He needed to find ways to accept both parts of himself, as well as to honor his vision of his future (cf. Waters & Lawrence, 1993). He wanted to feel that he belonged, although he was afraid to risk possible rejection from the people who meant the most to him, his aunt and mother.

Being empathic and sometimes taking a person's unstated point of view often helps us identify clients' strengths. To do this we "must find the person in [our] client and what is meaningful to that child, adolescent, man, or woman" (Ivey et al., 1997, p. 383). Why would Jackson behave as he did if he was not connected to his family? Sometimes, being involved and empathic means to be objective and to identify attributes that a client has overlooked. Rashelle's strengths jumped out at everyone, except her. Sometimes, as with Mervyn and his negative view of the future, being empathic means being able to step back and look at the broader picture. He *could* grieve for his son, yet find ways to be connected to the people in his life.

Willard (see table 8.6, p. 182) was moderately depressed as he anticipated retirement. He could directly control some problems (e.g., creating a financial plan), and he could influence others (e.g., communicating and establishing roles and expectations within his family). However, many of the issues that made retirement difficult were cultural and contextual factors over which he had little control. These included the Depression, the age of his friends, a youth-oriented culture, and the death of his father and brother shortly after their retirements. His therapist addressed the changeable, but also referred him to other agencies for additional help (see table 11.5, particularly Goal 3). He also encouraged Willard to become flexible in how he approached the unchangeable (see Goal 1). Although Willard could not change the uncontrollable, he could change how he perceived it. Most importantly, Willard could identify options that he previously had ignored while in crisis. In fact, as long as he did not see these options, he remained in crisis.

A MODEL FOR MAKING MEANING

Most meaning making occurs spontaneously and without professional help. People enter therapy only when they feel stuck and do not know what to do. Sometimes, many of the strategies that the lay population uses under these conditions (such as dismissing feelings and concerns, giving advice, and using distraction) are not helpful (Halonen & Santrock, 1997). The following discussion describes the meaning-making process that is part of good therapy.

TABLE 11.5 PROBLEMS AND INTERVENTIONS FOR TREATMENT OF WILLARD WHO IS MODERATELY DEPRESSED AS HE APPROACHES RETIREMENT

Willard
1. Willard finds it difficult to understand that a person can be retired *and* happy.
   a. Challenge beliefs that being retired leads inevitably to physical and psychological decline and deterioration.
   b. Identify peers in the community who have retired and have been successful in the transition into retirement. Encourage discussing the transition with at least one peer in order to identify strategies that can create a successful retirement.
2. Willard reports no hobbies and cannot imagine how he might spend his time during retirement.
   a. Brainstorm ideas about how to spend time in retirement.
   b. Explore at least three of these ideas and begin to put them into practice.
3. Willard is concerned about whether he and his family will have enough money to live on.
   a. Refer to financial planner in order to develop a plan to live comfortably on a reduced income.
   b. Monitor implementation of plan as needed.
4. Family relationships are rocky, and they increase his stress as he faces retirement. New roles and responsibilities are unclear.
   a. Discuss pending retirement with family members and identify expectations for the future.
   b. Practice successful communication patterns with family members.

Note: See chapter 8.

Accept Clients' Meanings First

Meaning making and problem solving cannot occur before the other person believes that his or her experience has been accepted and understood (Ivey et al., 1997; O'Hanlon, 1999). This was seen in the first exchange between Andor and Jalyse in chapter 9, where Jalyse attempted to push Andor toward change before she really listened to his story. Her goals made sense, but without the foundational understanding, her interventions fell on unfertile ground. Ivey (1984, as quoted in Ivey et al., 1997) worked with Martin, who described his fears after being trapped in quicksand. Ivey used a reflection of meaning to accept the past and his interpretations of those events, but moved Martin toward a new reframe of his experience:

> IVEY: *Is there anything positive? I know it sounds like a totally negative experience. Was there anything you could see that was positive about what happened? (Closed question, reflection of meaning, closed question)*
>
> MARTIN: *Well, it sure felt good when they saved me. I was scared, and I felt guilty, but at least they came and got me* (p. 384, client's name and therapeutic leads inserted for clarity and consistency).

Without first accepting his client's experiences in the statement ("I know it sounds like a totally negative experience"), Ivey (1984, as quoted in Ivey et al., 1997) would likely have found that his client would refuse any

Think about a place in your life where you are stuck. What sort of "stories" do you tell yourself about this? Are they hopeful, respectful, and compassionate?

Imagine you are your best friend or someone else who likes you. What would this person say to you in his or her most compassionate moments? If you are a religious person, what message would you receive from Jesus, Allah, Buddha, or other spiritual figure? How would this person or figure view you and your situation (O'Hanlon, 1999)? If you have formed a good picture of this conversation or message, how do you feel afterwards?

reframing of his experiences and perhaps would respond with "Yeah, but . . . " (see table 9.2, p. 203). But because Ivey listened empathically first, then accepted Martin's view of his experience, Martin was willing to consider alternative views of his experience.

Develop Positive Meanings

In early childhood, depression is best predicted by negative life events (Nolen-Hoeksema, Girgus, & Seligman, 1992). By late childhood, children's style of explaining events and the meanings they draw more fully explain the development of depression. Given this relationship, we as therapists must find ways to improve the explanatory style and meaning-making process of our teenage *and* adult clients.

Beck (1991) suggests that four factors are strongly predictive of negative thought patterns. Depression and anxiety most frequently occur when the data that could be brought to bear on the problem are:

1. Not immediately present in the here and now
2. Abstract
3. Central to self-esteem
4. Ambiguous

Unfortunately, as seen in the next example, culture-influenced mental health problems often share these problems.

Lenny, a gay man living in a small town, had been fired after his boss had made numerous off-color jokes about his sexuality and had put increasing pressure on him about his productivity. His employer denied that Lenny's sexuality had any influence on his decision. Lenny was confused and depressed. Although his job and his career in banking had been very important to him and his being fired had been devastating, his decision to be "out" was also important to him. Although he wanted to believe that his sexuality had not been a factor in the decision, his conclusions shifted almost hourly. With the important data ambiguous and unrecoverable, Lenny was unable to resolve this quandary. What, if anything, could he do to prevent anything similar from happening again? Would becoming more productive make a difference in future jobs? Was being fired an inevitable consequence of his affectional choices? Was he a worthy and acceptable person or did he deserve to be discriminated against?

Tori, in working with Lenny, first validated his perceptions of himself and his work and gave concrete reasons for why she believed his interpretation of events.

TORI: *Lenny, I wasn't there, but based on what you say, I think your boss's actions were the actions of a homophobe and unjustified. What I find telling is that two months after he finds out that you are gay, he fires you, saying that you had chronically bad interactions with your colleagues. You admit that your interactions with him were troubled, but that you had very positive relationships with your other colleagues, which matches my observations of you around town, your stories, and my experience with you in this room. You are an easy person to be with, someone who genuinely cares about the people around you . . . (Pause) What do you think about this? (Self-disclosure, influencing summarization, feedback, open question)*

With this intervention Tori quickly (albeit not immediately) addressed the concerns Lenny raised over several sessions and shifted his sense of meaning about these events. In doing so, she responded to the concerns identified by Beck (1991) that are predictive of depression and other negative thought patterns. Specifically, she pulled together concrete and unambiguous evidence from here-and-now observations to support her conclusions. He could use her intervention to develop a more supportive sense of meaning about his loss of job.

Ivey (1984, as quoted in Ivey et al., 1997, p. 384) does this even more gracefully with Martin when he asked, "Was there anything you could see that was positive about what happened?" By having Martin provide his own reframe, Ivey could both assess his willingness to accept a reframe and ensure that the reframe that was generated would be one that Martin could accept willingly.

Balance Responsibility with Control

While externalizing responsibility without sugarcoating the situation, Tori also began to return Lenny's sense of purpose. He could get another job and be successful. He could apply for other jobs without having all of his future employers also be homophobes. He could choose to file a complaint. Or he could go on with his life without allowing these events to overwhelm him.

Although the Truth was unrecoverable, Lenny could do some things to begin to make new meanings in his life. He talked to sympathetic coworkers to develop an objective stance about the requirements of the job. He began to think about what distinguished him from other tellers, only one aspect of which was his sexual orientation. After considerable thought, he decided to file a grievance against his supervisor, but only when he had concluded that he would use this action to get justice rather than determine Truth. Although the grievance was denied, he was able to be philosophical about it and find positive meaning. He felt good about the decision to start creating a paper trail for other GLBT employees. He took his life into his own hands rather than responding helplessly and hopelessly. He accepted responsibility for his own sense of self-worth. Although he concluded that life was sometimes unfair, he decided he did not need to accept the winds of fate as reflections on his own worth. With each of these changes, his depression began to lift. He looked for and found another job at which he was both happier and more successful.

Lenny's developing sense of meaning was one that placed the responsibility firmly on his boss's shoulders where it belonged, without denying the pieces that were his own, including the low productivity, poor timeliness in completing paperwork, and interpersonal problems with his employer. In the process of their work together, Tori and Lenny discussed things that he could do to avoid running into similar problems in the future *without* sacrificing his sense of self or his openness about his sexuality. In doing so, he regained a sense of control with its concomitant psychological advantages (Bradley et al., 1992; Delahanty et al., 1997; Shapiro, 1989).

Translate Insight into Action

Developing a sense of positive meaning in the face of the traumatic and overwhelming is often difficult. Insight alone can be therapeutic, because some clients naturally put their insights into action. However, some clients need to be reminded to translate insight into action. Lenny could not simply focus on his own failings or his employer's without doing anything about them. His meaning must be translated into different interactions with himself or others or with his changed values and goals. Prochaska (1999) summarizes these concerns, agreeing that balancing insight with action is important:

> [M]any patients . . . tend to substitute thinking and reflecting for acting. They can be very comfortable with clinicians who prefer contemplation-oriented processes. . . . But encouraging such clients to go deeper and deeper into more levels of their problems can be iatrogenic; that is, the treatment itself can produce negative outcomes, such as feeding into their problems of being "chronic contemplators." At some point, action must be taken. (p. 476)

Similarly, while some people are unable to translate insight into action, others are unable to translate action into insight that can generalize into action in other situations. Waters and Lawrence (1993) suggest that therapy should do more than just "fix" current problems, but also "heal" patterns that continue to get people into trouble. Although fixing can occur through paradoxical interventions and without insight, healing must combine insight *and* a different pattern of behaviors than ones used in the past. Dionne's therapist, for example, gave her family a behavior chart to get her children more active and cooperative around the house. Dionne's children met task goals, but Dionne never felt comfortable in applying this knowledge to other situations. She did not understand what made it successful or what she could do to use it in other situations. They ended up back in therapy two years later because they did not "own" the tools or feel comfortable using them. Dionne's first round of therapy had fixed her problems without healing them.

HOPELESSNESS AND COURAGE

Coping with life and problems requires considerable courage. It is often easier to pretend to be gruff and strong than to admit the presence of a problem and do something about it. This can be complicated by the reactions of family, friends, and acquaintances who have a difficult time distinguishing between acts of pseudocourage and real courage (see table 11.6). A woman who is crying after the breakup of her marriage may be more courageous than her husband who denies that there is a problem *if* she uses her fears to mobilize positive changes in her life.

This dialogue from a therapy session clarifies the relationship between failures of courage, hopelessness, and blame (Waters and Lawrence, 1993):

BONNIE: *You don't understand anything!*

IAN: *I understand that you want to run the family and avoid yourself. (Interpretation)*

BONNIE: *I don't! You're so stupid! That's not what I want. I just want to be left alone.*

IAN: *To have your way and avoid your feelings. (Interpretation)*

BONNIE: *No! (Confused) Just to protect myself and feel OK.*

IAN: *Protect yourself from what? What are you afraid of? (Open questions)*

BONNIE: *(Briefly tearing up) Nothing . . . Just leave me alone!*

IAN: *It's not nothing. I think you're scared to death. This is all a cover-up. (Feedback, interpretations)*

BONNIE: *(Starting to cry) I cannot stand the feelings I get! I just want to get the werewolf off my back.*

IAN: *The werewolf is the feelings you get if you can't protect yourself? (Closed question)*

BONNIE: *I hate it. It's so awful! You don't understand how those feelings are.*

IAN: *No I don't, but I want to. And your mom wants to. You've been hiding those feelings by being a tyrant, and it's not working. Have the courage to try something else: Let your mom and me in on this with you. We'll help you with those feelings. (Self-disclosure, interpretation and feedback, directive, self-disclosure)*

BONNIE: *(Sobbing) You don't know how bad they are!*

TABLE  **DIFFERENCES BETWEEN DISPLAYS OF PSEUDOCOURAGE AND REAL COURAGE**

Failures of Courage	Pseudocourage	Real Courage
Recognizing Feelings and Thoughts Becoming overwhelmed by feelings and thoughts without moving beyond them.	Denying the existence of bad feelings and thoughts.	Admitting and coping with bad feelings and thoughts.
Identifying Problems Seeing weaknesses only instead of also identifying coexisting strengths.	Pretending there is no problem; withdrawing from or compensating for the denial.	Facing and resolving a problem.
Interacting With Others Attempting to be what you believe others want you to be and entertaining or placating them.	Hiding insecurities and fears by presenting a gruff or unblemished exterior.	Interacting in an honest and authentic manner with others; asking for help; admitting real fears and insecurities.
Needing Help Asking for help even when unnecessary, especially as a way of maintaining relationships and resources.	Refusing help or any need for it.	Acknowledging that no one can do everything. Asking for help; disclosing the real number and extent of one's concerns.
Coping With a Problem Not coping; giving up; feeling helpless and defeated.	Using the same solutions over and over again, perhaps even harder, louder, or faster.	Conceding that old solutions have been unsuccessful and trying something new.
Searching for a Solution Not looking for a solution because it feels hopeless.	Making decisions rapidly, especially without thought; potential solutions identified dichotomously.	Considering the real pros and cons of all possible solutions and making a decision after examining these. Dichotomous solutions are rejected in favor of possible "grays."

IAN: *You're right. But I know they can't be as bad as the terror you live in, protecting yourself the whole time by fighting for control. Try to let go. (Feedback, reframe, directive;* pp. 99–100, italics in text, behavioral descriptions simplified from original text. Ian's name and microskills included for consistency.)

As long as Bonnie felt hopeless and could not see other options, she behaved in an angry and defensive pseudocourageous manner. When Ian was unable to see her situation from her point of view, his interpretations were blaming. As soon as he was able to fill in some context for her reactions (that Bonnie was overwhelmed and afraid, probably because of the very real stressors in her life), he was able to respond in a less pathologizing manner. At that point, he was able to take a more courageous stance with Bonnie and help her mother do so also. Bonnie's mother and Ian were able to begin to step outside of the "dance" they were engaged in and, rather than add more fuel to Bonnie's fears, help her hope that things could be better.

Hope *and* hopelessness are contagious. Ian's later interventions challenged Bonnie's belief (that change was impossible) by reframing her assessment of the losses she might face if she changed. The catastrophizing and stabilizing views of her situation ("It's so terrible, and there's nothing anyone can do to change it") were also addressed as she began to consider possible changes and potential benefits.

Because admitting a problem takes courage, some people may pretend that there is no problem. This helps them save face and maintain apparent courage. Others may admit that they do not have courage and may give up (see table 11.6). Instead of attempting something different, they conclude that a successful solution is impossible ("So why should I even try?").

Several problems lead to this kind of failure of courage and hope. Making change requires people to know where they want to go and to recognize how they can get there (Waters & Lawrence, 1993). More importantly, however, it requires believing that things can be different and gathering the courage to take the steps needed. Because of her cultural and religious background, Manuela (chapter 6, p. 124) had a difficult time believing that she could separate from her husband and *still* be loved by her family and accepted in her culture. Rather than thinking dichotomously about her husband and family, Manuela began to think about ways to meet her goals while staying connected to her family and culture. By choosing to recognize that she could be both autonomous *and* connected to her family, she was able to make a more sophisticated and courageous decision than choosing either one alone (see table 11.6).

Visions of the Future

This vision of the future is part of what is being assessed in contextual genograms. In the best of all possible scenarios, people will enter therapy with a hopeful and more or less achievable picture of their future (Waters & Lawrence, 1993). Rather than seeing what they *don't* want, they must develop a concrete picture of what they do want. "I want to listen to my children and support them in their decisions" is better than "I don't want to end up just like my mom." This picture of the future should be something that clients can control, rather than one that they must wait to have other people actualize (Walter & Peller, 1992). Although Manuela might prefer that her husband and family accept her unconditionally, she cannot change them. Her vision should be under her control, yet within her own personal, familial, and cultural values.

Many people enter therapy without a hopeful vision of the future, however (Beck, 1991). Like Mervyn, they are pessimistic and just want the pain to stop. People who feel hopeless about their future have no vision that can motivate them to take risks within the therapy experience and outside of it. They often become mired in ruminating about the past and present, rather than in planning the future.

Developing a vision for the future involves (1) challenging real and apparent obstacles in order to change and (2) developing a realistic picture of what the future might be (Prochaska, 1999). Sometimes, this can start relatively easily, as with the flip comment to Shaundra in chapter 8: "I've helped people much worse off than you." This touchstone kept her going through the next months of difficult therapy and allowed her to risk deciding where she wanted to go.

Clients may not have a vision of where they want to go, but therapists often have a failure of vision themselves (Waters & Lawrence, 1993). This seems especially true for work in the community mental health system, where indigent clients with a long history of problems also come with the tag, "I don't think you can do anything here." As long as we believe this, it will be true. Believing Shaundra could be helped (no one else had been able to) was the first step to being able to do so.

Conclusions

Our meanings of events direct the ways in which we live our life. When we perceive our life as damaged after a traumatic event, we experience negative outcomes. However, positive meanings and post-traumatic growth are possible. We can help our clients choose positive stories to tell about their lives. These stories can recognize strengths and courage and can attribute appropriate amounts of responsibility to the appropriate people and circumstances, all the while helping the client discover control. Rather than leading to a sense of isolation, their stories can leave them feeling connected and supported.

Therapy must provide a vision, but it also needs to nurture a sense of self-efficacy for meeting goals and developing the pathways for getting there (Bandura, 1997; Waters & Lawrence, 1993). If translating the vision into action is relatively easy, the first two steps are often the most difficult (Prochaska, 1999). Developing a positive sense of meaning can begin to build this sense of vision and self-efficacy. The struggle many people have with identifying the pathways for change is discussed in the next chapters.

BLAME, RESPONSIBILITY, AND CONTROL

Mrs. Shelton was a Native American mother of four, very overweight, and unemployed. Her three teenage children had already missed significant amounts of school. The school contacted Child Protective Services (CPS) to file a complaint about these absences. CPS, in turn, threatened to take custody of Mrs. Shelton's children if they did not go to school. When

Mrs. Shelton's family therapist contacted the family's caseworker, it became clear that the caseworker didn't like Mrs. Shelton and her children, had assumed that Mrs. Shelton did not see school as important, and had concluded that Mrs. Shelton might be causing their illnesses.

Unfortunately, the caseworker had not considered other options that might explain the children's truancy and the mother's attitude about it. In effect, the caseworker assumed that Mrs. Shelton did not care about her children, apparently because she was obese, had several missing teeth, was unemployed, and had been living in one of the poorer sections of town. The seven hypotheses in table 12.1 explain the initial data on the truancy and other issues, but they do not explain other pieces of the Shelton story equally well. In other words, some are not *comprehensive* hypotheses, even when combined with other explanations.

Mrs. Shelton was unemployed, but she worked hard. She took care of her four children, cleaned five houses a week, and clearly valued hard work and education. She also studied for a high school equivalency in the evenings after her children went to bed, and she preached the importance of school to her children whenever she could.

Every morning, she would get her children ready for school and send them out to the bus stop. She would then leave the house at 7:30 a.m. to clean houses until her children came home from school. Because she was gone during the day, her children pretended to take the bus to school and would often go back home to sleep or to spend time with their friends. Until the school called her and talked to *her* rather than to her children, she was unaware of the truancy problem. Even though she knew, she had a difficult time getting her children to school consistently—they would disappear in the morning and return after she went to work. Her caseworker was right in at least one instance, however. Mrs. Shelton frequently took them to the doctor for relatively minor and vague symptoms.

Mrs. Shelton's caseworker assumed that the school attendance problems were related to Hypothesis 1 and Hypothesis 4 (see table 12.1). However, their family therapist gave a more comprehensive and respectful assessment and concluded that the behavior was definitely *not* related to Hypothesis 1, because Mrs. Shelton *did* value education. Also, the therapist was unable to support Hypotheses 2 and 4 because the doctor visits, although frequent, were not for severe or unusual illnesses. There was significant support, however, for Hypotheses 5 and 7. Although it appeared that Mrs. Shelton was an effective parent when she had time and energy, she had a difficult time parenting at other times (partial support for Hypothesis 6). Therefore, the therapists focused on ways to reduce stressors and assist her in taking a consistent and firm parental stance.

Consider a problem in your own life or in the life of a client. Generate as many alternative explanations for this behavior as possible. Go back over them and think about which ones are blaming and which ones are unlikely. Why do you put them in these categories? What are the implications of the explanations for you or for the treatment? Are some more helpful? Are some more likely to build up or break down the relationship with the other person?

TABLE 12.1 HYPOTHESES TO EXPLAIN PROBLEMS IN THE SHELTON FAMILY

	Predictions	Interventions
Hypothesis 1 Mrs. Shelton doesn't care about her children's education or see it as important.	Mrs. Shelton does not attempt to find other ways to support her children's education, does not pick up her children's homework when they are absent from school, and will not attend school functions.	Identify ways to help Mrs. Shelton see school as important to her children's future employment opportunities and to her ability to retain custody of her children.
Hypothesis 2 Mrs. Shelton's children are sickly.	Children will have a series of well-documented illnesses and effective treatments if these are normal childhood illnesses. However, some illnesses such as chronic fatigue syndrome, allergies, and cancer may not be diagnosed as rapidly. There is often a lag time of as much as five years or longer for some illnesses to be diagnosed.	Get children good and consistent medical care and support effective preventive medicine.
Hypothesis 3 Mrs. Shelton is receiving secondary gain, such as help around the house and company, for keeping her children at home.	Children are more likely to be kept at home when she is under stress.	Identify source of secondary gain and remove it. Give positive attention for using effective parenting strategies. Remove identified stressors.
Hypothesis 4 Mrs. Shelton is receiving secondary gain, such as attention or sympathy, for keeping her children ill or in the sick role.	Illnesses will not follow any predictable pattern and will have vague symptoms. However, some problems diagnosed initially as malingering or fictitious disorders are later discovered to be rare and poorly understood illnesses.	Remove secondary gain to the degree possible. Provide attention for adaptive and growth-promoting behavior. Reduce identified stressors.
Hypothesis 5 Mrs. Shelton is too stressed to be able to get her children to school regularly.	Mrs. Shelton's children attend school regularly when her life is less stressful.	Help Mrs. Shelton identify ways to make their lives less stressful, such as developing effective coping strategies and improving the support system.
Hypothesis 6 Mrs. Shelton has a difficult time assuming a parenting role with her children. As a result, she has difficulty getting them to do anything they don't want to do.	Her children's school attendance is unrelated to stressors. Mrs. Shelton will have a difficult time getting them to come in for curfew, perform chores around the home, and go to bed on time.	Address family structure, supporting Mrs. Shelton in the parental role and in making parental decisions.
Hypothesis 7 Mrs. Shelton cares about her children and is, as a result, cautious about their health.	Mrs. Shelton will take care of her children in a variety of ways and is generally perceived as a good parent by her children and by outside observers.	Identify ways to help her keep her children healthy and to help her accurately identify when they are not. Support other ways of caring for her children.

Note: Hypotheses are not mutually exclusive. Several could be correct simultaneously.

HYPOTHESES IN THERAPY

Therapeutic hypotheses can be evaluated in many different ways. Many people prefer the normative way of explaining things ("This is the way it's always been done") but there are other, arguably better, ways of choosing explanations. Therapists should prefer parsimonious and comprehensive explanations that are helpful in therapy. They should also have solid research support, and they should definitely avoid blaming in their theorizing.

Science has generally used the law of parsimony to evaluate competing hypotheses, preferring the simplest, most economical, and streamlined of two *equal* hypotheses. Copernicus' description of the solar system did not explain the action of the stars any better than pre-Copernican systems. However, astronomers use this explanation because his system of elliptical paths around the sun was much more parsimonious than the complicated systems of circles within circles previously used to explain the paths of the celestial bodies. While Rube Goldberg's machines are entertaining, they are not useful because they require incredible expenditures in terms of time, energy, and material resources to accomplish simple tasks like opening the door or feeding the cat. Similarly, Bowers and Farvolden (1996) acknowledged that psychodynamic explanations may be helpful, but suggest that simpler, contemporaneous explanations may be more parsimonious and, thus, more useful.

A good therapeutic hypothesis should also be comprehensive. When choosing among the hypotheses that explain Mrs. Shelton's behavior, the preferred choice of explanations was one that explained a variety of behaviors, rather than only her children's nonattendance of school (refer to explanations in table 12.1). Some hypotheses could explain one or two pieces of her behavior, but none explained each piece equally well. Despite the fact that simpler hypotheses that explained parts of her behavior existed, a more complex hypothesis involving pieces of hypotheses 5, 6, and 7 was necessary to comprehensively explain (1) her parenting behavior under stress, (2) her children's health, and (3) their truancy.

These hypotheses were also therapeutically productive. It gave the therapy team insight into the mother's behavior and helped the group identify clear and specific things to do to resolve the Shelton family's problems. These family therapists helped Mrs. Shelton reduce stressors and take a firm and consistent stance concerning her children's behavior. They encouraged her to find new supports, after having lost others when she moved from the reservation to the city. They helped her work with the children's pediatrician to rule out some of the medical issues about which Mrs. Shelton was concerned, as well as to develop some simple guidelines for identifying when her children really needed to go to the doctor or should be kept home from school.

For the hypotheses used to guide interventions with the Shelton family to be useful in identifying a path for treatment, the treatment strategy should be associated with theory and research that support it. For example, a hypothesis that the Shelton children are out of balance and therefore need to spend six hours a day standing on their heads is a relatively simple, comprehensive, and even productive hypothesis. However, no theoretical or empirical evidence suggests that this intervention would be helpful. Without such support, it is unclear why one hypothesis should be chosen over another. The lack of theory and research has plagued many interesting and novel therapeutic approaches.

Finally, unlike scientific hypotheses, a good therapeutic hypothesis should avoid blaming clients and pathologizing their behavior. Besides having no redeeming qualities, blaming another person serves as a barrier to good communication (Alexander, Waldron, Barton, & Mas, 1989; Halonen & Santrock, 1997; Lussier, Sabourin, & Wright, 1993), and it disrupts therapeutic rapport. However, when therapists are optimistic and focus on "what works" or the exceptions in a problem, families also become more optimistic and hopeful (Alexander et al., 1989; Melidonis & Bry, 1995). When therapists are hopeful, treatment periods are also briefer (O'Hanlon & Weiner-Davis, 1989).

BLAME

Traditional therapeutic models generally focus on individual and intrapsychic issues at the expense of context. Even behavioral models, which consider situational issues much more extensively, tend to focus more narrowly on situational and environmental factors, time of day, and perhaps emotions and cognitions. Cultural values, group identification, and historical factors are largely ignored, despite the fact that each of these may strongly influence how a situation is perceived. When these factors are overlooked, the causes of behavior are underexplained. When behavior is poorly explained and situational causes are ignored, the therapist is more likely to blame the client, pathologize his or her behavior, and feel less empathy (Becker & Lamb, 1994).

Therapeutic Blame

Western values emphasize independent and autonomous approaches over relationship-oriented, interdependent, and contextualized ones. This decontextualized stance maintains blaming. Middle- and upper-class North Americans, in particular, believe in the individual's ability to lift up himself or herself by their "bootstraps." The unspoken assumption is that any

Read your last assessment or treatment plan. Imagine being your client(s). How would you feel about the assessment? Would your clients feel that you understood them if they were to read your reports? Would they think that you were being respectful?

How do you feel about the idea of sharing your reports with your clients? Why? How does your verbal feedback differ from your written report? Do your reports come from a strength-based or problem-focused perspective (Powell & Batsche, 1997)?

success is due to the person alone, just as is any failure. Because of this focus on the individual, most therapists recommend that clients focus on changing their own behavior rather than trying to change someone else's. In these cases, Walter and Peller (1992) suggest that therapists ask, "What are *you* doing?" or "What are you *doing?*" This style of questioning focuses attention on things clients *can* control (it's considerably more difficult to influence people not in the therapy room). Unless done well, however, these questions can place the *responsibility* for the problem on the client. This is a tricky dilemma for both therapist and client ("How can we help people recognize control without blaming them?").

Consider the dilemma Willie faces with Macy. As part of their work together, Willie asked Macy to pay attention to the situation and think about what she is doing before her partner blows up. She needs to discover ways to reduce the probability of violence, but if Macy believes that Willie was implying the domestic violence was her fault, he did her a disservice. Therapy needs to avoid even unintentional blaming and should help clients exercise the control that they *do* have.

Most therapies focus on client weaknesses rather than strengths (Powell & Batsche, 1997; Saba & Rodgers, 1990). These models are more likely to identify and discuss problems in parenting than its successes. They may recognize maladaptive coping or relational styles instead of adaptive ones. Problematic boundaries and structures are more likely to be identified than helpful ones. Saba and Rodgers (1990) note that the Joint Commission on the Accreditation of Hospitals, for example, requires that client charts include a problem list. A list of client strengths is not similarly required. The idea that strengths and successes may be key to identifying solutions is foreign to most therapists.

The assumption that therapists should focus on problems has face validity. Because our job is to resolve problems, many believe we should focus on problematic behaviors (Waters & Lawrence, 1993). In taking the approach described here, we are attempting to bypass problems. This is illustrated in the old story about the woman searching for her keys under the streetlight. She is asked, "Where did you lose your keys?" She responds with, "I lost them down the street, but there's more light here." Although the metaphor makes considerable sense in that situation, it makes only a little sense here. As Albert Einstein noted, "The significant problems we have cannot be solved at the same level of thinking with which we created them" (as cited in Moncour, n.d.). Focusing on problems not only maintains the blaming and conflictual stance within the family, but it is often a source of the problems (Alexander et al., 1989).

How do you feel about the idea of focusing on strengths rather than weaknesses in therapy? How do you think it can be helpful (or unhelpful)? If you had to guess what proportion of change seemed to be attributable to more hopeful intervention strategies, what would you guess?

The Criticism-Blame-Shame Cycle

Waters and Lawrence (1993) argue that many therapists are caught in a criticism-blame-shame cycle and have a difficult time interrupting it. Suicide attempts are often derogated as "attention seeking" rather than "cries for help" or expressions of a desire to make things different. Therapists often describe work with people with borderline personality disorder as chaotic and countertransference-provoking (Becker & Lamb, 1994; Rockland, 1992). But, Bachelor and Horvath (1999) report that problems in therapy are better explained by the style of therapeutic responses—critical and blaming, rather than honest, open, and respectful—than by the client's relationship history. G. Greenberg (1997) goes further and highlights the roles that people's individual and cultural values play in our diagnosis of borderline personality disorder.

What stops therapists from adopting optimistic and non-blaming sets in therapy? The parenting literature argues that we need to believe that being respectful and hopeful is important *and* to have faith in our ability to behave in this manner (Perozynski & Kramer, 1999). Generally, mothers and fathers in this study identified positive, child-centered strategies such as communicating, negotiating, compromising, and problem solving as the most effective approaches for handling sibling conflicts. Despite this, parents often did not use positive approaches. In fact, they tended to use negative patterns that included controlling, punishing, threatening, withdrawing privileges, or using passive nonintervention strategies. Their use of more positive methods was related to their possession of child-centered skills and their ability to see these strategies as unambiguously credible.

Perozynski and Kramer (1999) ask whether or not people have the skills to act in a strength-based, as opposed to a blaming, manner. For therapists, the answer is a definite "yes." Most of these skills are taught early on in graduate school therapy courses, before the "important" classes like model-specific therapy. Other strength-based skills can be easily taught and learned.

Do we believe that these strength-based skills are credible and account for a significant proportion of therapeutic change, as seen by Perozynski and Kramer (1999)? Probably not. Although most of us believe in the importance of active and respectful listening, many of us probably see it as relatively unimportant compared to the contributions of the therapeutic model. Lambert (Asay & Lambert, 1999; Lambert, 1992), however, suggests that model-specific interventions account for only about 15% of the variation in therapeutic outcomes, while the remaining 85% is attributable to common factors consistent with strength-based approaches—identification of client strengths and supports outside of therapy, 40%; the therapeutic relationship, 30%; hopefulness and expectancies, 15%. The field tends to minimize the contributions of strength-based approaches to clients, attributing change to model-specific factors despite significant evidence to the contrary (Hubble, Duncan, & Miller, 1999b).

An Example: Aaron, a Child with Tourette's Syndrome

Consider Aaron, a 14-year-old boy diagnosed with Tourette's syndrome, a neurological disorder characterized by motor and vocal tics (T. Thompson, 1999). His parents' struggle with the issues raised by this disorder, especially his anger, highlight the concerns discussed here. His parents ask, "How much of Aaron's behavior is evidence of his illness and how much is his responsibility?" (p. Z12). The parents are, because of their differing conclusions, split on issues of discipline. His older brother, also diagnosed with Tourette's (although a much milder case), comments on his parents' question:

> Even if [Aaron's anger is] not caused by the disorder in and of itself, one thing affects another. . . . But I think without the Tourette's, he would not have such severe problems, and maybe none at all." (p. Z12)

The problems Aaron's family faces are common ones in North America, a culture that emphasizes autonomy and personal responsibility, yet also looks to excuse behavior outside personal control (Seligman et al., 2001). Although we do not hold a man criminally responsible when voices order him to kill his wife and children, we do hospitalize him until he is no longer a threat to himself or to society. When an intoxicated woman loses control of her car and kills someone, we hold her responsible, but she may be charged with involuntary manslaughter rather than murder. If the prosecution were able to demonstrate that she knew what she was doing and that she controlled her actions, and perhaps even planned them out beforehand, she would be charged with murder.

North American psychology is immersed in the cultural ideals of autonomy and personal responsibility. It has tended to hold people responsible for their actions and has tended to focus on intrapsychic factors leading to their irresponsible behavior. But therapists can overlook cultural and contextual factors influencing a problem, unless they are directed to see them. So, where does this approach leave a child like Aaron? If we choose to blame Aaron or to excuse his responsibility, Aaron as well as his parents remains caught. Blaming holds him culpable for behavior outside his real control, which leads to greater anxiety and self-hatred as he internalizes failures. Excusing his behavior may maintain his self-esteem, which may come at the cost of keeping him a child and ignoring the things he *can* do.

His family's handling of his competitive diving may be a good example of a successful solution to this dilemma. When a ticcing episode interfered with a dive, Aaron asked his father to talk to the judges about Tourette's, and the judges allowed him a second dive. Afterward, his dives were judged on their own merit. Aaron is given the help needed to level the playing field, but his performance is evaluated for what it is.

Unfortunately, other Tourette-related situations are not as easily handled. Vocal and motor tics can be identified readily, but what if Aaron's tantrums are a kind of emotional tic? What if they occur when people expect him to handle more than he can? What if this leads to his becoming stressed and overwhelmed? Perhaps tantrums would be reduced if he were given shorter and less stressful school periods during which he does not need to suppress tics to avoid being teased. Should he, as a 14-year-old, be expected to control these factors perfectly every time? Although he should be given good situations as much of the time as possible, he should also be held responsible for his tantrums, as well as for any physical damage caused at these times.

Invisible Handicaps

If attributing responsibility is confusing when we talk about physical problems or illnesses, it becomes even more complicated when we talk about "invisible handicaps." These are things that we may not even see, but that oppress individuals or limit their options. To what extent should their families, friends, and therapists accept excuses for problematic behavior? Should everyone agree that Patricia's drinking is merely a function of her genetic background, which was shaped by her alcoholic mother, grandfather, and aunts, and thus is not her fault? Would it matter if her drinking occurred only when she was severely depressed rather than only when she went dancing on Friday nights? What if Kyle's spending binges, which resulted in more than $45,000 in debts, occurred during manic episodes? Would you react differently than if his spending binges seemed unrelated to a mental health diagnosis?

Excusing people or holding them accountable is a difficult question. One example is Eugene, a man with mild left hemiplegia resulting from a birth injury, who had a history of depressive and manic episodes. During the depressive episodes, he would hear a cacophony of screaming voices that told him he was worthless and that he should kill himself. He was moderately cooperative with his psychiatrist and took a mood stabilizer regularly. He hated his antipsychotic medication, though, and took it only when the voices became overwhelming. He said he had a "chemical imbalance" and could not do anything about it. Also, he was puzzled and angry when his psychiatrist referred him to a psychologist.

When we examine Eugene's psychosocial history, it becomes obvious that many things were going poorly in his life. On one hand, he was under-employed and poverty-stricken and had medical problems, family stress, and a history of abuse (see table 12.2). On the other hand, he had

TABLE 12.2 EUGENE'S PSYCHOSOCIAL HISTORY

Problem

Current symptoms
Reports a history of infections and other relatively minor, but extremely bothersome illnesses occurring over the last two years. These have led to his taking one brief medical leave.

Beliefs about symptoms
Saw symptoms as primarily medical in nature, but willing to consider his physician's suggestions.

Personal history of psychological disorders
Although a "well-behaved child," he reports being seriously out of control beginning in his teens. He has abused alcohol and a range of legal and illegal substances. He has been hospitalized on numerous occasions for suicidal ideation, generally during depressive episodes. He reports hearing voices during manic and depressive episodes and having difficulty trusting others.

Family history of psychological disorders
Family of origin is chaotic and has a positive history of affective disorders and substance abuse.

Current Context

Recent events
Reports significant stressors, but these are no greater than others that he has reported in the past. Stressors, however, include health problems, poverty, chaotic relationships with his partner and their children, and a history of physical and emotional abuse.

Physical condition
Has some left hemiplegia from an injury incurred at birth. His seizures have been under control for the last 32 years, and he no longer takes medication for them.

He is 20 pounds overweight, does not exercise, and tends to eat a fair amount of junk food,

Drug and alcohol use
Has a history of significant polysubstance use and abuse during his 20s and 30s, but has been abstinent for the last ten years except during several major crises.

Intellectual and cognitive functioning
Has above-average intelligence. He maintained a high college GPA despite not having the time to study or read his textbooks. His children are in gifted programs at their school.

Coping style
Takes his antidepressant medication regularly and his antipsychotic medication as needed. Otherwise, he reports that there is nothing he can do and locks himself in his room when he gets overwhelmed. He listens to music sometimes when he's upset and tends to work harder when stressed.

Self-concept
Appears very competent and composed, yet describes himself as "a fraud" and expects to be "found out" at some point. Self-esteem is very fragile during depressive periods.

Sociocultural background
Identifies with the "underdog" and goes out of his way to make people who are "different in any way" feel comfortable. Because he lives in a largely Euro-American community, most of his friends are, as he is, working-class Euro-Americans.

Religion and spirituality
Was raised a Baptist and continues to think spirituality is important. He has not gone to church regularly in seven years, because of his differences with the minister over handicapped access to the church and affirmative action issues.

(continued)

TABLE 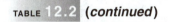 **12.2** (*continued*)

Resources and Barriers

Individual resources
Is very bright and has good social skills, especially with acquaintances. He is a hard worker and moderately hopeful, although not optimistic, about getting major stressors resolved in the future. He likes to putter around the house, but the house requires more work than he has time or money for.

Social resources, such as friends and family
Has a number of friends for whom he is often a significant support and resource. However, he does not disclose himself to them, nor does he ask them for help when he runs into problems.

His female partner of 12 years has significant mental health issues, has been diagnosed with borderline personality disorder, and is often very reactive when he has a depressive episode. She generally becomes depressed at these points, and he needs to take care of her. Their relationship is rocky at best.

Their three children from previous relationships do not get along with one another, and they get along even less with their respective step-parents. Evenings together are often disrupted by screaming and tears.

His family of origin continues to be verbally abusive at times and only minimally supportive.

Work
He is a college graduate, but is underemployed and looking for a better position. He continues to qualify for food stamps.

He would like to get his master's degree so he can get a better job, but he needs more pay to be able to afford to go back to school.

Community resources
Has an antagonistic attitude toward his daughter's school, which he believes does not provide either a good education or adequate services for her needs.

His family income is just above the poverty line, but is low enough that he is still eligible for food stamps. His family has received services from Child Protective Services, although he does not believe that the workers listen to his concerns.

He has a very positive relationship with his psychiatrist, but he is afraid that she will hospitalize him if he honestly discloses the depth of his suicidal ideation. His partner's therapist sees *him* as "the problem."

Community contributions
Has been active with two groups in the community that address issues for people with disabilities.

Mentors and models
Has several people in his field within the community who have been very supportive and have mentored him actively during his career. He tends to see them as qualitatively different from himself. He believes that he will be unable to do the things they have been able to do in their lives.

Obstacles to change
Sees his problems as "biological" and beyond his control. He tends to fight any implication that he has any control over current events because he might then be blamed for them.

Therapeutic relationship
Likes both his therapist and psychiatrist and is open with his therapist about the range and severity of his problems. He is afraid to disclose suicidal ideation to his psychiatrist because he feels he might be hospitalized as a result.

significant, often overlooked strengths such as his empathy for and support of others, which was a good, (albeit underutilized) support system. Other strengths included a willingness to make changes in the community in order to make his life better, his work around the home, his intelligence and commitment to education, and his work ethic. As these findings were discussed in therapy, he was able to acknowledge that these strengths and skills could be used to cope with problems in other parts of his life. He began being more empathic toward his teenage children when they were stressed, a skill that came naturally whenever he talked to friends and acquaintances, but which initially clashed with his beliefs about good parenting (see Perozynski & Kramer, 1999). He began to notice how his children were calmer when he talked to them empathically.

Eugene was also able to look at some of his weaknesses and think about making small, but helpful, changes. He began to make three changes in his life. Just like people who receive less social support in their lives experience more emotional conflict (Emmons & Colby, 1995), he began talking proactively to people in his wide, but underutilized, support system whenever he became depressed. He had previously waited until he was severely suicidal before attempting to find help. His family also began to work on developing a healthier communication style with each other, which decreased the amount of negatively expressed emotions (Simoneau, Miklowitz, & Saleem, 1998). Finally, he began to work on developing a wider array of coping strategies and self-soothing behaviors whenever he became stressed or depressed, such as listening to soothing music, reading books, lighting candles, and walking in the woods. Together these interventions significantly decreased the chaos in his life and the fluctuation of his moods. He continued to take medication to regulate his moods, but his suicidal periods decreased significantly in both duration and intensity, which were clearly linked to major life stressors. His psychiatric hospitalizations, previously at one or two per year, stopped completely.

Because Eugene's mood fluctuations seemed to have a biological component, he responded well to medication. However, accepting that he had no control over his moods, as he had initially tried to tell his psychiatrist, underestimated the role that his environment played in his moods and in his ability to control his mood stressors. Although he had often felt that he was at the mercy of his own biology, he now felt more powerful and capable. This improved self-concept, in turn, influenced his actions in other parts of his life. He found a better job, ended his present relationship, and eventually moved in with a more stable and supportive woman.

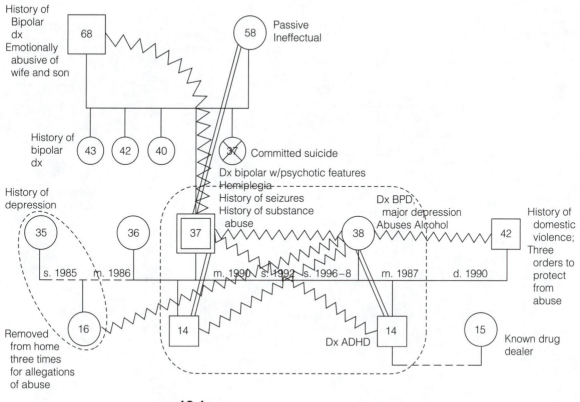

History of
Bipolar
dx
Emotionally
abusive of
wife and son

Passive
Ineffectual

History of
bipolar
dx

Committed suicide

Dx bipolar w/psychotic features
Hemiplegia
History of seizures
History of substance
abuse

Dx BPD,
major depression
Abuses Alcohol

History of
domestic
violence;
Three
orders to
protect
from
abuse

History of
depression

s. 1985   m. 1986

m. 1990 s. 1992 s. 1996–8   m. 1987   d. 1990

Removed
from home
three times
for allegations
of abuse

Dx ADHD

Known drug
dealer

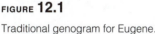

FIGURE 12.1

Traditional genogram for Eugene.

Strength-based Genograms

Traditional genograms are useful in identifying problem areas (McGoldrick et al., 1999). They can identify the things that are going well, although they often include conflict lines, patterns of substance abuse, mental illness, deaths, suicides, and enmeshments at the expense of anything healthy.

When Eugene entered therapy with a previous therapist, they did a traditional genogram, part of which is included in figure 12.1. As might be expected, this genogram focused on the mental illness and conflict within his family. During a period of frustration with the negativity in his family ("You must think we're all nuts!"), he asked to look at some of the strengths in his family as well. This had been something we had been doing for him, but he had been avoiding these strengths. His new genogram looked, in part, like that seen in figure 12.2.

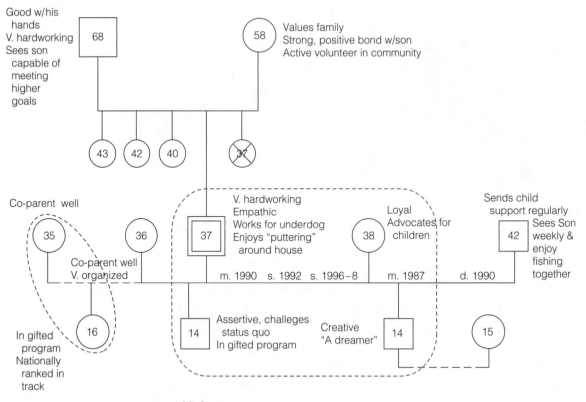

FIGURE **12.2**

Strength-based genogram for Eugene.

Preparing this strength-based genogram was often difficult for Eugene, because he tended to believe that he was from a "crazy" and dysfunctional family. The strengths of his birth father and stepfather were initially mixed compliments. He had difficulty identifying *any* strengths for his father. Although the dysfunction was still there when he completed his genogram, he was more hopeful about his ability to change at the end. Rather than being an anchor around his neck that would inevitably drag him down, he began thinking about his family more hopefully and as a source of support and strength. Furthermore, rather than the changes he hoped for coming out of the blue, now he saw these as based in family strengths that he could choose to develop. He concluded that it was unlikely that he would be like them in every way, but that he could be like them in positive ways, including his work ethic and concern about community action and change, rather than only negative ones.

Countertransference

Our blaming is often related to countertransference, which is all of our reality and nonreality-based reactions to clients. Countertransference can be influenced by our developmental histories, values, and current struggles. Kia commented that she was uncomfortable with inviting certain kinds of clients, especially those with poor hygiene, into the privacy of her office. After some work on this issue, she began to acknowledge that she wanted to distance herself from the poverty of her own childhood, something that still felt very close. Les' partner was struggling with the sequelae of sexual abuse. He found it difficult to work effectively with perpetrators because he kept fantasizing about doing the things to them that he wanted to do to his partner's father and uncle. He imagined his clients' abusive acts in detail, but found it difficult to think about other parts of their lives. For him, they *were* the abuse, and he had difficulty seeing them objectively and empathically.

Knowing ourselves and our limitations is an important piece of our preparation to do therapy. Kia decided to tape her work with welfare clients and specifically discuss this work in the course of supervision. Les realized that sexual abuse was still a hot issue for him. Although his first response was to avoid work with perpetrators, he realized that his reactions also contaminated work with survivors, a group that was a significant part of his agency's clientele. He decided that he needed to work through his own issues as part of a partner's group.

Both Kia and Les recognized their issues and, with some discomfort, decided to work on them. However, the issues that cause countertransference are such a normal part of our experience that they can be difficult to identify and challenge. Karl could not admit his own blind spots in his work with Luci, a poet of Italian extraction, who tended to look at her life from many different points of view and poke at it as part of her own spiritual and psychological growth. She was emotionally expressive in her descriptions of concerns, a common response style among Italian Americans (Giordano & McGoldrick, 1996). However, as a result of his gender and cultural background (both of which valued emotional restraint), Karl, a Euro-American man of German extraction (Hinawer & Wetzel, 1996), found it difficult to see Luci's style of self-disclosure in a positive fashion. Instead, he wondered what she wasn't telling him ("If she's willing to show this much, how much more is there?"). This conclusion also fit with his early training in psychodynamic techniques, which influenced his tendency to see things from a pathology framework. Luci stayed in therapy with Karl for a while, but struggled with him when she recognized that he pathologized parts of her that she liked and that she thought were effective. After she dropped out of therapy with him, he began to challenge his interpretations of her behavior and his identifications of "normal" and "healthy" behavior.

STRENGTHS

Normal Social, Developmental, and Cultural Constraints

Context is easy to overlook. When we ignore it, even the normal can be pathologized. For this reason, it is important to understand normal development, typical cultural values and norms, and common responses to stressors. Yalom (1989) described his reaction to a grieving mother's coping mechanisms as being initially appalled that she maintained her dead daughter's bedroom intact and even slept in her bed, until he interviewed other grieving parents and saw that her responses were common. O'Hanlon and Weiner-Davis (1989) explain it this way:

> Grieving follows a loss, chaos thrives in homes filled with children, major adjustments follow the birth of a child, tension and worry characterize financially unstable families, and so on. Sometimes, external events create challenges that are difficult to overcome. (p. 99)

People will call their therapist days after a funeral (while grieving is still within normal limits) concerned about a parent who is "crying all the time." Of course, it would be different if the parent were suicidal, but labeling the "normal" as "abnormal" is not helpful when it is not maladaptive. Normal grieving helps people come to terms with their losses, and labeling normative and adaptive behavior encourages people to blame themselves. Rather than resolving the problem, it adds to it without helping the afflicted recognize the role of external events in their lives (O'Hanlon & Weiner-Davis, 1989). Understanding the typical often allows therapists to empathize and respond without pathologizing.

For a period of more than 35 minutes in 1964, Kitty Genovese was stabbed to death in front of 38 neighbors. Their failure to act or to call the police created a huge public outcry. Latané and Darley (1968) eventually suggested that this failure to intervene over such a long period, while appalling, was not surprising. They attributed the witnesses' behavior (or lack thereof) to a diffusion of responsibility in an ambiguous situation and suggested that their failure to help was precisely because there were so many people observing the murder.

Latané and Darley (1968) described the bystanders' behavior as normal and understandable, but they did not excuse it. In fact, subsequent research focused on bystander apathy and factors that exacerbated the failure of people to act altruistically. Similarly, our job as therapists is to recognize whether or not behavior is normal or typical, to challenge it when maladaptive, and to encourage our clients to choose healthier patterns of living. We also need to recognize and nurture our clients' strengths.

Distinguishing the normal from the pathological is also a problem with developmental issues (Waters & Lawrence, 1993). When is it unusual and problematic for a child to be afraid of the dark? Is it unusual for a five-year-old to be playing doctor? What about a nine-year-old? When is telling stories more than that, and how can you tell the difference between stories and lies? A good therapist will know and understand these developmental norms. He or she will also understand how these norms depend upon contextual issues such as culture, religious background, and intelligence. As with "normal" group phenomena, our goal is to understand behavior without excusing it and to find the healthy and competent goal in the midst of the unusual or problematic behavior (Waters & Lawrence, 1993). Tyrone, age four, frequently wrote his name on walls, then denied it despite the irrefutable evidence. He also hid behind and under furniture, forcing his single mother to search frantically. When Arlene pointed out that Tyrone was bright, competent, and searching for attention the only way he knew how, Tyrone's mother was able to identify more positive ways of giving him attention. She was soon being amused by her son's creativity.

As Karl belatedly discovered in his work with Luci, cultural issues also influence our understanding of the normal. A large and enmeshed family setting might not be normal for British families, but would be comfortable and adaptive for Italians and Maltese (McGoldrick et al., 1996). Conversely, British families would feel cold and distant to Italian and Maltese observers. Although Jews tend to identify, discuss, and agonize over emotional and physical pain, people with Irish backgrounds tend to repress and deny it to a point that they not only fail to express the pain, but also cannot identify its location (McGill & Pearce, 1996).

Awareness of "typical" behavior is not enough, if typical means typical for middle-class Euro-Americans. Laotian families, for example, tend to be relaxed in terms of sleeping, eating, and parenting strategies relative to middle-class U.S. families (Zaharlick, 2000). Rules are often not explicitly stated, and children are expected to learn by example. They are also expected to eat and sleep when hungry or tired. Food is given to fussy children as a culturally appropriate response to emotional problems. Elisabeth, an upper middle-class African American working with a Laotian couple and their angry adolescent son, was surprised at the relative laxness of rules in this family. Their rules were generally functional and culturally normative, but she focused instead on the family's acculturation patterns and how the family's style worked for them. Rather than asking whether a behavioral pattern is normal, perhaps therapists should consider first how well it works or doesn't work for the individual and the system.

Strength-based Approaches

Within the last 15 years, strength-based approaches have become especially prominent among providers of services for children (Bean et al., 2000; Berg, 1994; M. H. Epstein, 1999; Powell & Batsche, 1997). They are commonly used among those working with families and adults (O'Hanlon, 1999; O'Hanlon & Weiner-Davis, 1989; Waters & Lawrence, 1993). In part, this change in the field is the consequence of the civil rights movement, when treatment decisions were questioned as biased against the groups out of power (Powell & Batsche, 1997). It is also based in the long tradition of Afrocentric social work that has been practiced since the beginning of the 20th century (Carlton-LaNey, 1999).

Problem-focused and strength-based models adopt different approaches to therapy. Generally, problem-focused models explore the problem situation and motivations for behaving in the problematic way, while strength-based models explore the exceptions to the problem and when things are successful. Good coaches may briefly acknowledge the "problem" an athlete is having in competition, but then focus on what works and how to get there (Waters & Lawrence, 1993): "Try holding your racket a little closer to the head." We can be more like coaches than problem-focused therapists.

Strength-based approaches acknowledge that people vary significantly in their values, goals, and behavioral patterns. Our clients' values may be different from the norms of the majority culture, but they are not necessarily less valid. This may mean that we need to become aware of other cultures and values and consciously view a situation from multiple viewpoints and valuing systems (Yi, 1995). Furthermore, strength-based approaches presume that every person, family, or community has resources and strengths, no matter how notable the problems. Sherene's work with Rashelle (see chapter 4, p. 79) was based on this premise. As a result, she mentored Rashelle and drew out her leadership abilities, believing they were there. Similarly, Jackson's therapist (see chapter 3, p. 51) recognized that even problems often stemmed from healthy intentions. Thus, she saw Jackson's social withdrawal as an attempt to create distance from relationships that were very important to him and that he was afraid of losing. In the second dialogue, rather than attempting to solve Andor's problems, Jalyse (see chapter 9, p. 202) stopped to listen to him. She prompted him to keep going even when he felt stuck. Because she believed he could get there, he continued longer than he thought he could and thus earned positive results. These strategies, as well as others discussed in this book, are outlined in table 12.3. Because strength-based approaches pay attention to often-overlooked strengths and resources, they often feel more respectful to both parties. When we assume clients have resources and strengths, co-

TABLE **12.3** **STRENGTH-BASED ASSUMPTIONS AND WAYS TO INTEGRATE THESE INTO TREATMENT**

Assumptions	Actions
There is something hopeful toward which to work.	Be hopeful about the client and his or her future.
The client has something to contribute to therapy and can be an active agent of change.	Strive for an egalitarian and empowering relationship.
Strengths may be an asset to the change process. The whole person includes both strengths and weaknesses.	Expect strengths and build on them without covering up or denying any weaknesses.
The client is trying to solve a problem rather than being "broken" or "bad."	Recognize the healthy intention in "the problem." Consider whether "symptoms" may be maladaptive ways of coping.
Problem behavior may not be "a problem" from the client's individual or cultural set of values. It may appear to be a problem at the junction between the individual and the dominant culture.	See "problematic behavior" from the client's own individual and cultural valuing stance and challenge knee-jerk responses to pathologize.
The client has attempted to solve the problem in the past and may be able to do so now with support.	Listen to problems without blaming or jumping in prematurely to solve them.
The client is partially solving the problem already. Partial solutions can be used as the basis for a solution.	Listen to and expect solutions, or partial solutions, to the problem. Ask questions such as "When do you . . .," "Where do you . . .," "What is right about this?" and "How can this be useful?"
The client is partially successful in solving the problem already. The client is not "broken" or "bad," but sometimes has bad or problem behaviors.	Use situation rather than trait language to describe the person and problem, especially when talking about maladaptive rather than adaptive behaviors.

Note: From Gelso, 2000; Waters & Lawrence, 1993.

operation and empowering interventions are more common (Clark, 1998; Waters & Lawrence, 1993).

Regardless of the severity or apparent frequency of the problem, strength-based approaches assume that natural solutions already occur. Although Jace reports that she is *always* jealous of her boyfriend, we can ask whether she was jealous when they first began dating (see figure 12.3). What was different last Thursday when she reports they had a good day? What is different in the therapy relationship, which is relatively calm and supportive? Acknowledging these exceptions in her behavior allows Jace to recognize that her behavior is changeable and that she already has the resources to change. These questions can also be the beginning of developing a vision about what she will be doing when her relationship is back on track.

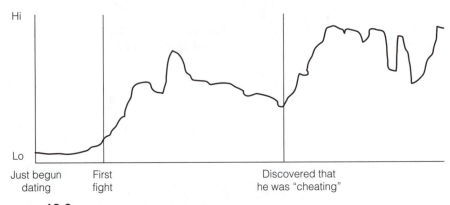

FIGURE 12.3

Changes in the strength of Jace's jelousy with her boyfriend across time.

Strength-based therapy begins by identifying strengths and natural solutions and believes that this attitude alone can be a healing reframe. The fact that Ella assumes that Jace is sometimes able to be trusting allows Jace to step around the self-blaming stance of the trait approach she had adopted ("Am I a jealous person, *or* am I jealous under certain conditions?"). The latter is a much more hopeful belief, because situational factors are more readily changed than central traits.

Although pathology is assumed to underlie problems in a problem-focused or deficit model, strength-based approaches believe problems are the result of healthy intentions gone awry (Waters & Lawrence, 1993). Jace's jealousy is problematic, and it interferes with her relationships. However, it arose from a healthy core—the desire for a stable and committed relationship with a person who is very important to her. In fact, when she began looking at when problems occurred and when they did not, she noticed that they did not occur when she felt that her boyfriend was being open and honest with her. Unfortunately, her current approach to resolving this problem was unsuccessful, because the more she attacked him for being unfaithful, the more he tended to shut down and hide things that he thought might bother her. This became a self-perpetuating cycle, until they began to work on developing a more open and honest relationship in the safety of the therapy room.

Strength-based approaches are different from problem-focused approaches on a number of dimensions (see table 12.4). This style of work is especially adaptive with people who have less power or feel different from societal norms, and thus is especially useful in the work described in this book. People in minority groups often expect that dominant-group members will devalue cultural patterns and adaptations and turn them into discrimination and oppression rather than accept and value them (Carlton-

Remember a time when you were blamed for something that felt outside your control. How did you feel? What did you think about yourself and the person who made these accusations? Did you later learn some ways of controlling these "uncontrollable" thoughts, feelings or behaviors? How do you view this time now?

TABLE 12.4 DIFFERENCES BETWEEN PROBLEM-FOCUSED AND STRENGTH-BASED APPROACHES

	Problem-focused	Strength-based
Focus	Focus is on understanding when and why problems occur.	While therapy is problem-driven and identifies treatment goals, the focus is on assets, strengths, and potential solutions that can solve the problem.
Fixed or Mutable	Problems are the result of fixed and unchangeable traits.	Problems are part of everyone's continuing attempts to adapt and change. Problems are often viewed as thwarted attempts to meet goals.
Normal or Abnormal	Problems are manifestations of individual pathology.	Problems are part of the difficulty in meeting life's goals. Contextual issues, including family functioning and cultural variables, may make the behavior more understandable.
Holistic or Reductionistic	Problems and psychopathology are the most important things to understand in order to change.	The problems are important, but so are the strengths. Problems are seen in a larger cultural, developmental, and contextual framework.
Essential Questions for Therapy	How did I get into this mess? What causes the problem?	How do I get out of this mess? When did the problem not occur? What was different about those times?
Relative Importance of Insight?	Insight is often very important, with the assumption that people cannot do things differently without understanding why they got themselves into trouble in the first place.	Action is often more important than insight. Exploring the past may be most important in helping a client feel understood, but it is not necessary for change.
Therapeutic Relationship	The relationship is often hierarchical in nature, with the client taking a one-down stance.	Generally, the relationship is relatively egalitarian, respectful, and cooperative in nature. Therapist assumes strengths, as well as problems, and thus emphasizes empowering interventions.

Note: From Bean et al., 2000; Clark, 1998; Powell & Batsche, 1997; Waters & Lawrence, 1993.

LaNey, 1999). Adolescents, especially those in the juvenile justice system, often anticipate being blamed and misunderstood, as the other adults in their lives do (Clark, 1998). It is also essential for productive work in highly stressed situations, including interagency work (Bean et al., 2000). Listening, understanding, and valuing are essential parts of helping others make effective change.

RESPONSIBILITY

A problem's cause can be attributed internally or externally, and the source of the solution can be attributed to the person of the larger system or community. These attributions can be judgmental ("Why didn't you handle your stress better?") or nonjudgmental ("It's been a difficult time of year for you, hasn't it?"). In this section, we'll look at behaviors that cause therapists to blame clients, as well as the consequences of blaming. Finally, we'll consider ways to stop blaming our clients and, instead, work with them productively.

Responsibility Versus Blame

Strength-based approaches do not deny responsibility for problems. In fact, they avoid blaming while also holding people accountable for making changes. What is the difference between being held responsible and being blamed? Blame occurs when we feel that there is insufficient justification for a behavior, as in "You could have . . . ." (Lussier et al., 1993). For example, while Eugene may excuse his behavior as having been caused by his affective disorder, his partner can both accept the legitimacy of this explanation *and* still hold him responsible for his mood swings. She must believe there are things that he can do to keep his moods more moderate. Nonaccountability stories ("There's nothing I can do about it!") are just as problematic as blame stories ("He is just a moody slob!). Neither helps the person grow or change (O'Hanlon, 1999).

Objectivity about a situation and its contributing factors are necessary for attributing responsibility accurately. Without an awareness of context and culture, we are like visitors to Alber's painting *Homage to the Square,* who see two different purple squares on red and blue backgrounds rather than the squares' true nature (see chapter 9, p. 206). Looking beyond the problem to its greater context allows us to understand behavior and avoid blaming, while also providing a perspective on what we can do differently.

Although objectivity is important, a subjective understanding of the situation is also necessary to work empathically and to join with clients (May, 1967). As we begin to see the goals of their behavior rather than just the problematic consequences, the therapeutic alliance is strengthened and shame decreases (Waters & Lawrence, 1993). This dual perspective of objectivity and subjectivity also helps us identify previously overlooked strengths. What do clients see as their real strengths? Many people are unable to identify their own strengths, but comparing their behavior to developmental and cultural norms can be very helpful in finding them.

Waters and Lawrence (1993) state that "health-hunting requires a strong level of engagement; for us, pathology-hunting occurs most readily when we are least connected" (p. 117). When stuck in supervision or during a consultation it is useful to ask, "What do you like about this person or family?" This question moves us out of the criticism-blame-shame cycle and helps us join with our clients toward an effective alliance. Kia, who had difficulty working with people with bad hygiene, was able to identify other things that she liked about them. Les had been stuck thinking about perpetrators only in terms of the abuse. He was able to admire the emotional bond between Lorna and her aunt, even as he helped them identify other ways to show their love.

Some therapists working with people accused of crimes ignore the crime in their attempt to accept and understand their clients (Zhang, 2003b). However, some people doing forensic work believe that they cannot effectively hold their population accountable for crimes if they pay attention to what is likable about the person (Clark, 1998). This is the dilemma: How can we join with our clients *and* hold them responsible for their behavior? Masterful work requires attention to both sides of this tricky dichotomy.

Although interpretations and reframes can be blaming, they can be at the core of challenging blaming and shaming processes (Ivey et al., 1997). A reframe can take old, stuck inferences about behavior and shift them to help a person change. Arlene, for example, was able to suggest that Tyrone's drawing on walls and hiding were not obstinate and oppositional, but playful, attention-seeking behaviors. Tyrone's mother could relax and appreciate the positive aspects of his behavior, while helping him find healthier ways to get attention.

Responsibility Versus Irresponsibility

The United States has consciously chosen not to punish or imprison people whose behavior is outside their control (Schlenker et al., 1994). Six-month-olds should not be punished for wetting their pants, although older children might be. Insanity pleas in criminal cases have been handled in a similar manner. For example, the American Law Institute (1985) concluded that a person should not be held responsible when "as a result of mental disease or defect, he lacks substantial capacity either to appreciate the criminality (wrongfulness) of his conduct or to conform his conduct to the requirements of law." The exception recognized by ALI is when the "abnormality is manifested only by repeated criminal or otherwise antisocial conduct" (p. 62), behavior that is presumed to be willful. Insanity defenses and other approaches to excising responsibility are used far less frequently and are far less successful than many people think (Silver, Cirincione, & Steadman, 1994). This finding is consistent with the fundamental attribution error discussed in chapter 1 (Gilbert & Malone, 1995; J. Greenberg et al., 1982; Jones, 1979; Zuckerman, 1979).

What happens when we hold clients accountable for things such as seizures, sexual abuse, and racism that are outside their control (see table 12.5)? What if, on the other hand, we fail to hold them accountable for things they *can* control? They can, for example, take their seizure medicine, decrease the stress in their lives, and get enough sleep. We need to broach

TABLE **12.5** CONTROLLABLE AND UNCONTROLLABLE BEHAVIORS

	Uncontrollable	Controllable
Voluntary	No direct voluntary control.	Under some direct voluntary control.
Responsive to External Stimuli?	Does not vary in response to external stimuli.	Varies in response to controllable external stimuli, including medication, social support, lighting, noise, and the like.
Role of Stress?	Does not impact the nature or severity of the problem.	Worse when under stress.
Voluntary Behaviors and Influence on Behavior?	Voluntary behaviors do not directly influence the magnitude of problems.	Behaviors under voluntary control can amplify or decrease the severity of problems.

this dilemma. Paraphrasing the Desiderata, how can we recognize the things our clients can control, as well as those they cannot and, more importantly, how can they gain the wisdom to recognize the difference? How can we avoid either being naïve and *excusing* behavior, or perceiving spurious controls over a person's behavior and *blaming* them for the dilemmas they face? How can we recognize the contributions of an abusive childhood and a life filled with discrimination, yet still encourage our clients to discover the ways they *can* change and control their relationships (Bowers & Farvolden,1996)?

Few problems are completely controllable or uncontrollable. As Eugene discovered, many behaviors that initially appear "uncontrollable" become manageable when controllable intervening variables such as stress, fatigue, noise, and diet are identified. Cancer, for example, often responds to medications and other treatments. Even biological and uncontrollable problems, like depression, appear to be under the control of unidentified factors, including self-care, sleeping and eating habits, and self-talk.

Multiple Determination of Problems

A farmer was milking a cow while sitting on a three-legged stool. A tourist stopped and watched the farmer for a while, fascinated by the whole enterprise. Finally, she asked, "Which leg is the most important?" The farmer said, "They're each important. Without each one, the stool would fall down."

Most problems have multiple causes and would disappear without each contributing factor (Kettl, 1999). What causes youth violence? High testosterone levels? Low serotonin? A weak bond between parent and child? Absence of other mentoring figures? Too much unsupervised time? Media violence? Shame and loss? Peer pressure? While there is significant evidence that each of these is a contributing factor, the truth is that most teenagers are not violent, and people with fewer of these factors are less likely to be violent.

What does that mean, then, for our clients? Although they are ultimately responsible for the decisions they make, regardless of the other factors that play a part in a problem's etiology, we as therapists must also acknowledge the extraneous agents and the role they play. This has the potential of allowing us to take a more empathic and realistic stance in our work. Luisa (in chapter 1) must develop academic skills and will be held responsible if she is unable to do so. However, we will make different recommendations depending on whether we believe she is having problems concentrating because of the domestic violence between her parents, her depression, attentional problems, or simple defiance. We are negligent when we fail to address the domestic violence or when we blame her for her response to it. Similarly, Jackson (in chapter 3, p. 51) is responsible for his decisions to use drugs and to skip school, but our culture is also responsible for failing to nurture its youth and for creating huge material desires without developing teens' hopefulness about the future. His community must create an atmosphere that can help him succeed within adaptive channels.

Other-Blame and Self-Blame

Blame is a difficult and complex construct. In reviewing outcomes following threatening events, Tennen and Affleck (1990) report that blaming others (although not the situation) was associated with negative outcomes in 15 of 25 articles. Blaming others was associated with positive consequences in only one article. They conclude that blaming others removes one's perception of control and interferes with adaptive coping. It challenges cherished worldviews and weakens support systems, without replacing them with something positive.

Tennen and Affleck (1990) conclude that self-blame, on the other hand, has positive attributes that can help a person cope with a situation. Janoff-Bulman (1979, 1992) extends these ideas by suggesting that not all self-blame is adaptive and by distinguishing between behavioral self-blame ("I shouldn't have walked there") from characterological self-blame ("I'm too trusting"). Characterological self-blame is maladaptive and should be discouraged because it suggests a stable and unchangeable approach to the problem, but *behavioral* self-blame is adaptive because it allows people to think about what they can do to prevent problems in the future.

Although Janoff-Bulman's (1979, 1992) suggestions on the advantages of behavioral self-blame are provocative, the support for their ideas is

---

TABLE 12.6 **QUESTIONS TO ASK FOLLOWING TRAUMA TO ASSESS ATTRIBUTIONS OF SELF-BLAME AND CONSEQUENT DEPRESSION OR ANXIETY**

How did the person's behavior contribute to the event?
- Could the person have reasonably known about the event?
- Did the person have the skills, knowledge, or authority to prevent the problem?
- Did the person engage in behavior that put him or her at greater or lesser risk?

Is someone else at least partly to blame?
- Was someone else present?
- Did the other person have greater authority, knowledge, or ability?
- Could that person have done something to prevent the problem?
- Did the relationship between the two people create some responsibility for the event on the other person's part?

How does the person's attributional style contribute to perceptions of the event?
- Is the person generally optimistic or pessimistic? Is he or she trusting or paranoid?
- Does the person generally have an external or internal locus of responsibility? Does the person generally have an external or internal locus of control?
- Does the person's thinking style while under stress versus normal conditions support dichotomous and extreme responses or intermediate ones?

What are the attributions of other-blame and self-blame?
- Can the person do anything to cope with the stressor?
- Does the person possess effective coping skills?
- Is the person's social system supportive?
- Do attributions interfere with cherished beliefs?

Note: Based on Tennen & Affleck, 1990.

---

mixed. For example, women who used more behavioral than characterological self-blame after having an abortion ("I should have said no!") were less depressed and had coped better following the abortion (Mueller & Major, 1989). People who were addicted to opiates were more successful in preventing a relapse when they attributed problems to behaviors rather than to stable parts of their character (Bradley et al., 1992). However, rape survivors *and* women who were recently diagnosed with breast cancer experience greater amounts of depression and anxiety when they engage in either kind of self-blame (Frazier, 1990; Glinder & Compas, 1999).

Perhaps the advantages of self-blame depend, at least in part, on the nature of the stressor and what is done with the self-blame. If the self-blame, regardless of type, isolates or shames a person and functions as useless rumination, then anxiety and depression will increase (Nolen-Hoeksema & Morrow, 1991; Tennen & Affleck, 1990). See table 12.6. Some types of behavioral self-blame, although it may identify a controllable problem, may not lead to a solution. The person may still need to identify different behavioral strategies of intervening and feel that it is okay to act. In other words, a woman may clearly believe that saying "no" would be helpful when her partner wants to have unprotected sex, but she may not know how to do so without antagonizing him or her—and she may not believe that she has the right to have an opinion on the matter.

When behavioral self-blame motivates change, anxiety and depression will be lower. Mueller and Major (1989), for example, reported a modest but positive correlation between behavioral self-blame and self-efficacy. The modest nature of this correlation is not surprising given the difficulty some people may have in identifying solutions to the problems they have identified. Furthermore, some problems may require a normal course of grieving before adjustment, as with any kind of significant loss.

Conclusions: Finding a Balance

Blame and criticism are rarely useful, and they often serve as barriers between two parties (Halonen & Santrock, 1997). Similarly, excusing someone from all responsibility is a barrier to change and is disempowering (O'Hanlon, 1999). Therapy needs to acknowledge a problem and its effects on a person, while simultaneously recognizing the things that can be done to make a significant and positive impact. Although responsibility for a problem may be correctly assigned as external to the person, *controllability* must be attributed internally whenever possible and appropriate. Nevertheless, identifying control where it does not exist can be pathologizing.

Ponterotto (1987) described his work with a Mexican American male who was frustrated in dealing with an Anglo agency that had no Spanish-speaking caseworkers. He also experienced significant anxiety and somatic symptoms stemming from these conflicts. Ponterotto chose a multimodal intervention strategy that unambiguously exemplifies the ideas in this book. Most important, he specifically addressed oppressive and blaming environmental influences in three ways.

1. He acknowledged oppression in the client's environment.
2. He developed a plan to pressure the agency to hire members of the Spanish-speaking community.
3. He looked for referrals to other comparable agencies that had more culturally relevant services.

By acknowledging the oppression in the client's environment, Ponterotto (1987) squarely placed the blame for the problems on the shoulders of the Anglo agency. In doing this, however, he also challenged his client to accept that he was not helpless and that he could do things to change this difficult situation. Similarly, Elligan and Utsey's (1999) African American men's peer support group (see chapter 11) suggested that Carroll's program director's statement was prejudiced and unfair *and* that there were things he could do to challenge it. This group and Ponterotto attribute the problem elsewhere, but they empower each person to recognize the real control that they have, or can regain.

For these externally ascribed problems, the goal is for the client to recognize an external locus of responsibility while retaining an internal locus of control. Obviously, therapeutic goals are different when the client is believed to be responsible for the problem or the problem is outside the person's ability to control. When the problem is primarily individual, therapeutic goals may emphasize developing the courage to make responsible changes. When it is primarily external (e.g., anxiety stemming from racist attacks), acknowledging the problem and changing systemic and cultural factors are in order. When the problem is caused by value conflicts between people, their home culture, and the dominant culture, therapy should attempt to explore this value conflict and identify ways to resolve it.

FINDING NATURAL SUPPORTS: OUTSIDE AND IN

Andrea Yates, a 37-year-old mother, apparently calmly and with premeditation drowned her five children in the summer of 2001 (Roche, 2002). Many people decried her humanity, asking "How could anyone kill her children in such a cold-blooded manner?" However, with more information we can draw a more complete picture of her.

The available information suggests that Mrs. Yates was not a monster, but had been (prior to the incident) an exceptional and loving mother (Roche, 2002). She homeschooled her children and was creative and thoughtful in raising them. She was a deeply religious woman, with a spiritual base that suggested "bad children come from bad mothers" (p. 48). She became deeply depressed after the births of each of her children and grew more and more convinced that they were being tainted by their contact with *her,* as well as with the *materialistic world* in which they lived. Nonetheless, she and her husband agreed that having children was a sacred act, despite the fact that additional children would put her at risk. Andrea's delusional depression increased, and at some point, she came to believe that killing her children would be an act of love.

Mrs. Yates was clearly a woman with many strengths, although it appears that she did not recognize them in her deepening depression (Roche, 2002). She was very bright and hardworking and had even been valedictorian of her graduating class in high school. She was a deeply committed fundamentalist Christian; a devoted, nurturing and creative mother; a loving daughter to her father (who had been diagnosed with Alzheimer's); and a good wife.

She also appeared to have a number of supports within her family and community, including her husband Rusty, various relatives, and a few neighbors. However, her husband was described by some as "lacking empathy" (Roche, 2002, p. 44). Also, her psychiatrists were accused of failing to recognize the severity of her depression, and members of her family grew increasingly concerned about her psychiatric state, but stayed at a distance. The more depressed she became, the more she tended to distance herself from these supports.

Identifying the "cause" of therapeutic change is difficult. The strengths a person brings to therapy—a motivation to change, sense of humor, or extra-therapeutic influences—are believed to account for as much as 40% of the change made in therapy. This is more than any other factor, including model-specific therapeutic techniques (Asay & Lambert, 1999; Lambert, 1992; Tallman & Bohart, 1999). If such a percentage of all change is attributable to factors *outside* the therapy process, then it makes sense that we actively intervene with clients and help them to access systemic supports, so that these contributing factors can become as strong and healthy as possible. Although not the only contributing factors, harnessing Andrea Yates' considerable strengths and helping her support system work more effectively might have prevented the murders.

Community and family resources predict how a person will do and how well they will be able to respond to stressors. This is an underlying dynamic in the psychosocial histories throughout this book. Every case study in this book has someone who was poorly supported initially. When a person was followed across the course of therapy (see Rashelle in chapter 4 and Lu in chapter 11), social support always increased. Would Lu's goals have been met were she unable to receive greater support from inside *and* outside her family? Did the increase in support enable Rashelle to accept herself, overcome the past, and attempt things outside her grasp? Did her ability to accept herself and succeed cause the increase in support?

> How might the lives of Andrea Yates' family have been different had she perceived and been given consistent, effective support from her husband, friends, family, and psychiatrists? What might be different had her religious beliefs been supportive of her roles as a woman and mother? What if her intellectual and caretaking strengths had been nurtured better?

The causal relationship probably goes in both directions. As Rashelle collected support from the people around her, she became more self-confident, she tried new things, and she gathered new friends. Furthermore, as she did these things, the positive changes fostered additional growth, and she became more self-confident in important areas of her life.

COMMUNITY SUPPORTS

Stress is a natural part of life. Most studies of social support report advantages, regardless of their forms, these can include active helping, provision of information, and emotional attachment (cf. Cutrona, 1989). Most of the studies discussed in this chapter do not make distinctions among these kinds of support, however.

Nature of Support

Experiencing stressors does not lead inevitably to increases in perceived stress. Consequently, many researchers have examined predictors of more positive outcomes. A person's stressors can increase with time, without that person experiencing increased perceptions of stress (Goode, Haley, Roth, & Ford, 1998), or be equivalent across two groups, despite one group experiencing significantly less stress than the other (W. Haley et al., 1996; Ituarte, Kamarck, Thompson, & Banacu, 1999). These differences have been attributed to race, social support, attributions about stressors, and expectations about life. For example, Goode and her colleagues report that caregivers of people diagnosed with Alzheimer's disease reported no change in perceived stress over the course of two interviews, each one year apart, even though their stressors were significantly greater at the second interview. In addition, African Americans report more stressful life events than Euro-Americans, but no greater perceived stress despite an equivalent amount of perceived social support (W. Haley et al., 1996; Ituarte et al., 1999). This suggests that some variables cause psychological resilience in the face of stress, something that Greene (2000) described for many people who are culturally different.

Although the importance of community, systemic, and family supports has generally received approving nods from the psychological community, these supports are frequently overlooked in therapeutic assessments and not formally incorporated into DSM-IV formulations (American Psychiatric Association, 2000). However, Frances and his colleagues (Frances et al., 1991) suggest that assessments of community support will be integral to future versions of the DSM.

Draw your community genogram (as in figure 2.3, p. 21) or complete the community parts of your psychosocial history. What do you learn about your support system? Do you have enough supportive people in your life? Are your relationships primarily supportive, conflictual, or challenging? What do you want out of these, and are you getting what you want?
Now draw a picture of your ideal community genogram. Identify at least one step you can take to make your real community genogram look more like your ideal.

Consider a time when you had a major shift in the amount of support you received. It can be either an increase or decrease. What was this like for you? If your feelings about yourself and your attitudes toward life changed, did they become more positive or more negative?

Consequences of Support

Social support predicts positive outcomes for both psychological and biological problems. A strong network of social ties can provide tangible and emotional resources that aid in coping with stressors. But, those who are socially isolated are at increased risk for heart disease, in particular (Ituarte et al., 1999), and have greater health problems, in general (Goode et al., 1998). Schiller and Bennett (1994) describe Schiller's coping with psychosis and her ultimate recovery in the following excerpt:

> It happened over the summer when I was working on this book, dredging up old memories of the time between my first two hospitalizations. It was a particularly difficult period in my life and very painful to recall. At the same time, other stressful things were going on in my life: My brother Steven had married and moved with his wife Ann to South Africa. I missed him and was anticipating missing Mom and Dad, who were retiring and moving to Florida. I was feeling abandoned by my two other supports as well: Dr. Doller was taking a maternity leave, and my caseworker Jacquie was returning to school. At the same time, Dr. Doller and I were experimenting with lowering my medication. It was all too much for me. (p. 268)

Consider the support you've received from two different people. If the outcomes of these experiences were different, what distinguished the two? Did the people offer different kinds of support? Did they intervene too often or not enough? How did they offer their support?

Schiller and Bennett (1994) clearly described the results of losing the psychological, personal, and medication supports. Nonetheless, Schiller recognized that stressors do not invariably stress her, because the ways she responded to these "losses" kept her on track:

> Such a psychotic episode could have easily spun out of control. It didn't. What stopped it? I did. I knew something was wrong. The illness had seized a portion of my brain, but it hadn't seized all of it. I knew I needed help. I raised my medication back up to its normal level. I called Dr. Doller. I talked to my parents. At first, I scorned what they said. My Voices and I knew better. But I never became completely consumed. Over the years I had learned to trust Dr. Doller. So if she said I was experiencing a psychotic episode, then I probably was, no matter what the Voices told me. (p. 268)

Differential Consequences of Support

When supports are perceived to be greater, psychological adjustment is also generally better (Aquino et al., 1996; S. L. Brown, 1991; T. Elliott et al., 1992; T. Elliott & Shewchuk, 1995; Kurdek, 1988; Zemore & Shepel, 1989). Stressors are less overwhelming, and change is easier. However, when support is weak or absent, people often have fewer resources for coping with stressors. Consequently, physical and psychological pain are often greater, and change is more difficult (Beattie & Longabough, 1999; N. S. Robinson,

1995; Weisberg & Clavel, 1999; Zimmerman, 1991). Unfortunately, many people enter therapy with few supports in place, and do not have other options. People do not enter therapy when their natural supports are effective, but rather because their resources are insufficient at that point in time.

Trauma can cause a sense of personal inadequacy, diminished feelings of control, increased feelings of vulnerability, and a sense of confusion (Helgeson & Cohen, 1996). Social systems can increase feelings of being damaged or may intervene to ameliorate this sense of damage. Marsh, who was heard and supported by his friends after he was assaulted, had fewer and milder symptoms than Krys, whose mother asked what he had been doing to cause the "problem." Forced optimism, avoidance, marginalized concerns, and physical care in the absence of emotional support lead an already victimized person toward a growing sense of isolation and depression (Helgeson & Cohen, 1996; Nolen-Hoeksema & Davis, 1999). But, acknowledging concerns in an atmosphere of empathic understanding increases the perception of emotional support.

All support is not alike, however. Although social support generally has positive consequences, consequences are not exclusively positive. Disclosing problems can either stigmatize a person—especially when the disclosure goes against social norms—or it can marshal a person's support system (Chin & Kroesen, 1999). When the disclosure may bring shame to the group, members of collectivistic cultures often have greater difficulty disclosing, but they may also feel an increased sense of isolation (Mason, Marks, Simoni, Ruiz, & Richardson, 1995; Simoni, Mason, Marks, Ruiz, Reed, & Richardson, 1995). Both attitudes toward one's culture and levels of acculturation can influence disclosure rates, in this case, of HIV status (Chin & Kroesen, 1999; Mason et al., 1995; Simoni et al., 1995). Mason and her colleagues, for example, have reported greater disclosure of HIV status among English-speaking Latinos, than in Spanish-speaking Latinos who presumably are more collectivist in orientation and hold fewer North American cultural attitudes.

Beattie and Longabough's work (1999) with an alcohol-dependent population asserted that the nature of the supports present makes a difference in predicting abstinence from alcohol. While abstinence-specific social support predicted positive outcomes, regardless of the level of general social support, outcomes were best when general social supports *and* alcohol-avoidance supports were present. Conversely, general social support's importance in predicting a person's ability to abstain from alcohol was greatest when very little *specific* support for abstinence existed. In this case, general support seemed to make up for abstinence-related support.

Similarly, T. R. Elliott and his colleagues (1999) suggest that, at least for a population with spinal cord injuries, it is not just the amount of social support that predicts psychological adjustment and physical health, but the na-

TABLE 13.1 CULTURAL BELIEFS ABOUT SUPPORT, CONSEQUENCES OF BELIEFS, AND IMPLICATIONS FOR THERAPY

Attitudes	Consequences	Implications for Therapy
Individualistic Cultures • Tend to believe that others should solve problems on their own. Value autonomy and achievement to a greater degree than collectivistic cultures.	• Less likely to offer support and are often suspicious of offers of support, especially when the offers are pervasive or unnecessary. More likely to offer physical than emotional support.	Therapy should: • Offer or engage support while fostering client's sense of autonomy and self-efficacy.
Collectivistic Cultures • Tend to expect and prefer support from others. • Often see their problems as shameful and stigmatizing.	• Tend to offer and expect social support. Are less threatened when they must offer support for longer periods. • Tend to withdraw from others when behavior goes against cultural norms and values.	Therapy should: • Focus on engagement and support more than autonomy and self-efficacy. • Assume the presence of shame and challenge it when clients withdraw from others in their support system. Intervene in public settings or with family members to repair connections and challenge inappropriate shame.

Note: From Chin & Kroesen, 1999; Goode et al., 1998; W. Haley et al., 1996; Mason et al., 1995; Simoni et al., 1995.

Consider how your family or culture supports its members. If you can, contrast this with how other families and cultures support their members. Think about who tends to offer support, what kinds of support do various members offer, and when and how do they do it.

ture of that support (T. R. Elliott, Shewchuck, & Richards, 1999). People with caretakers who had weak and impulsive problem-solving skills tended to be less accepting of their injuries one year later regardless of their adjustment immediately following their injury. Their support system was not very "supportive."

Cultural Differences

Culture plays a role in how stress affects groups. It also influences the kinds of social supports that different groups seek (see table 13.1). Different groups look to different members of their system for support. Gays and lesbians, for example, receive a greater percentage of their support from friends than heterosexuals do (Kurdek, 1988). Groups that value autonomy and achievement, such as Euro-Americans, are more likely to look to friends and coworkers for support than are groups where *familism* is valued, such as in the Latin American culture.

Expectations about stressors, which can sometimes be a cultural variable, also influence responses to stress. Culturally normative and accepted events are less stressful than those that fall outside cultural norms. For example, African American caregivers report less stress and depression and appear more resilient when caring for a relative diagnosed with Alzheimer's (W. Haley et al, 1996). These caregivers seem to do better than Euro-American caregivers because taking care of an elderly relative is culturally normative, and they use more positive reappraisal to cope. They also see themselves as more capable in handling this stressor (Goode et al., 1998; W. Haley et al, 1996).

The converse is also true. Some stressors are outside the norm for a group and, as a result, are poorly tolerated. Returning to Seligman's model of learned helplessness (Alloy & Seligman, 1979; Seligman, 1968; Seligman, 1975), individuals or groups who feel that they are unable to challenge a particular stressor can be expected to be less likely to do so. However, individual or group successes engender additional striving against identified injustices and, presumably, greater self-efficacy and less stress.

Different Kinds of Supports

Cutrona (1989) describes various kinds of social support as (1) active helping, (2) provision of information, and (3) emotional attachment. Each one may be accessed to support a person in crisis. Assets can be *financial,* such as when a family pays for a woman's visit to an attorney to press charges against an unfair school system. The assets may also be *physical,* as when her partner searches the Internet to identify the laws about school suspensions and expulsions. They can be *emotional,* too, as when her friends simply listen to her as she vents about how unfair the principal is. Family, partner, and friends are readily apparent sources of support, but others are less so and are noted primarily by their absence. This can be seen in three superficially similar scenarios (see table 13.2) in which parents have been struggling with active, often impulsive preschoolers. In each scenario, the children were removed from the home after their parents hit them and left bruises.

Generally more supports are better than fewer ones (Beattie & Longabough, 1999; Brewin et al., 2000; T. R. Elliott et al., 1999; Nolen-Hoeksema & Davis, 1999). Because of this, Nita, who received supports from a variety of resources, was in a better situation than Bernard who had few pre-existing supports. For instance, both his friends and his family were highly critical of him and the actions that led to his children being removed from the home. However, different types of "supports" can have markedly different consequences (Nolen-Hoeksema & Davis, 1999). Nita's support system was enabling and disempowering. Her supports believed that she had a problem, and they worked to solve it for her. This action can be a form of discrimination, as when a Latina is presumed to be incapable of solving her own problems without help (Saba & Rodgers, 1990). The balance refused to admit that she was part of the problem ("The system's out to

Look at your community genogram again. Rather than simply focusing on the number of people in your system, think about *how* they support you or fail to support you. While others may tell you that a person or group is or is not supportive, do you see their support in the same way? Why or why not?

TABLE 13.2 COMMUNITY SUPPORTS FOR THREE PARENTS STRUGGLING WITH AN IMPULSIVE CHILD, EACH OF WHOM WAS REFERRED TO CHILD PROTECTIVE SERVICES (CPS) FOR HITTING A 4-YEAR-OLD CHILD

Bernard	Nita	Kevin
Cultural Factors		
Sociocultural background		
• Lives in a Euro-American community distant from where he grew up and feels isolated.	• A single Latina and lesbian in a mixed-raced community that is tolerant, but not accepting, of her sexuality. Some community members believe children should not be raised by lesbians.	• Lives in the close-knit African American community in which he grew up. He has always liked the fact that he could go out for dinner and be greeted warmly by half of the restaurant's customers.
Religion and spirituality		
• Bernard's minister is unforgiving and tells him that his wife should have custody of their children.	• Nita's church members encircle her during this crisis and arrange 24-hour respite for her children.	• Kevin's minister asks him what he needs during the crisis. He tells his minister that he would like his forgiveness and prayer. They develop a plan whereby he can be forgiven.
Resources and Barriers		
Social resources, such as friends and family		
• His friends and neighbors are angry, and they withdraw from him.	• Nita's friends tell her that it is not her fault and that her son "deserved it."	• Kevin's friends are supportive of him, but they encourage him to identify strategies for changing his parenting approach to a more effective one.
• Bernard's family lives three hours away from him. He does not tell them about the charges.	• Nita tells her family about the allegations, but they ignore the issue and try to change the subject every time she brings it up.	• While Kevin's family is upset about the charges, they are more upset that he did not ask them for help earlier. They work out a plan for respite when he is stressed or the children act out.
• Bernard's children are angry, and they refuse to talk to him.	• Nita's children are parentified. They call home every evening crying, but they end up reassuring her that it will be all right.	• Kevin's children, while initially angry, agree rapidly to begin working on things to make the family work better.
Work		
• Bernard's boss does not know about the charges. He is warned that he will lose his job if he misses another day of work (for meetings with CPS).	• Nita's coworkers know about the charges, although they do not know how serious the charges are. They talk about her behind her back, and she feels increasingly "paranoid" at work.	• Kevin's employer has a liberal family-leave policy and lets him rearrange his work schedule in order to make CPS meetings. A close friend at work who has been listening to him, suggests alternatives when Kevin is stuck and has been very supportive.
Community resources		
• Bernard's caseworker tells the foster family that she does not think he will be able to regain custody. She sets meetings when Bernard has said that he cannot be there. She believes his absence from some meetings means that he does not care about his children.	• Nita's caseworker is cooperative, but he makes all of the decisions regarding placement.	• Kevin's caseworker likes Kevin and his children, but warns him about his drinking. When Kevin's children are placed in foster care, the caseworker asks Kevin about their food preferences, bedtime routines, and chores.

(continued)

TABLE 13.2 *(continued)*

Bernard	Nita	Kevin
• Bernard's children are placed in foster care with a couple that is openly hostile toward Bernard. The two receive his family rules, but they think he's "too tough" and apply their own rules. They are told that Bernard will lose custody of his children and that they will have first crack at being considered as the children's adoptive parents.	• Nita's children are placed in foster care with a couple that blames the children for the abuse. Her children call home every evening wanting to come home.	• Kevin's children are placed in foster care until the crisis decreases. Their foster parents agree to the rules and follow them, even though they are different from what they would use with their own children. They refuse to talk badly about Kevin in front of his kids.
• Teachers and staff at his children's school think he is "the problem." They take an openly hostile approach in inter-agency meetings.	• Teachers and staff at Nita's children's school think her children are "little hellions." They tell her, "Don't worry. We have it all under control."	• With him and other agencies, teachers and staff at Kevin's children's school develop a truly collaborative plan for handling school problems.
Community contributions • None: "Why should I?"	• None: "What would I have to offer?"	• Kevin has volunteered at his children's school, and they see him as a good and competent person.
Mentors and models • Bernard is unable to identify anyone who has believed in him. His friends think he should do whatever he can to "screw the system."	• People have been kind to her, but she cannot identify anyone who has believed in her.	• Kevin would like to be like his employer, who seems to be both a *harried* and *successful* single parent.
Obstacles to change • Bernard has few social supports. Most prior supports have withdrawn from him, although he has also withdrawn.	• Few people have asked Nita to take responsibility for her behavior. Few believe she can be an active and competent parent.	• Kevin recognizes that it was his "fault" and is concerned about whether he can change. He also acknowledges that he is a good parent in many ways.
Therapeutic relationship • Bernard had an individual therapist in the past who was pessimistic about his ability to keep his children.	• Nita's therapist sees that she is overwhelmed. He talks to other agencies for her, but does not share "the bad stuff."	• Kevin had not been in therapy, but readily contacted a therapist and began working with her on individual and family issues that put the family at risk. Goals and intervention strategies were identified in a cooperative fashion.

get you."). They failed to encourage her to make changes or to hold her accountable.

The truly collaborative work of Kevin's system, a system that believed in him, supported him, *and* held him accountable for his actions, was the only one that encouraged effective change. Kevin's interactions with his system were hopeful, collaborative, and empowering, while Nita's and Bernard's interactions seemed hopeless, unilateral, and disempowering. Unfortunately, the treatment that Kevin received is typically reserved for

TABLE **13.3** CONSEQUENCES OF PARENTING STYLES ON CHILDREN

	System's Interaction Style	Consequences for Child
Authoritative Systems	Warm, encouraging, and supportive without being enabling. Values communication and open, democratic resolution of problems. Makes reasonable limits and expectations on behavior.	Self-confident, self-reliant, socially competent, responsible, and able to plan for their future successfully.
Directive Systems	Restrictive, cold, and punishing. Makes decisions in an autocratic and hierarchical manner. Does not assume that other members of the system have as much to contribute to decisions.	Anxious about social comparisons and has difficulty planning and initiating independent actions. Has poor communication skills and a low degree of autonomy.
Indulgent Systems	Highly involved and warm, but places few demands, controls, or expectations.	Has poor self-control and handles independence poorly.
Uninvolved Systems	Uninvolved, with low levels of warmth and communication. Places few restrictions, demands, or controls.	Has difficulty controlling behavior and learning respect for others.

Note: From Baumrind, 1991; Gauvain & Huard, 1999; Wentzel, 1997.

middle-class consumers. Poor and lower-class individuals and families tend to get less of this treatment, which can be just as successful with families that are generally seen as "high risk" (Motter et al., 1999; Powell & Batsche, 1997).

Support systems that are authoritative, warm, encouraging, and supportive without being enabling (like Kevin's, see table 13.3) are more effective than those that are

- Authoritarian—restrictive, cold, and punishing
- Indulgent—highly involved with few demands
- Uninvolved—indifferent with few restrictions (Baumrind, 1991; Gauvain & Huard, 1999; Wentzel, 1997).

These ideas are seen in Greif's research (1998) on fathering by academically high-achieving African American males. Although the fathers were generally described as unconditionally supportive, they also held consistently high expectations. Many reported an extensive range of community supports, including the church, school, and extended family. Although an unusually large number of the boys in this sample had highly involved fathers, those who did not generally had other community supports, which often included a family member who served as a tutor or mentor. A supportive and functional support system seems to be extremely important for making change and maintaining a positive adjustment in the face of adversity (Beattie & Longabough, 1999; T. R. Elliott et al, 1999; Greif et al., 1998; Jarrett, 1999; Wentzel, 1997).

Culturally Appropriate and Creative Supports   Social supports must be culturally appropriate. LaFramboisie (2000), for example, describes formal helping patterns as the "servant" of natural supports. Different groups have different natural helpers and helping strategies. Regardless of how well-intentioned our offerings of services, we cannot assume that Native American peoples, for example, will turn to formal helping systems if these systems are not compatible with their community and informal support system.

In her report of successful parenting strategies in the inner city, Jarrett (1999) describes parenting techniques that are useful in any neighborhood and consistent with the ideas raised in this chapter. These include accessing effective community schools, tutors, and after-school programs and using in-home enrichment strategies. She also points out that parenting in high-risk neighborhoods often requires significant creativity, especially when resources are limited. Ethel, for example, spent her (rare) free time ferreting out the best schools, tutors, and after-school programs for her four children. Despite her best efforts, her daughter Quita began to run into problems. To keep her out of trouble, Ethel sent Quita to live with Quita's grandmother across town while she searched for a school that offered services that would work well with her.

Although Jarrett (1999) described identification of effective resources as an essential parenting strategy, she also emphasized that highly effective parents closely monitored their children to prevent them from being exposed to dangerous or subversive influences. Again, she described successful parents as creative in meeting their goals. Ethel, for example, could not be around her children at all times, especially because she often needed to work the second shift, but she refused to let her children run wild in her absence. When LaToya wanted to spend time at her boyfriend's house, Ethel would agree, but only if LaToya's brother Washington joined them. Washington would inform Ethel whenever LaToya did anything dangerous.

Although Ethel's strategies weakened typical family boundaries with Quita and subverted typical age hierarchies with LaToya, the strategies were effective for the family at that point in time. Note that these actions were *at Ethel's behest* rather than because her children were independently deciding what action should be taken to keep their siblings under control (cf. Boyd-Franklin, 1990). Ethel retained her powerful place at the top of the family's hierarchy, and her children served as her arms and legs rather than as her head. In addition, her strategies were culturally relevant *and* personally relevant, and fit this African American family well. Evaluating family structure means asking what works, rather than what might be "right."

At the top of the list to be considered are culturally relevant definitions of family, strategies of accessing community resources, and individual family needs. For many culturally different families, extended family plays a much larger and more important role than it does with Euro-American families. This point is often overlooked because most theories have been written by Euro-American practitioners for Euro-American clients in the United States and Europe (Guthrie, 1997). In addition, a disproportionate number of caseworkers and therapists in the United States are White or socialized and trained in upper middle-class Euro-American values in school. To assume that African American grandmothers should not be actively parenting their grandchildren would be culturally insensitive. However, failing to question the grandmother's involvement, especially when boundaries, responsibilities, and roles are ineffective, is equally insensitive (Boyd-Franklin, 1990). In our example, Ethel's mother and son each served parenting functions with her children, yet Ethel was the one who made the decisions. When her children attempted to undermine her authority by pleading their case to another "parent" she insisted that all parents work together. If they failed to do so, problems could be expected.

Even culturally relevant ways of asking for and receiving support should be considered. For example, although traditional psychotherapy is generally done behind closed doors, most Native American healings are done in an open setting surrounded by friends and family (Tafoya, 1990). On one hand, therapies like network therapy emphasize publicly stating the problem so that community resources can be mobilized, which is much more culturally relevant for Native Americans. On the other hand, therapies that force a client into public admission of a problem to his or her Native American community may be premature. Some people may choose a non-Native American therapist as a way to preserve privacy. This decision should be respected, at least initially.

Formal and Informal Supports

Return to your community genogram. Think about which of these supports are advisors, professors, therapists, caseworkers, and the like whose function it is to support you. Think about which ones are supportive without it being a primary function such as friends, siblings, or neighbors. What patterns do you notice? Has this changed over time? If it has, how and with what implications has change occurred?

Formal and informal supports are important, and people often comment about the importance of the informal or natural supports in their lives (cf. Richie et al., 1997). When we turn to the people and systems that are naturally around us such as our family, neighbors, friends, school, work, and church, we often continue to feel strong and competent even when we ask for help. Often when we turn to formal supports such as therapy or social service agencies, it is because other informal strategies have been less successful. Regardless of the helper's real intentions or actions, the person who is being helped often feels less competent and capable simply because he or she needed help.

At his first session, Justin confessed that needing to go to therapy made him feel "weak." Meiping acknowledged the validity of his concerns, "It would be nice if you had had sufficient resources in place so this bump in the road didn't throw you. But, it takes real strength, real courage, to recognize a problem, admit it and address it."

Why do formal helping strategies seem to undermine a sense of competency, while informal systems can leave someone feeling strong? Probably part of the difference comes from the typical style of each kind of relationship. When Justin entered therapy, it was unlikely that Meiping expected to receive anything (other than payment) from him. It was also unlikely that Justin expected to be able to offer anything to her. When he turned to his minister for help with clothing and housing after a fire, Justin knew that these came from a natural network of support and service that he had contributed to in the past and expected to continue to contribute toward in the future. As a result, he felt more comfortable receiving this help.

Healthy natural supports generally feel at least adequately balanced, with "withdrawals" more or less matched by "deposits." People who deposit more than their share may either expect that they are "saving" for their future or may feel taken advantage of. Most parents of young children do not feel like they are being taken advantage of by their toddlers' demands. On the other hand, parents of teenagers and young adults can become resentful when their children maintain the same level of demands. This is perhaps because their children's requests often seem unnecessary and because their own needs are unlikely to be met in the future. People who tend to withdraw more than their share frequently feel dependent and unable to resolve problems on their own. This seems especially true for those people who feel like they have no choice but to accept help from others.

Traditional social service systems have significant disadvantages relative to the natural supports that many people have used in the past. When people turn to someone who does not also ask them for help, they are often left in a dependent state by the nature of this inequity. Many social service agencies, while building a network of care for those without other resources, can also build a culture of dependency and can undercut feelings of self-efficacy. Rather than encouraging individuals to feel powerful and capable or facilitating their development of skills to deal with future stressors, networks can encourage a sense of dependency and powerlessness by shielding them from stressors (Bandura, 1997). They may "do for," like Nita experienced, rather than being offered the kind of support and encouragement that Kevin enjoyed. Rather than proactively engaging resources, they may encourage active reliance on others to resolve their problems. As discussed in chapter 10, these feelings of powerlessness can continue into the future if we as therapists do not consciously do things to recognize and re-build our clients' power.

Are these differences necessary aspects of the differences between these helping systems? No. In issues raised in chapter 10, we can also imagine formal helping systems that can recognize and rebuild power and informal systems that rob power. The following examples may clarify these distinctions. Consider how each interaction could be redefined so as to increase the client's self-efficacy and sense of self.

- Latitia was an in-home family therapist working with the Malachi family. Over the course of a particularly problematic session, Mrs. Malachi repeatedly complained about how difficult it was to get her son to clean up around the house. Latitia took Timothy into his bedroom to help him clean the room.
- The Brown family was concerned with how they would look at the start of the new school year in last year's clothing and wanted new school clothes. Without asking the Browns, Tessa asked her administrator for a voucher for clothing from the community's discount store.
- Suzie struggled with her math homework. She had particular difficulty with solving fractions. Her father, frustrated at the end of a long day, took her paper and filled in the answers.

In each of these cases, the helper took the easiest route and solved the problem *for* the person or family. In none of these cases did this solution solve problems over the long term. In fact, these solutions can undermine the person's or family's self-esteem and self-efficacy.

ETHICAL ISSUES

What might you do in each of the previous scenarios to help the family meet its short- *and* long-term goals? Do your solutions meet other ethical prerogatives, including competency, professional and personal integrity, respect for the dignity of others, concern for people's welfare, and social responsibility (American Psychological Association, 2002)?

Clearly, effective community supports are more or less bi-directional and empowering, but therapeutic attempts to meet these goals can violate ethical standards (American Psychological Association, 2002; American Counseling Association, 1995; National Association of Social Workers, 1999). If not done carefully, our attempts to be respectful, empowering, and caring can lead to dual relationships with the potential for exploitation (Slattery, 2000a).

Empowering interventions result from a complex interplay of warmth, respect, caring, recognition of individual, family and community resources, and cultural awareness. When any one of these is missing, the relationship can go awry.

This issue is explored in an essay written by a psychologist we'll call Dr. Anon. He was brought before his licensure board on ethics violations (Anonymous, 2000). Dr. Anon had worked with a client who, shortly before dying, asked him to take care of his wife Edna and their children. In his attempts to meet this promise to his client, Dr. Anon:

- Accepted Edna into therapy to resolve her grief issues
- Arranged for her to transcribe his notes and correspondence in exchange for therapy.
- Hired her as a secretary in his office.
- Gave her jewelry as presents.
- Had an affair with her.

His account of their interactions sounds like he *tried* to do the best he could for her at all times. But his actions were counterproductive in the long run. Eventually, she felt used, exploited, and abandoned. He was left feeling confused about why she felt the way she did.

Dr. Anon's good intentions were in vain because he failed to think about their relationship from a contextual viewpoint. He correctly identified that Edna had a variety of unsatisfied financial and emotional needs (Anonymous, 2000). But, he assumed that *he* needed to be the one to meet them. His decision to accept her as a client, although well-intentioned, may have underestimated the resources that she had available at that point in time and certainly did little to nurture those resources. Rather than encouraging her to strengthen her support system such as by turning to family, friends, neighbors, and her minister, he narrowed it by suggesting that he was the only one who could meet her needs emotionally, financially, and sexually. He reported that he and his colleagues became her family. Who else could listen to her and support her through her grief as well as they did? While their actions were kind, did she need help or just *feel* that she needed help in the typical period after a crisis when everything seems to be falling apart? Did she have the personal resources to work through these feelings? If she needed therapy, were there ways to get it that would not have required that they enter a potentially problematic dual relationship? Were there others who could listen to her and support her? If not, why not?

Dr. Anon's view of this situation was narrow and dichotomous (Anonymous, 2000; Slattery, 2000a). He seemed to feel that Edna was able only to receive help from him or fall apart completely. How could this viewpoint empower her? How could it help her recognize other options? How could it nurture her personal and systemic resources? His decisions, although apparently well-intentioned and caring, were motivated by the same stress-limited morass that she apparently felt stuck in. Perhaps this morass also mirrored his concerns for his mother after his father's death. As May (1967) describes, empathy in therapy without objectivity can be dangerous—and the converse is true as well.

Effective therapy should consider the short- and long-term costs and benefits of interventions beforehand. Dr. Anon's actions were responsive to

TABLE 13.4 **BENEFITS AND COSTS OF DR. ANON'S ACTIONS WITH EDNA IN THERAPY**

Benefits	Costs
Providing therapy in exchange for transcription services Therapy available when it otherwise did not feel available.	May feel exploited by bartering process, especially if her time is not priced equal to his.
Edna and her son stabilized as a result of having therapy available.	Did not need to learn to identify other ways of solving problems when her initial approach to the problem was blocked.
	Was not forced to accept responsibility for ways that she blocked options (i.e., by refusing to accept *pro bono* therapy).
Giving jewelry as a gift Her contributions around the office were acknowledged with a gift that she enjoyed.	Their relationship was further sexualized because in their culture jewelry suggests romantic intentions.
Entering a sexual relationship with her Both found a romantic and sexual partner who met their needs at that point in time.	Alternative romantic avenues were intentionally or unintentionally discouraged when she identified her therapist as a possible sexual object.
This relationship may have served to equalize their power and helped her to acknowledge the very real things that she could give to someone whom she valued.	Romanticized the former therapeutic relationship. Because of his loss of objectivity, removed it from the realm of possibility if the need for therapy again arose.
	Sex and intimacy were confused, which, if this was related to her initial presenting concerns, could create problems both in this relationship and in future relationships.
	Because of the preexisting inequities in power and because of the prior therapy and work relationships, one or the other members may have felt taken advantage of.
	Sexualized the former therapeutic relationship. His loss of objectivity precluded future therapy.
	More than other romantic relationships, this one may have been motivated by factors that had the potential of confusing the parties about their own motivations and those of their partner. What acts were part of therapy? What was the sexual relationship?
	When the relationship ended, both may have felt taken advantage of in ways that amplify the typical problems at the end of a relationship.
	Did not need to learn other ways of interacting with other people that did not depend on sexualizing themselves and others.
	His wife and family may feel abandoned as he attempted to meet Edna's needs rather than theirs.

Note: From Anonymous, 2000.

TABLE 13.5 **BENEFITS AND COSTS OF MODERATE LEVELS OF TRANSPARENCY AND OPENNESS IN THERAPY**

Benefits
- May be culturally relevant, especially in cultures where disclosures only occur in the context of a relationship.
- Can normalize "crazy" periods by indicating that someone who is respected has experienced something similar.
- "Vulnerability" in therapy can access some aspects of the therapeutic consequences of being able to help someone else.
- As transparency often occurs in a trusting and safe environment, it is often more strength-based. Acknowledging clients' strengths can help clients recognize them.
- Transparency can create a safer therapeutic environment and may shorten the periods of effective therapy as a result.
- Can create a more egalitarian and empowering relationship, thus fostering a client's self-efficacy.

Costs
- Can undermine perceptions of expertness if not used carefully, especially in cultures where ability to help depends on perceptions of perfection.
- May interfere with the development of transference. Any strong transferential responses may be particularly important, however.
- Therapy has the potential to be for the therapist rather than for the client if the therapist is not careful.
- The assumption is that the client has skills that foster growth and that the client can make healthy decisions.

her immediate needs for emotional comfort, therapy, family, friendship, and sex (Anonymous, 2000), but these actions did not consider long-term consequences of this behavior on this client, other clients, his colleagues, and his family (see table 13.4). Feelings of betrayal and abandonment were predictable. Because Dr. Anon failed to see this act contextually, he concluded that, "I failed because I didn't know how to limit care" (Anonymous, 2000, p. 3). Rather than being problematic because his actions failed to *limit* care, they were inappropriate because they attempted to provide care directly rather than provide it through a nurturing system and resources. Instead of attempting to be the only one to meet her needs, he could have met her needs and their goals more successfully by helping her identify ways of meeting her needs *outside* their relationship.

Contrast Dr. Anon's dilemma with the decision to be open and transparent in therapy. As in any other decision, there are advantages and disadvantages to any option taken (see table 13.5). Here, however, the advantages of openness are more significant and the disadvantages are much easier to avoid, depending on the particular therapist-client pair. This pragmatic type of cost-benefit analysis, in which the consequences of behavior are considered and where "coloring outside the lines" may or may not meet the client's goals, is an important aspect of the contextual approach to therapy. In looking at the costs and benefits, we acknowledge that all clients are not alike and that some individuals (especially those with difficulties trusting others) may profit from approaches tailored to them (Zhang, 2003g). Nonetheless, because straying off the beaten path can be risky and self-serving, therapists should surround themselves with people who can serve as their sounding boards and can force them to recognize the hidden disadvantages of their ethical decision-making behavior and encourage them to consider other approaches.

REAL VERSUS PERCEIVED SUPPORT

Think about the people in your life. Are there any who perceive less support than others might think they have? If so, what effect does this have for them and the people around them?

In determining levels of general support, some research has simply counted the number of common supportive relationships (Beattie & Longabough, 1999). Although support is important, levels of perceived and real support are not identical. Most studies reporting the stress-buffering effects of social support have found that *perceived,* not *received* support best predicted social support's ability to protect against stress (S. Cohen & Wills, 1985; Hagerty & Williams, 1999; Hagerty, Williams, Coyne, & Early, 1996, but see Cutrona, 1989, which finds good correlations between reports from self and others). People who felt that they belonged did better socially and psychologically, regardless of the size of their social network (Hagerty & Williams, 1999; Hagerty et al., 1996). Cohen and his colleagues (L. Cohen, Towbes, & Flocco, 1988) also argued the opposite end of this argument when they suggested that when people are depressed, they tend to remember more negative life events and perceive less social support, even when there is no real drop in social support. In fact, exposure to chronic stressors, something rarely studied, seems to erode perceived support and cause greater problems (Lepore, Evans, & Schneider, 1991).

Support may be assumed or inferred based upon others' reactions to their disclosures. For example, a rape survivor's ability to report a rape to her family is predictive of positive outcomes. They have less depression as adults, more successful marital relationships, and higher self-esteem (Palmer, Brown, Rae-Grant, & Loughlin, 1999). When survivors refuse to tell family and friends, it is often because they expect negative reactions, criticism, and blaming. In some cases, however, survivors still expect a negative outcome, even though they would be believed, and when they receive considerable support once the rape is finally reported. As described earlier, perceived support predicts outcomes better than the amount of available real support.

Nolen-Hoeksema and Davis (1999) reported that people who tended to ruminate about problems were more likely to access social support after the death of a loved one than people who worried less. Perhaps because they were more likely to worry about their problems, they were more likely to reach out to others and profit more from social support. However, perhaps because ruminators tend to have a high need to talk and to be understood, they often underestimate the strength of their support network. Their need to talk about the trauma long after culturally sanctioned grieving periods have passed may also leave them feeling unsupported. Others may feel that the person should "move on" in her life (and they may even withdraw).

Although Melba, a typical ruminator, had considerable support throughout her life, she did not perceive it (see table 13.6). In fact, for any number of reasons, she focused on the stressors affecting her support system and believed that her needs were greater than her system could handle. Her family and friends worked on being honest in their communications with her. They continually asked her whether and when she needed help, and they let her know when they were truly overwhelmed. However, these changes were gradual both for Melba and her support system. She had to learn to accept their offers for what they were, and her family and friends needed to learn to respect their own needs and limitations and to communicate these accurately.

Why did Melba assume that no one would be there for her, despite considerable support from family and friends? This might be due to one of two factors:

- Her response could be a projection of her own feelings about being overwhelmed by the stressors in her life.
- She may have incorporated our culture's attitudes about rape and rape survivors.

That both of these played a part in her feelings of being alone is supported by two observations. When she felt more stressed, she felt more alone (cf. L. Cohen et al., 1988). She felt more supported when her stress levels dropped, although her real support did not change. In addition, she became more self-accepting and felt less alone as she began to recognize and accept that *some* people had victim-blaming attitudes and others did not.

Internal Supports

How do you support or care for yourself? How does this change when you are stressed? If it does change, what consequences does the stress have?

External supports clearly are important, however for the stressed individual it is especially so in Western (and individualistic) cultures. Melba can ask for support from others, but she must also learn to support herself. This can be seen in Schiller's descriptions of how she learned to cope with psychosis (Schiller & Bennett, 1994). She depended on the support of family and friends, but she also began to accept responsibility for those things that she could control:

TABLE 13.6 MELBA'S PERCEIVED AND REAL SUPPORT WITHIN HER COMMUNITY

Perceived Support	Real Support
Cultural Factors	
Sociocultural background	
Is a traditional Native American living in the city. Feels isolated, different, alone.	Has an extended family network both in the city and on the reservation.
Perceives people who are raped as "bad," "damaged," and "broken." Does not know how she can practice as a nurse given her history of sexual assault.	A large number of people with a history of sexual assault have entered the field. Her therapist and the local community assure her that she can survive and grow rather than be destroyed by the rape.
Religion and spirituality	
Is not currently affiliated with a church. Believes God would damn her because she was raped.	Ministers in her community do not take a blaming stance toward rape and that several have gone through rape crisis training.
Resources and Barriers	
Individual resources	
Spontaneously identifies few strengths or coping strategies.	Is a voracious reader who attends a large number of musical and cultural events even when they are at great distances away. She is organized, persistent, creative, and empathic. Her leadership skills are exceptional, and she is willing to work extremely hard.
Social resources, such as friends and family	
Does not think she can talk to her friends about the rape or the problems she has been having coping.	Has an unusually large and supportive group of friends. Her friends have been universally supportive of her since the rape, but not of the things she has been doing to cope with flashbacks and self-blaming.
Refuses to talk to family members about how she's doing because she does not want to "overwhelm" them.	Has very close relationships with her extended family, especially with her mother, uncle, and younger sister. Her mother, in particular, is a calm and nurturing person who is not rattled easily, and she responds readily to Melba's calls for help.
Sees her husband of 11 years as sometimes supportive and believes that he is getting tired of her depression.	Has a supportive husband, although he does not know what he should do for her when she's depressed.
Has two children (ages 8 and 5) whom she loves dearly and for whom she goes the extra mile. She recognizes this is reciprocated.	Loves her children and they love her. Her eight-year-old has increasingly adopted a parentified role in the relationship.
School and work	
As a nontraditional student earning As, she is afraid that she will be "found out." She begins each term thinking that she will "fail" all of her classes.	Is an A student who has received multiple awards within her department (and outside of it) for her service, academic accomplishments, and research.

(continued)

TABLE 13.6 *(continued)*

Reports that her supervisor is very critical of her and has unreasonable expectations for her work.	Has a supervisor who is generally viewed as one of the nicest men in the university. He has been very flexible during periods when Melba has been depressed.
Community resources Sees a number of physicians, but does not believe that she can be helped or that they are helpful.	Sees a number of physicians who have helped her with her significant health problems. Some have given her medicine samples because they know that she cannot afford her prescriptions.
Community contributions Admits that she has been active in the nursing association, but dismisses the importance of her contributions.	Has been very active serving in her university and community at large in numerous ways for which she has recently received a service award.
Models and mentors Has a very supportive mother and uncle.	Has strong relationship with her mother and uncle.
Obstacles to change Sees her problems as stable in orientation and unchangeable: "I am broken." She identifies an internal locus of responsibility and an external locus of control for these parts of her life.	While the kinds of issues she presents with often can be resistant to treatment, there are things she can do to cope better and to reduce the probability of a second rape.
Therapeutic relationship Often does not view her therapist as supportive or as understanding of her.	Has a therapist (Dena) who is generally seen as especially gifted. She likes Melba and has changed her schedule on several occasions for her.

I still hear the Voices from time to time . . . . I distract myself, lecture myself, and focus on the outside world. I have taught myself to use a little mantra when they reappear: "These Voices are not real. Don't be frightened. Don't get upset. They are not real. Don't let them overcome you. Try to think of what happened just before you heard them. Is there some emotion you can isolate that will explain why they are here now? They are not real. It's okay. Don't be afraid."

When I hear the Voices, I shake myself back to reality by using all my senses. If I'm riding the train to Manhattan, for example, I concentrate on the taste of the Diet Coke and the smell of the perfume I am wearing. I look out the window at the changing view, and listen carefully to the sound of the conductor collecting tickets. I feel my own ticket flipping back and forth between my fingers. (p. 269)

None of these strategies is, by itself, magical. However, when Schiller is successful in one situation, she is more likely to attempt to use these same skills the next time she has a problem. Accepting that she *can* do something to challenge the Voices increases her sense of self-efficacy (Bandura, 1997). Her self-esteem will likely increase, as her sense of hopelessness decreases.

Schiller (Schiller & Bennett, 1994) cannot change on her own, but neither can her family, friends, psychiatrist, and caseworker. Even her medication cannot do it *for* her. As the actions of her supports became coordinated and she worked with them effectively, she improved.

SERVING COMMUNITY

Consider how you serve your community. Think about your service in broad terms and include both your service to the local domestic violence shelter and your shoveling of your neighbor's sidewalk. What do you get out of this service? Does it strengthen and support your sense of self or undermine it?

Volunteering meets personal and social needs for many people. In general, people who volunteer are more adjusted and satisfied with life (Aquino et al., 1996; Dorfman & Moffet, 1987; D. Hoyt, Kaiser, Peters, & Babchuck, 1980). Giving to one's community has the potential of moving a person from a powerless stance to a more powerful one. It can be empowering, and it can improve one's self-esteem, especially when actions are successful and when they contribute to a valued part of the self-concept (S. Epstein, 1973). Giving in this way can strengthen one's ethnic identity and make it more positive (Horenczyk & Nisan, 1996).

Volunteering was one aspect of Rashelle's work (from chapter 4) that was especially therapeutic for her. She initially saw herself as worthless and having little to contribute to others. But as she began to peer-critique her friends' papers and after she started an informal support group for minority students, she started to see herself as more powerful ("I have something to contribute!"). She also felt more supported, a second valuable outcome of her experience also reported in the literature (Aquino et al., 1996; Omoto & Snyder, 1995).

This was not Melba's experience, however. Melba had a difficult time incorporating her community contributions into her self-esteem and often dismissed them as meaningless acts. This evaluation was consistent with her depressive thoughts, as she tended to minimize her accomplishments and become overwhelmed by any apparent failures.

Most people internalize their accomplishments more rapidly than Melba did. Perhaps Melba viewed what she already did as normal. As with social support, contributions are not always objectively self-evaluated. Some people seem satisfied with fairly small contributions while others, like Melba, dismiss significant contributions. In general, the amount that contributions must increase in order to positively impact self-esteem probably depends on the amount currently performed. When pre-treatment contributions are small, a relatively small difference can be effective. When a person is already an active volunteer, whether or not they internalize this identity, a much larger change in their behavior will be necessary in order to incorporate this change into their self-image. With people who are already very active in the community, therapeutic interventions should focus elsewhere.

Furthermore, before making the decision to focus on community contributions as a source of fostering self-esteem and self-efficacy, we need to consider its potential for impacting self-esteem. The largest improvements in self-esteem occur when a person's strengths and competencies match their values (S. Epstein, 1973). Think about poor Lisa Simpson from *The Simpsons* television series. She's a very bright, musically gifted, and generous-hearted girl living in a home that barely recognizes her gifts and often ridicules them. As long as she accepts her family's values and compares herself to them, she is likely to feel depressed. Conversely, we can expect that her self-esteem will rise as she rejects her family's values and chooses a set that matches her skills and achievements, or moves to a home or community that values her competencies.

While many people feel more competent and productive when they are contributing to others (Aquino et al., 1996; Dorfman & Moffet, 1987; D. Hoyt, Kaiser, Peters, & Babchuck, 1980), this is an idiosyncratic value, not a universal one. Providing service to others or the community should not be recommended for everyone. People who are socially isolated, but socially interested, may not be currently volunteering in any capacity and may expect that some type of personal gain from their actions will profit most.

CONCLUSIONS

Support is given, as well as received. Helping others *and* receiving help can decrease stress and increase self-esteem. However, as the chapter notes, not all kinds of help are equally useful. In general, helpfulness depends on the nature of the help received, the pervasiveness of the help, and the implicit messages about the person being helped. For example, Bernard received too little help, but Nita received too much. Both felt that others were disappointed in them and that they had let them down. Kevin, on the other hand, received no more help than he needed and his system asked him to specifically identify the kinds of help he wanted. As a result, he felt supported and powerful. He believed that others believed that he would be able to handle things in the future.

As in other chapters, events and circumstances foster our sense of meaning about ourselves and others. Too much help or too little may encourage maladaptive meanings. Nonetheless, like Melba, we may conclude that we have less support than we really do. In these cases, we need to help them recognize and access the supports that *are* available.

Volunteering is obviously helpful for the persons being helped, but it is also useful for the person volunteering. It builds healthier connections with others in the community, increases self-esteem and self-efficacy, and redefines the person's role in the community. For these reasons, volunteering can be an important part of the therapeutic process.

BRINGING IT INTO THE COMMUNITY: GROUP IDENTITY AND GROUP TRANSFORMATION

They were young black men preying on other young black men. They had been informed, successfully, that they were worthless, and everyone who looked like them was equally without worth. Each sunrise brought a day without hope and each evening the sun set on a day lacking in achievement. Whites, who ruled the world, owned the air and food and jobs and schools and fair play, had refused to share with them any of life's necessities—and somewhere, deeper than their consciousness, they believed the whites were correct. They, the black youth, young lords of nothing, were born without value and would creep, like blinded moles, their lives long in the darkness, under the earth, chewing on roots, driven far from the light (Angelou, 1981, p. 81).

Imagine that you were asked to intervene with the members of this gang. What would you do? Like Angelou (1981), we might suspect that the gang felt hopeless about themselves and their future. They attacked other Blacks, people they saw as equally worthless. As they did so, they chewed on their own "roots," undermining their own sense of self and that of other Blacks. Without individual and group pride, they were "like blinded moles . . . driven far from the light." If success was impossible through "normal" channels, they redefined success to make it possible.

This chapter, then, focuses on the sociopolitical aspects of individual change. When we fail to recognize the real barriers that some members of our society face, we fail in empathy. Without challenging those barriers, individual change can be difficult. Tearing down barriers can empower individuals and redefine how they see themselves. In the process of, and simultaneous with the previous changes, therapy should focus on developing a positive sense of culture, and thus self. This approach is relatively brief and action-oriented, but the goal is not just a quick fix, but a solution that decreases the probability of additional problems (cf. T. Robinson & Ward, 1991; Wachtel, 2002).

PERSONAL AND CULTURAL SELF-ESTEEM

How do you feel about your culture and community? When you meet someone who says, "Oh, you're from . . . " how do you feel—proud, defensive, some other response? Do you deny your racial, ethnic, or community ties? If so, when?

When you visit other racial or ethnic communities, how do you feel about these groups? How do you feel about your own? How would your feelings influence your work with members of any of these groups in therapy?

Psychology has tended to focus on personal self-esteem and its consequences on the individual, while failing to pay attention to *cultural* self-esteem. This is the sense of worth drawn from being a member of a particular group. Research on the cultural and personal self-esteem of culturally different group members has been inconsistent and controversial (Oyersman et al., 2002; Twenge & Crocker, 2002). What is most clear, however, is that the same variables have not affected all culturally different groups in the United States. Although some groups have lower self-esteem than Euro-Americans, others have higher self-esteem (Twenge & Crocker, 2002). It appears that sociocultural influences often define the ways in

TABLE 14.1 CONTEXTUAL FACTORS RELATED TO PERSONAL SELF-ESTEEM

Individualistic worldview	Individualistic attitudes are related to more positive self-esteem.
Collectivism	Messages valuing self-effacement are related to lower self-esteem.
Identification with group	Strong, positive identification with group predicts positive personal and global self-esteem.
Racial identity	More sophisticated statuses, such as internalization, are especially predictive of positive self-esteem.
Socioeconomic status (SES)	Generally higher SES group members have higher self-esteem.
Gender	This seems to depend on group and temporal issues, with African American women generally having a more positive self-esteem than African American men, and white women having a less positive self-esteem than white men (although the latter difference has decreased recently).
Cultural and political events	People who were children during periods of positive group-defining attitudes have high self-esteem.
Group density within area	People from areas and schools with a high density of group members have more positive self-esteem.
Group-valuing educational process	People exposed to group-valuing and group-centered curricula and cultural messages have more positive self-esteem.

Note: Summarized from Twenge & Crocker, 2002.

which groups and members of those groups value themselves. As we will discuss later in this chapter, these variables suggest important ways of intervening.

In recent studies, African Americans are reported to have a more positive personal self-esteem than that of other groups. Euro-Americans are generally intermediate between Blacks and other culturally different groups (Gray-Little & Hafdahl, 2000; Rotheram-Borus, 1990; Twenge & Crocker, 2002). This pattern has been attributed to several factors (see table 14.1).

Collectivism and Individualism

Individualism refers to an emphasis on personal responsibility, freedom of choice, actualization of one's potential, and respect for others' autonomy. Collectivism emphasizes the importance of maintaining mutual connections and building harmonious relationships and often requires emotional restraint and modesty to maintain this harmony. It also involves working toward the common good—two ideas that are not mutually exclusive (Oyserman et al., 2002). As seen in figure 14.1, African Americans, on average,

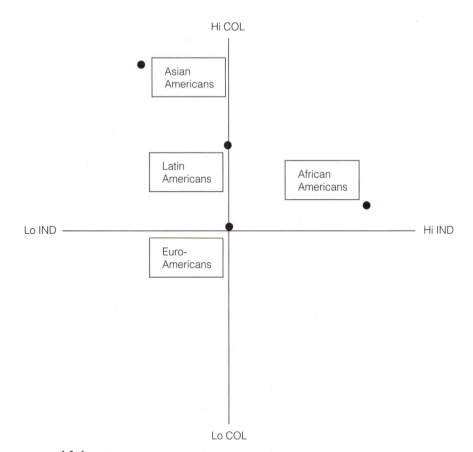

FIGURE 14.1

Degree of individualism (IND) and collectivism (COL) relative to Euro-Americans (modified from Oyserman et al., 2002). This study did not look at Native Americans, however, Twenge and Crocker (2002) hypothesize that Native Americans would be very similar to Asian Americans.

are as individualistic as Euro-Americans, and they have fewer collectivistic attitudes. Latin Americans, on average, are more collectivistic in orientation than Euro-Americans, while Asian Americans have both fewer individualistic and more collectivistic attitudes.

People from more individualistic cultures, on average, have higher levels of self-esteem than those from less individualistic cultures (Twenge & Crocker, 2002). Self-effacing attitudes, characteristic of more collectivistic cultures, are negatively related to self-esteem, while person-oriented attitudes and goals are positively related to it. Lily, an immigrant from China, focused much more on her Chinese community, church, and her family than did her granddaughter. R. J. rarely thought of herself as a Chinese

American, dated a Euro-American man, and attended a school with few Asian Americans. Not surprisingly, Lily and her granddaughter also derived their self-esteem from different sources: Lily from family, church, and other residents of Chinatown and R. J. from her relationships (her boyfriend and friends) and her ability to paint beautiful and challenging abstract images. Lily tended to take less credit for her accomplishments, because her culture frowned on it.

Given the relatively high individualistic attitudes of African Americans and their relatively low collectivistic attitudes, it is not surprising that African Americans have especially high levels of global self-esteem. The differences, however, are much smaller when academic self-esteem is factored in (Gray-Little & Hafdahl, 2000). Conversely, less individualistic and more collectivistic attitudes place Asian and Latin Americans at greater risk of lower self-esteem. It must be noted, however, that self-esteem is less likely to be an important value for Asians and Asian Americans than for African Americans and Euro-Americans, because the self is not as important a construct.

Group-centered Attitudes   Pride in self and in one's culture and community are often reported to be interconnected and are believed to be important pieces of personal identity (Bianchi, Zea, Belgrave, & Echeverry, 2002; Bloom, 1998; Parham & Helms, 1985; Poindexter-Cameron & Robinson, 1997; Pyant & Yanico, 1991; Tsai, Ying, & Lee, 2001; but see Rowley, Sellers, Chavous, & Smith, 1998). It is difficult to be self-accepting or to cope well with stress when one perceives the cultures one identifies with as "bad." Bianchi and her colleagues (2002), for example, report that black Brazilian men who devalue their racial group and embrace the values and standards of Whites have more negative self-esteem.

By meeting culturally valued outcomes, one fosters self-esteem (Oyserman et al., 2002). Therefore, thin, young white women often feel better about themselves than do white women who are overweight (Stice, Presnell, & Spangler, 2002). African American women, who tend to value thinness less, are less likely to have their self-esteem depend on their weight (D. Sue et al., 2000). However, meeting the norms and values of each group fosters self-esteem in people who have significant contact with two cultures. Tsai and her colleagues (2001) report that Chinese American students who are proficient in both Chinese and English and who value the Chinese community and maintain ties and contacts with it have higher personal self-esteem than those who do not. Similarly, numerous authors report that Helms' internalization status—a status in which people value both their own group and others'—is associated with positive cultural and individual self-esteem (Bianchi et al., 2002; Walters & Simoni, 1993).

On average, African Americans who were raised in the South or are attending historically Black colleges have significantly higher self-esteem than those raised in the North or in areas with lower concentrations of Blacks. Feeling included in a critical mass of people of one's race seems to affirm self-value and a sense of worth better than frequent contact with out-group members. Furthermore, historically Black institutions are more likely to provide an Afrocentric educational experience that fosters Black self-esteem. Rashelle's self-esteem (see chapter 4), for example, improved as she came into greater contact with other African Americans. She even began to feel a sense of belonging. In addition, her service projects encouraged her to see and recognize Afrocentric strengths, as opposed to only equating Good with White.

Roles of Racial Identity and Culture   Twenge and Crocker (2002) reported that age and self-esteem are correlated for many groups. They attributed these age-related changes to the development of racial identity; that is, older people are more likely to be able to think about themselves as racial beings in ways that help them maintain their self-esteem.

Although having pride in one's community and ethnicity is important, this pride does not need to be simplistic or to paint group members with a stereotyped brush. Helms (Helms & Cook, 1999) acknowledged this in her racial identity models (see tables 14.2, also 7.3 and 7.4). She described earlier ego statuses as being more primitive and stereotyped in their views of self and others. People with primitive statuses that are dominant are more likely to see other racial or cultural groups (Conformity) or their own group (Immersion-Emersion) as good and other groups as bad. People with the dissonance status as a prominent characteristic may fluctuate between these extremes, being uncomfortable with either stance. Because this good-bad distinction is overly simplistic for each of these three statuses, self-esteem can be fragile and rigidly defended. As group members begin to see themselves and their group as positive, even when mistakes are made, self-esteem is also likely to rise.

With later statuses of the Racial Identity Model (especially the Internalization and Integrative Awareness statuses), there is greater recognition of the complexity of human nature. Also, "goodness" is not defined by color (Helms & Cook, 1999). Furthermore, in these later statuses, people of color are able to challenge and overcome internalized racism in order to accept and embrace their race and themselves as members of it. In so doing, they begin to define themselves in personally meaningful ways, rather than in terms of self-limiting stereotypes. As Krech (1999) warns, both positive and negative stereotypes of one's cultural group are "ultimately dehumanizing . . . [and] they deny both variation within groups and commonalities between them" (p. 26). The cognitive changes associated with later statuses entail moving beyond stereotypes and the dichotomies of race, as seen here:

TABLE  **ATTITUDES TOWARD ONE'S OWN RACIAL OR CULTURAL GROUP AND THE DOMINANT GROUP AT EACH STATUS OF THE RACIAL IDENTITY SCALE FOR PEOPLE OF COLOR**

	Toward One's Own Group	Toward the Dominant Group
Conformity	Is accepting of societal prejudices.	Recognizes and admires contributions made by this group.
Dissonance	Recognizes that their treatment is unfair; uncomfortable accepting group as valid members of society.	Continues to admire members of this group and their contributions.
Immersion	Is uncritically idealizing.	Is uncritically denigrating; anger toward group is prominent.
Emersion	Is uncritically idealizing; positive connections with group are prominent.	Is uncritically denigrating.
Internalization	Has positive attitudes toward self and group.	Makes attempts to see members of this group as individuals.
Integrative Awareness	Has positive attitudes toward self and group. Able to see individual members of group as either good or bad.	Has positive attitudes toward group and is able to see strengths and weaknesses of individuals.

Note: Based on Helms & Cook, 1999.

I like living in this community, and I like being Choctaw, but that's all there is to it. Just because I don't want to be a white man doesn't mean I want to be some kind of mystical Indian either. Just a real human being. (quoted by White, 1990, as cited in Krech, 1999, p. 228)

More sophisticated racial identities are associated with an increased perception of control (Martin & Hall, 1992), and stronger coping mechanisms are associated with less stress (Klein, 1981, in Diller, 1999; Siegel, Yancey, & McCarthy, 2000; C. P. Thompson, Anderson, & Bakeman, 2000). Klein (1981, in Diller, 1999) also argues that "struggling with and resolving conflicts in identity release tremendous energy formerly stifled by ambivalence and disaffiliation. This energy can be a potent source of self acceptance and acceptance of one's own kind" (p. 222). His description of the effects of accepting his Jewish roots matches Moya-Gutierrez's description of her experiences of moving between Harlem and media images of American culture:

I was so anxious to assimilate, to blend in, that I started to forget who I was. Suddenly I was listening to Pearl Jam instead of Kinito Mendez and trying to shop at J. Crew. There's nothing wrong with listening to Pearl Jam and wanting to wear J. Crew. It was just when that was *all* I wanted to do it became a problem. I just felt it wasn't cool to be a poor Latina girl from Harlem. It was better to mosh than to merengue and to be able to go to a country home on the weekends. I almost forgot who I was and where I came from, and it's important not to do that. Remember, you come from beautifully vibrant cultures filled with rich music and traditions. Share that. Enlighten others with *your* history. . . . Try new things but don't forget the old. . . . Remember who you are. (Lahr, 1997, p. 41–42)

As long as Moya-Gutierrez believed that she was better when she passed as White rather than as a Latina, she struggled. When she was able to accept herself and her culture for what they were, and even as she tried new things, she was able to experience real pride in herself.

Culture-specific Development of Self-Esteem

Cultural values and attitudes also play a role in the development of self-esteem, since not all cultures show the same relationships between age and self-esteem. Although African Americans' self-esteem tends to increase with age (and presumably with more sophisticated views of self and race), Asian Americans' self-esteem tends to drop in adolescence (Twenge & Crocker, 2002). In addition, Asians in Asia tend to have lower self-esteem than either Asian Americans or Euro-Americans, suggesting that greater exposure to North American culture impacts Asian Americans' self-esteem. One possible explanation for this finding is that the self-enhancing tendencies typical of North American culture are less common in East Asia. This can be seen in R. J.'s and Lily's responses to being complimented on their artwork. R. J. accepted the compliment, and Lily attributed her skills to her teacher, while also suggesting that her work was not very good.

Culture-specific Self-Esteem

The differences between African American and Euro-American self-esteem are smaller when academic self-esteem is included (Gray-Little & Hafdahl, 2000; Twenge & Crocker, 2002). African Americans are less likely to base their self-esteem on achievements or others' opinions than are Euro-Americans, and their global and academic self-esteems become increasingly independent of each other in adolescence. Steele (1998) suggests that this may be related, in part, to the apparent incompatibility between succeeding in school and being an African American. Arroyo and Zigler (1995), however, conclude that teens of all races have difficulty reconciling achievement and their sense of self. For many, achievement

Over the next week, monitor the factors that seem to be especially related to your self-esteem. How do your mood, your successes, others' comments, and media images influence the way you see yourself?

is a competitive activity that conflicts with the more relational goals of adolescence.

It is important to note that different cultural groups derive their sense of *value*, which is perhaps a better term when referring to less individualistic groups, like Asian Americans, from different behaviors. Low self-esteem in academic, physical appearance, and relational areas does not mean that a person or group has a low sense of value, especially when the person or group does not value that particular attribute.

DEVELOPING CULTURAL SELF-ESTEEM

Self-esteem is not stable and unchangeable, but rather it fluctuates both across days and over longer periods. Given this fluctuation, there must be things we can do to influence it. Most descriptions include exploring and coming to terms with one's race and culture, while perhaps simultaneously working to change weaknesses. These interventions are described in the next sections.

Useful Attributions About Prejudice and Discrimination

In a review of the literature, Branscombe and her colleagues (1999) concluded that attributing others' actions to prejudice is something that most culturally different people attempt to avoid, since recognizing discrimination generally has negative consequences for psychological and physical health (cf. Landrine & Klonoff, 1996). Attributing others' actions to prejudice also implies a stable and unchangeable cause. While learning how to drive a car is something that a person can change, we cannot change our skin color or gender.

Stable and uncontrollable attributions "People are prejudiced, and there's nothing I can do about it," tend to increase depression (Seligman, 1975). Attributing problems to prejudice seems to have the most negative impact on self-esteem when people perceive the prejudice to be pervasive rather than occurring in isolated instances and when it is perceived as justified, such as when someone says, "I can't get anywhere in life because I am overweight. I agree; fat people aren't as good as other people" (Branscombe et al., 1999; Crocker, Cornwell, & Major, 1993).

However, attributing harmful acts to prejudice actually has a positive rather than negative impact for dominant group members (Branscombe et al., 1999). In this case, dominant group members appear to make external, unstable, and controllable attributions like, "That's not about me; some people are just unfair and have difficulty recognizing others' competence. I'll just show my work to someone else." This line of thinking suggests that therapists should maximize group identification, challenge the legitimacy of prejudice, and minimize the perception that prejudice is pervasive—something many minority group members already do—to strengthen personal and cultural well-being. Notice how Chad begins to meet these goals in the following dialogue with R. J., a Chinese American college student:

> R. J.: *I don't even know why I'm here. Mostly I'm doing pretty well. But . . . I've noticed that I feel like everyone is watching me all the time, expecting me to know everything. My math professor seems to think that I should know this stuff and that it should be easy. He keeps asking me to tutor other students in the class, and I don't like math! I'd be more than happy to help them in their art classes though . . .*
>
> CHAD: *Let me see if I have this right. It seems like your math prof and other people think that you should be good in math just because you are a Chinese American? (Paraphrase)*
>
> R. J.: *Yeah, that's it. I feel like everyone else thinks that I'm some sort of brainy nerd, but I'm not. They don't see me for who I am.*
>
> CHAD: *Who are you? (Open question)*
>
> R. J.: *Well, I am smart, but I'm also an artist and funny and lazy and hardworking. I could just sit and watch people all day. (Pause) I don't want to be just some sort of inscrutable Chinaman or dainty geisha.*
>
> CHAD: *You're pretty clear about who you are and who you aren't, but you seem to feel that everyone is pushing you into this box that you don't fit into. (Feedback, interpretation)*
>
> R. J.: *Yeah, that's exactly how I feel!*
>
> CHAD: *Everyone's this way? (Open question)*
>
> R. J.: *Well, not everyone. You, for example. You let me be me. So does my boyfriend . . . Still, I look different than most other students on campus and, while most of the time I like being the in-your-face artist, other times I'd just like to fit in. I hate it when I'm introduced to someone I've never met before—and they know me! It's like I have to be some sort of example all the time.*
>
> CHAD: *That's not fair. (Pause) Have you talked about this with other Asian Americans on campus? How do they handle it? (Feedback, open questions)*
>
> R. J.: *Good question. Most of the time I try to handle being stereotyped by not hanging with anyone who looks like me, but maybe I'm handling this the wrong way. Maybe spending time with other Asians would be helpful.*

Because R. J. is bright and already thinking in a complicated manner about herself, she is able to follow and extend Chad's ideas fairly rapidly. In fact, she seems ready to make her identity as a racial being as sophisticated

Remember a time when someone said something bad about you or some group. What did you think about yourself or the speaker and what were the short- and long-term consequences of this remark? Are there times when you have responded differently?

as that of the rest of her sense of identity. On the one hand, this task is limited by her lack of cultural knowledge, which may be showing in her comment about geishas. On the other hand, her comment may simply reflect her awareness that most people are ignorant about the differences among Asian cultures.

Black Is Beautiful

Banaji and her colleagues (1993) reported that people can express politically correct attitudes while still showing implicit prejudice. How can one change the underlying prejudice, when even its assessment has often been problematic? Dasgupta and Greenwald (2001), using the Implicit Association Test to assess automatic racial attitudes, demonstrated that increasing the salience of positive images of group members (e.g., Denzel Washington) was useful. Exposure to positive images caused drops in implicit racial bias.

Dasgupta and Greenwald's (2001) work is consistent with other research that suggests that exposure to positive messages about a group can have positive effects on global and cultural self-esteem. Twenge and Crocker (2002) noted that African Americans who were children during the Civil Rights movement, and those born afterwards, had higher self-esteem than African Americans born earlier in the 20th century, but were assessed at the same ages. This, in combination with the association between locale and self-esteem—African Americans in the South or at historically Black institutions have, on average, greater self-esteem—caused Twenge and Crocker to conclude that civil rights movements and Afro-centric education have positive consequences on self-esteem. Furthermore, they conclude that this may be one important explanation for why African Americans have *higher* self-esteem relative to other culturally different groups *and* Euro-Americans, despite experiencing *more* racial stigma. African Americans have been more likely to receive Afrocentric educational programs and to attend historically Black institutions, while members of other groups have not received such advantages as frequently.

As we will discuss later, these changes can be made at a cultural level, but they can also be made at an individual level. As Chad encourages R. J. to learn who she is as a Chinese American woman and to self-explore with other strong Asian Americans, he is also helping her to appreciate her culture and herself as a cultural being. With a woman who tends to think about herself in a relatively complicated manner and who is open to doing so with others, the fact that Chad is a Euro-American male seems to have little negative impact on this process. However, we should keep in mind that a person's racial identity can either help or hinder this process.

Acknowledging the Bad While Accepting Self

Moya-Gutierrez (Lahr, 1997) talks about how rejecting one's culture can be a symbol of self-hatred as well as an action that maintains it. In general, people at lower racial identity statuses that tend to reject their own group in favor of the dominant group also tend to have lower individual self-esteem (Bianchi et al., 2002; Parham & Helms, 1985; Poindexter-Cameron & Robinson, 1997; Pyant & Yanico, 1991). People at the Immersion and Emersion statuses reject the dominant culture without having significant contact with it. Rejecting the dominant culture without having first explored it may be a kind of defensive self-protection, like an oppositional child who decides who she is by doing the opposite of what her mother wants. See, for example, the Racial Identity models (Helms & Cook, 1999), described in tables 7.3, 7.4 and 14.2. Conversely, people at the most complex ego statuses tend to have higher self-esteem. Healthy self-esteem is developed by exploring values and goals in the context of one's culture, while also opening oneself to other possibilities. It involves accepting both the strengths and weaknesses of your own group and other groups.

The self-destructive nature of this connection with one's culture can be seen in Hegi's (1997) autobiographical writings. Hegi, a German born shortly after World War II and now living in the United States, struggles with how one can identify with a culture in a positive manner while hating parts of it and its history:

> . . . I keep redefining the boundaries in my struggle between preserving my personal vision as a writer and being part of a community. A lot of that depends on how much we identify with our community of origin. I envy the Chickasaw writer Linda Hogan and the Inupiaq educator James Nageak . . . who both come from cultures they regard with admiration and loyalty, whose personal visions reflect those of their communities.
>
> But I spent the first eighteen years of my life within a culture that has a history of oppression and violence—I can neither trust that community nor identify with it. I feel no loyalty to preserve the secrets of that community—only the loyalty to myself to tell the truth as I perceive it, regardless of how flawed my vision might be. And to preserve the integrity of my vision, I have to risk not belonging to any community. (p. 41)

Hegi (1997) has worked to free herself from her culture, but she remains connected by the Holocaust. Working free leaves her without the emotional support that could be provided by her community. She plaintively complains that she does not feel German, but does not completely feel like she belongs in the United States either. While her vision is not comfortably mirrored in her culture's, stepping back to examine her culture and her new home means that Hegi earns several positive outcomes. Honest attempts at objectivity can nurture the senses of loyalty, truth, integrity, and risk-taking, regardless of "how flawed [our] vision might be" (p. 41).

How can we encourage people to develop a more sophisticated racial identity? Especially when clients paint themselves in a completely negative fashion as members of a group (e.g., victims of sexual abuse), our job is to enlarge this picture. Is it true that they *only* have negative attributes associated with this group membership? Are there also positive ones? Is it true that all members of this group are bad? Have there been positive members and important contributions also? How, for example, is being a survivor of sexual abuse different from being a victim? How has being sexually abused led to some of her strengths?

CHANGING THE COMMUNITY'S MEANINGS

In chapter 11 we talked about making personal kinds of meaning from traumas that cannot be problem-solved or fixed, such as when a family member is murdered. When wars, discrimination, and natural disasters have traumatized whole groups, however, we need to find ways to change both the individual's and the group's meanings about the event. Bloom (1998), for example, argued that personal or group traumas should be converted into community assets, rather than only a personal catastrophe or, if post-traumatic growth has been successful, only personal growth. She further argued that such diverse and apparently unrelated events as the Nuremberg trials, political demonstrations, black humor, and artistic works are attempts to do just that.

Communities have the power to accept traumas as inevitable and destructive or to see them in a different light altgether. In accepting the dominant culture's views of an event, we can be defeated. By challenging this definition, we can begin to change our community and ourselves. This is the goal of memoirs like *After Silence* (Raine, 1998) and *Telling* (Francisco, 1999). In talking about her decision to talk about her rape Francisco said,

> I have kept writing because I want rape to be unacceptable, not in polite conversation, but in our lives . . . I don't want the details of this old story to be kept private any longer. I want a different world for women, for men, and the children who inherit what we make of it. (p. 3)

Telling this story is also personally therapeutic, as one woman says, "'Every time we tell our story it helps take away the power this experience, and its subsequent shame, have over us'" (quoted in Raine, 1998, p. 5).

Weine, Kulenovic, and their colleagues (1998) reported that Bosnian refugees experienced similar beneficial effects from giving "testimony"

Step back. Think about the way that your community has seen events that have been important in your life, such as a first menstruation, graduation, marriage, and retirement. How have these and other developmental landmarks affected how you see yourself? If you know families or cultural groups that celebrate these events differently, what differential impact have you seen?

How has your community perceived political events that have had an impact on your community such as war, the Holocaust, unemployment rates in your city? How does the story your community tells affect you or other members of the community?

about war-related trauma, and their PTSD symptoms stemming from these traumas. Talking about their experiences in a way that made sense within their social contexts and meanings returned both a measure of control and a sense of positive self-worth. Talking about their experiences in a way that contributed to other refugees allowed them to accept therapy that otherwise would have been unacceptable.

Telling is therapeutic, but telling should eventually lead to more positive consequences, including acceptance, a sense of transformation, or individual or social change. This can be seen in a high-achieving woman's description of her history of discrimination (Richie et al., 1997):

> I think many people would feel that it's been a challenge . . . being a female. It's been a challenge being Black. . . . It's been a challenge, many people probably think, being from the South. But . . . I really think that I've turned those challenges into assets for me, and made them work for me instead of against me. (quoted in Richie et al., 1997, p. 139)

Secondary Victimization

Consider how others' feedback during a difficult time in your life either increased or decreased your pain during that period. What other effects did it have?

As Raine (1998) commented, being able to tell one's story and be believed can be very therapeutic. But, this is not a typical reaction. Many people are victimized directly, then a second time indirectly by their friends, family, and greater cultures (S. L. Brown, 1991). We victimize when we don't believe, when we don't want to hear, and when we dismiss the pain that someone feels ("Well, it's not like you were hurt or anything . . . "). We are secondary perpetrators when we fail to stand up to say that something is wrong. We are secondary perpetrators when we talk about the crime—be it discrimination, oppression, rape, or assault—without understanding the victim's viewpoint.

Unfortunately, secondary perpetrators include family, friends, and neighbors who may fail to believe or to support (and may even be unaware of how they can support). Police officers, reporters, teachers, doctors, therapists, ministers, and lawyers revictimize when they ask questions that blame "What were you doing there anyway?" Secondary perpetrators, such as politicians, the media, and the legal system, may not even know the victim. Politicians victimize when they fail to create a system that is responsive to a victim's needs or that fails to prevent a problem from occurring. The courts victimize when they set up a system that is responsive to the accused's needs and rights without also considering the rights of people who have been victimized.

With people who think dichotomously, as many people do under stress, silence may seem like approval. Therapists must clearly (and sometimes frequently) say that oppression and oppressive acts are wrong. We must be vigilant for as-yet-unidentified ways that our culture has been oppressive and be willing to challenge our culture, our clients, and ourselves when we recognize these.

TRANSFORMING COMMUNITY

The Desiderata asks that we think about what we can control and what we cannot, asking for the wisdom to recognize the difference between them. Have you identified an injustice and done something to address it? What was the consequence of doing so? What happened if you failed to do so because of lack of skills, time, energy, and hope or other barriers?

Problems in living are less attributable to failings of individuals than to a "macrosystem that deprives them of power, justice, and opportunity" (Cowen, 1991, p. 407). Cowen noted the correlation between a history of disempowerment and problems in living. Albee (2000) argued:

> There are major political differences between a medical/organic/brain defect model to explain mental disorders and a social-learning, stress-related model. The former is supported by the ruling class because it does not require social change and major readjustments to the status quo. The social model, on the other hand, seeks to end or to reduce poverty with all its associated stresses, as well as discrimination, exploitation, and prejudices as other major sources of stress leading to emotional problems. By aligning itself with the conservative view of causation, clinical psychology has joined the forces that perpetuate social injustice. (p. 248)

Cowen and Albee conclude that changing society to empower the disenfranchised is an important part of therapy for client *and* therapist. Although our attempts to understand the inherently senseless are often primarily cognitive in nature (see chapter 11), many people also take action to convert their pain into a moral outrage and commitment that serves both the individual and the community. Encouraging Melba (chapter 13) to spend her time volunteering in a rape crisis center transformed her anger into something that served rather than undermined her.

Huey, a *Boondocks* character, is often angry about society's hypocrisy and injustices. However, his anger sometimes leaves him feeling like Don Quixote, alone and miserable, tilting at windmills. His grandfather reminds him that anger can be productive without hurting him (see Figure 14.2). Bloom (1998) details a number of ways in which people can transform pain into something socially useful. These include educating others to prevent the recurrence of similar problems in the future (Mothers Against Drunk Driving and Physicians for Social Responsibility), creating self-help groups (Alcoholics Anonymous), rescuing others (the Underground Railroad and Oskar Schindler), seeking justice (Mothers of the Plaza de Mayo), taking political action (Vaclav Havel), finding humor (Richard Pryor and Ellen Degeneres), or making art (Picasso's *Guernica*, Woody Guthrie's protest music, and Havel's poetry and plays). As these exemplify, anger is more

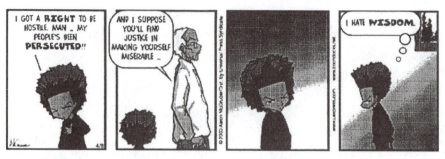

FIGURE 14.2

Huey's struggle to find a positive use for his anger (*Boondocks* © 2000 Aaron McGruder. Distributed by Universal Press Syndicate. Reprinted with permission. All rights reserved.)

than an act of defiance and can be transformed into a celebration of self and culture (Cotterell, 1999).

Justice and Forgiveness

Although a search for meaning can be individually transformative, each of the political and social acts described in the last paragraph also unequivocably holds the guilty parties responsible for their behavior. Boraine (1996), for example, movingly argued that failing to do so has significant consequences for a society and sends an ambiguous message about the morality of the offense. However, there are a number of ways to hold a culture responsible for terrorism and oppression (see table 14.3). Within the spirit of this argument, Pope John Paul II and President Clinton apologized to Jews and Native Americans, respectively, for crimes occurring before their tenure in office. Their acceptances of responsibility when words are translated into action, are first steps toward creating a more just and equitable society.

Forgiveness and acceptance may be important parts of the healing process (McCullough, Worthington, & Rachal, 1997), but they cannot happen before holding the perpetrating individuals or groups responsible for their behavior (Freedman & Enright, 1996). Premature forgiveness without first receiving justice, hearing an apology from the offending party, or experiencing justifiable anger may lead to self-blame and shame (Boraine, 1996). It can undermine one's faith in self and humanity. Therapy, then, needs to find a balance between accepting what happened, challenging its meaning, and taking actions that clearly demonstrate to self and others that the traumatic act was reprehensible. Lorri tries to strike this balance in the following dialogue:

> SAMUEL: *I keep thinking that it was my fault. I shouldn't have been there. If I hadn't walked in right then my mother might be alive . . . .*

TABLE CONSEQUENCES OF GRANTING AMNESTY OR OTHERWISE FAILING TO HOLD INDIVIDUALS OR SOCIETIES ACCOUNTABLE FOR THEIR ACTIONS AND INACTIONS

Allows the guilty to escape punishment.	Amnesty and premature forgiveness make it possible for people to escape without facing appropriate consequences or punishment, sometimes even without acknowledging their involvement. "Was he/she really wrong?" "Did he/she really commit the crime?"
Threatens our belief in a democratic society.	People who are responsible for their crimes against individuals and society are not punished, which creates doubts about fundamental democratic ideals and suggests that these do not apply to all members of the society. "Are some people above the law?"
Institutionalizes hypocrisy.	When amnesty is written into laws, hypocrisy is created and institutionalized. While one law prohibits violence, another allows wrongdoers of "protected crimes" to avoid a fair trial and punishment. "Is it okay to engage in 'certain crimes'?" "Why?" "What does this say about the victims of those crimes?"
Confuses and creates ambiguous social, moral, and psychological limits.	A society that allows crimes to go unpunished or uninvestigated fosters a lack of respect for laws and prohibitions and reinforces divisiveness among classes or groups. "Are some behaviors only 'wrong' if you're caught?" "Can people in power commit crimes with impunity?"
Invalidates and denies what has happened.	When people are allowed to avoid punishment, the real concerns of people who have been victimized are invalidated. Victims may blame themselves or excuse victimizers. Because victims' stories have not been validated, others (including victims) may question their memories. This reduces the ability to understand and to be understood. "Maybe no one did anything wrong?"
Affects people's beliefs in the future.	Impunity creates a culture of hopelessness. People are supposed to believe that things are fair, but are they? Without some sense of legal or judicial validation, people may fear that history will repeat itself and that society will remain unjust. "Can we perceive a future that will work for all people?" "Can we feel hopeful about the future and work to make it possible?"
Causes powerlessness, guilt, and shame.	Until the experience of events is validated in a respected realm such as by a parent, therapist, court, or legal system, many people feel powerlessness, guilt, and shame as a result of being victimized. These feelings can be handled in maladaptive ways whenever adaptive venues are blocked. "Am I a worthwhile person?" "Did I deserve this punishment?" "Can I do anything to stay safe in the future?"
Tempts people to take the law into their own hands.	When trials and justice are not carried out by proper authorities, people who have suffered are tempted to take the law into their own hands and carry out their own private vendettas. "The powers that be don't care. I'm the only one who will try to do anything to make it better."

Note: Modified from Boraine, 1996, paragraphs 41–48; see also Cheng, 1986.

LORRI: *It sounds like you're still blaming yourself for your mother's death 25 years later. Like you're rerunning the tape, trying to figure out what you could have done differently. (Reflection of feeling, low-level interpretation)*

SAMUEL: *You're right about that. I keep worrying about my woman, our kids . . . What if it happens to them? I'm gonna be ready this time!*

LORRI: *You sound very angry at them rather than you. (Reflection of feeling)*

SAMUEL: *You're right, there!*

LORRI: *That's good. You were little, and it wasn't your fault. I'm worried, though, about what you're talking about doing with that anger. (Feedback, self-disclosure)*

SAMUEL: *(Quickly) What you mean?*

LORRI: *It sounds like you're ready to pick a fight with me, with everyone. (Yeah.) Maybe we can talk about ways to be angry that won't end up hurting you or anyone else. (Yeah.) Maybe they could even help both you and your family . . . (Pause) You've been active in the Neighborhood Watch program for the last year. I wonder whether this might be a way of handling your anger. (Reflection of feeling, information, interpretation)*

SAMUEL: *You know, that's so cool! I've been working on the Watch and enjoying it. People look up to me. I feel powerful, not like that scared child, but I hadn't made the connection . . .*

At the beginning of this conversation Samuel still tended to think dichotomously, "I can hurt or I can be hurt. I can control or be controlled." Because Lorri has a good relationship with Samuel and frequently leads with a reflection of feeling to help him recognize that she understands him, she has the power to help him understand the implications of his apparent beliefs "Righteous anger should be expressed and destroy those who have destroyed me". At this point Lorri can encourage him to see options that will help him feel better about himself and his behavior over the long run. In doing so, Lorri avoids an unquestioning acceptance of Samuel's perspective, while remaining empathic, and empowers him to take healthy and adaptive steps (cf. Greene, 1985).

HELPING INDIVIDUALS CHANGE THEIR COMMUNITIES

D. W. Sue and his colleagues (1999) assert that, as psychologists, we must strive for social justice and its core values of justice, respect, fairness, equity, and dignity. And this must be done across our discipline and in our work with clients. It requires examining our individual actions and inactions *and* making a commitment to making changes in the community and profession that foster social justice. How have our actions (or inactions) moved us closer to or further from these core values?

Anger can often be a very destructive emotion to self and others. Destructive anger, such as self-mutilation or violence against others, often comes about when no adaptive means for solving a problem is identified (Levenkron, 1998). In the face of adversity, like Samuel, we can feel like we have no choices ("He *made* me angry!"). While anger is a logical reaction to many situations, it can take many forms—some productive and some destructive to self and others. It makes sense to be angry about racism, poverty, discrimination, and other environmental barriers, but this anger can be used productively such as in the cases of Martin Luther King, Jr and Mother Teresa, who transformed anger into positive action (Cotterell, 1999). Using anger in a destructive manner with assaults, substance abuse, and self-mutilation, allows aggressors to win a second time. The first time is when they were oppressors and perpetrators and, the second, when they got their victims to act out.

Ponterotto (1987) asserted that, "Given the many social injustices and prejudicial views confronted by Mexican Americans and other minorities, a change is needed not in the individual but in the 'system' in which that individual lives" (p. 308). Identifying and changing the deeply unfair aspects of our culture is a profoundly empowering and liberating response to societal and cultural problems. Rashelle's therapy (detailed in chapter 4) also took an activist's stance. As she began to identify her school and the greater community as oppressive *and* began to identify ways to change these problems (e.g., by developing a program on ethnic and minority authors and starting an internship program with minority businesses for minority students), her depression began to lift. This simple intervention can move responsibility for the problem from an internal locus to an external one, and simultaneously increase an internal sense of control ("I'm not helpless in the face of adversity"). Actions as varied as bra burnings, civil rights demonstrations, advocating for legislative and community change, developing social action programs, and writing a letter to the editor can be effective sources of change. They also tend to be very empowering for the individual making these changes.

> Identify a problem that seems unfair to you. Brainstorm as many ways of addressing the problem as possible. Change can be local and only affect you or more global and affect the larger community.
>
> If you remember a place where you have made community change in the past, think about the positive and negative consequences for you and your community.

Teaching Pigs to Fly

Sometimes, being active in the community and doing things to change it can feel as productive as attempting to teach a pig to fly ("It ain't going to happen no matter how hard we try"). That assumes, however, that our goal is to change community opinion directly rather than to create an atmosphere where we begin to challenge the acceptance of the unacceptable.

Recently, a local minister posted his sermon topic "The abomination of homosexuality" outside his church. I wrote several letters to him as part of my outrage about this oppressive act. Did I expect to change his opinion? Did I want him to change mine? No and no. The fact that I wrote my opinion and shared it with community members was part of my attempt to support the GLBT community. I wanted to say that his message and actions were unacceptable. Consequently, I wrote (in part):

> I believe that we should stand up to address inequities in our society and to make clear that injustice and oppression in all of its forms is unacceptable. If your sign had talked about women as "unclean," women and men would have walked against your church. If your sign had justified slavery based on its occurrence in the Bible, Blacks and Whites would have walked hand in hand to protest your words. In fact, most people, even if they believed those things, would not post them on a sign because they know that they would receive righteous indignation. It concerns me that you would think it was okay to post your sign, that it would be okay for your congregation to applaud your words, that it would be okay for you to allow them to do so, and that hundreds of people did not descend on your church to express their outrage. (Slattery, 2000b, p. 5)

I was afraid that if I kept silent I would seem to be expressing a tacit approval of his words and acts. Silence seems to suggest that the unacceptable is acceptable and that the perpetrator has enough power to commit a transgression with impunity. Isn't this what happened during Nazi Germany?

Silence does not necessarily indicate tacit approval, however. Sometimes, we are silent when we don't know what to say or how to react. Sometimes, we feel helpless to change the system. At still other times, we may be quiet because, as a colleague described it, it is the "nice thing" to do. Her mother had told her, "Be quiet if you don't have anything nice to say." Do we have to be "nice and quiet" when we see or hear something outrageous? Do we give away our power by doing so? Do we also become oppressors when we attempt to "keep the peace"?

Breaking the Silence

Taking action, both in the community and in the therapy room, can be an important step in challenging privilege and oppression. Rollo May (1989) does this powerfully in his work with Mercedes, a bi-racial woman who had been prostituted by her stepfather, and perhaps with her mother's knowledge. When she had difficulty expressing her anger toward people who had taken advantage of her, May did, and thus enabled Mercedes to develop a voice. She became aware of her anger and began to express it in more appropriate ways.

Becoming aware of oppression and choosing to do something to address it is a risk (L. L. Shaw, Batson & Todd, 1994). Acknowledging oppression can force us to make changes. It can also require admitting that life has been unfair and that we have received more than our fair share of life's resources. We may feel committed to expending considerable time, energy, and money to change the situation. Reputations can be gained or lost based on our actions and on the nature of the cause we attempt to address. Many people do not feel able to accept these costs. Depending on our circumstances, however, we may believe that the costs of identifying oppression and expressing our outrage are acceptable.

While some situations prevent us from raising our voices (L. L. Shaw et al., 1994), Latané and Darley (1968) have identified those situations where it is *easier* to behave courageously and altruistically. In particular, we are more likely to help others and to stand up for what we believe when we see others, especially those we admire, behaving altruistically. As a result, raising our voices against oppression can be useful, even when there is little hope that we will actually be able to teach pigs to fly.

Taking Over Their Voice

When we speak for someone else, there is a danger that, rather than giving their concerns a voice, we take over that voice in an action akin to Columbus "discovering" the Americas and "civilizing" the Native Americans. How can we express our outrage at injustice without becoming yet another oppressive agent? Was May (1989), for example, expressing his concerns and forcing Mercedes to think and feel in a particular fashion or was he encouraging her to recognize and accept her voice? How could we know the difference?

Mercedes entered therapy out of touch with her own anger, but aware of its absence. She often repeated a kind of prayer: "Let me have a child, let me be a good wife, let me enjoy sex, let me feel something" (p. 167). Across time, as May gently noted evidence suggesting that Mercedes was angry, she began to feel her anger and set appropriate limits with her family. Rather than stealing their voices, therapy should add to theirs in order to give them greater force. As May (1989) describes it:

> Far from toning down aggression, it is of the very nature of psychotherapy to help people *assert* it. Most people who come for therapy are like Mercedes, though less pronounced—they have not too much aggression, but too little. We encourage their aggressiveness provisionally, confident in the hope that, once they have found their own right-to-be and affirm themselves, they will actually live *more* constructively interpersonally as well as intrapersonally. (p. 173)

TABLE 14.4 WAYS TO IDENTIFY THAT PEOPLE HAVE GIVEN VOICE RATHER THAN STOLEN IT

	Stolen Voice	Given Voice
Frequency of speaking	People speak less frequently or more briefly over time.	People often begin to speak more over time.
Recognition of ideas and their worth	People often respond with "I don't know" in response to questions about their thoughts and feelings. Do not develop ideas even when asked.	While they may initially respond with "I don't know," they are more able to develop their ideas when given an opportunity.
Development of ideas	New ideas may be another futile attempt to be heard and may be dropped at any sign of opposition.	New ideas are generally developed over time.
Use of others' ideas	Thoughts expressed are only reiterations of therapist's ideas or are diametrically opposed to them. For example, "Yeah, but . . ." can be a common response in the latter case.	Ideas are expressed more thoughtfully. People are free to include and exclude their therapist's ideas.
Autonomy of voice	Actions are responsive to (or against) perceptions of others' wishes.	Initiative actions occur independent of, rather than in opposition to, others' wishes.

This type of understanding depends on an empathic understanding of our clients' worldviews. As with all additive empathy (Carkhuff, 1969), our actions should increase our clients' feelings of being understood and increase rather than decrease their awareness and sense of power. Their ideas should become unique and spontaneous rather than be made to fit a single mold (see table 14.4).

Cheng's (1986) description of life during the Cultural Revolution in China can help us see this distinction. When revolutionaries expressed a politically correct concern during coercive times, it was apparently embraced by other citizens, with the rank and file repeating it almost verbatim (rather than paraphrasing or developing it). If the revolutionaries had truly been returning the proletariat's voice, there should have been a proliferation of ideas and free critique of the pros and cons of these ideas. There were, however, "good" ideas and people that were above criticism and "bad" ideas and people that were dangerous to embrace.

If May (1989) truly empowered Mercedes, we would expect that she would become free to express both her anger at her mother and stepfather, as well as the deep ties to them that we might suspect are also present. Her ability to express her ideas would become more fluent and frequent. Rather than interrupting herself or otherwise dismissing her ideas, she would develop these more fluently. She would not be left feeling that there are some feelings and thoughts that she can have and others that she should not, although May might help her to find ways to express her ideas more effectively and more assertively. In fact, these conclusions are consistent with May's report.

Empowerment Versus Validation

Sometimes people attempt to address problems in their community in order to be validated. Although a positive response from the court system or the school board can be exciting, there can be real disadvantages to going through the court system (or any decision-making body) to make change. Specifically, many people assume that the court system determines "truth." Although identifying the relative fault of defendants and victims is one goal of the judicial system, it is only one. Another important aspect is to protect the rights of the accused by making sure that confessions are not unfairly coerced and that the body of evidence supports a guilty judgment. If the evidence does not support a guilty judgment, the judge or jury must pronounce the perpetrator "not guilty."

"Not guilty" sounds like "innocent" to most people. Especially for those people who think relatively dichotomously, a not guilty judgment for the defendant may feel like a guilty verdict for *them*. They may feel that the "problem" (e.g., incest, discrimination, sexual harassment, etc.) was their fault. It may feel like yet another person (or system in this case) failed to believe or support them. They may believe that others think that they were imagining the problem or misinterpreting others' actions. While it is disappointing to fail to receive the kind of judgment that you want, it does not mean that you are guilty, not believed, or misinterpreting others' actions. The conclusions described here seem to be based in emotional reasoning (Parrott, 1997), such as in "I feel guilty, therefore I am guilty."

Changing environments and creating positive change is important, but we should be cautious about determining our personal worth or innocence based on others' judgments. As therapists, we must help clients recognize the court's, school board's, legislative body's or employer's actions for what they are. They are decisions that are only based on the evidence presented, the judging body's ability to understand it, and limited by the level of proof required.

Even when significant physical evidence exists, which often is not available in social action cases, it may be difficult to obtain guilty verdicts because of societal beliefs and biases. Jurors who believe that only dirty, nasty strangers molest children are unlikely to convict the father who is an

Remember a place where you requested a ruling from an external source (a court, the school board, a parent, or a supervisor), but were not believed. How did you feel? What were you thinking that made you feel this way? What protected you? What did you do? How can you transfer what you have learned from this experience to your work with clients?

upstanding member of his community, regardless of the level of evidence offered. A judge who makes sexual comments to his staff is less likely to take a sexual harassment case seriously, unless the behavior is egregious. A parent's fair-haired child is unlikely to do anything wrong, despite evidence to the contrary. Life is not fair no matter how much we may wish it to be. We can, however, work to make it more fair.

Failing to Act

The Desiderata suggests that we identify those things that we can change and then change them while recognizing those things that we cannot change and then accept them. On a very local level this may be an important thing to do: to accept the fact that a rape has occurred, a child has died, a friend has been diagnosed with HIV, rather than denying their existence. However, even in these situations, it is often important to acknowledge the problem's existence and work to change it. Wiesel (1982) tells the following story about the individual and societal implications of action and inaction:

> One of the Just Men came to Sodom, determined to save its inhabitants from sin and punishment. Night and day he walked the streets and markets preaching against greed and theft, falsehood and indifference. In the beginning, people listened and smiled ironically. They stopped listening: he no longer even amused them. The killers went on killing, the wise kept silent, as if there were no Just Man in their midst.
>
> One day a child, moved by compassion for the unfortunate preacher, approached him with these words: "Poor stranger, you shout, you expend yourself body and soul; don't you see that it is hopeless?"
>
> "Yes, I see," answered the Just Man.
>
> "Then why do you go on?"
>
> "I'll tell you why. In the beginning, I thought I could change man. Today, I know I cannot. If I still shout today, if I still scream, it is to prevent man from ultimately changing me." (p. 72)

Recognizing a problem and not acting on it, despite our awareness of it, can be more than mere acceptance of an injustice, but a small death (Bergin, 1991). Making community change is not a completely altruistic act. Failing to speak out against perceived injustice and overlooking (and even accepting) the small horrors we see daily can kill our soul (Hardy, 2001). Keeping our eyes open and speaking out takes courage, but it is also individually revitalizing. However, our individual inaction destroys our communities by leading to a cynicism and indifference "as if there were no Just Man in [our] midst" (Wiesel, 1982, p. 72). This can lead to the bystander apathy that was, as discussed in chapter 12, an ultimate cause of Kitty Genovese's murder (Latané & Darley, 1968).

CONCLUSIONS

The ideas of this chapter and the last one can be summarized concisely in a model of Tatum's (2000). She suggests that three things must happen to help a culturally different person become healthy individually and a part of the community. These include: **A**ffirming identity; **B**uilding community; and **C**ultivating leadership. Identity is affirmed when we discover things that we like about our ourselves and our group identities. It is often useful to start to learn, practice, and value our unique "language" and differences in same-group communities. When we challenge oppression and appreciate people who are similar to us, we can begin to make social change (Watts et al., 2002).

Returning to Sherene's work with Rashelle (see chapter 4), Sherene helped Rashelle identify ways to see herself as a young black woman in a positive light. As she began to do so, Rashelle stopped trying to become something that she was not and accepted herself for who she was. Rather than ignoring or devaluing other African Americans in her largely Euro-American community, she began to connect to Blacks in positive ways. She strongly identified with Sherene, but also admired local African American business leaders and Afrocentric writers, while reconnecting with her family.

REDISCOVERING A SENSE OF BALANCE

I love raisins, but when I don't eat enough, I become anemic and dizzy, and I get headaches. When I eat too many, all sorts of nasty things happen in my digestive system.

This chapter is about balance. The assessments in this book are designed to help therapists identify places where clients might be out of balance, whether in their spiritual life, physical health, social relationships, or their connections to family and culture. Mervyn (from chapter 2), for example, was out of balance in several parts of his life. He had severed ties with his church, had few (and unsatisfying) relationships with friends and family, and was working long and overwhelming hours. In some areas of his life, he was "psychologically deprived," and in others, he received so much focus that he felt overwhelmed.

Saccharine used to be classified as a carcinogen, but now it's okay to consume it. Like so many things, of course, it is toxic in large amounts but fine in smaller ones. People in general and clients in particular run into problems when, like Mervyn, their work consumes their life or when, like Jackson in chapter 3, they spend their life with friends and avoid work, school, and family. Large amounts of these activities and decisions are problematic. Moderate amounts can be healthy and adaptive.

A Sense of Balance

One way to think about problems is to imagine having wandered off a path and gotten lost. People might also get out of balance by how they spend their time, as the Native American story suggests. People may be rigidly approaching solutions in a single-minded manner or thinking dichotomously about themselves, their families, and their "problem" situations. This chapter helps identify ways for people out of balance to get back on track.

Getting Out of Balance

A common way to get out of balance is to enjoy doing something, then do more of it, as though more were better (Watzlawick, Weakland, & Fisch, 1974). If one sports car is fun, then two will be better. If two are good, then four will be even better. This style of thinking is a form of positive reinforcement that is out of control. Uninformed by the laws of psychophysics, this thinking process fails to recognize that a larger absolute difference is needed to notice a change when starting with big stimuli than with small ones. This philosophy is especially problematic because it takes away time from doing the things that keep people *in* balance.

People also get out of balance when they are reinforced on a lean reinforcement schedule. Darby's daughter, Rae-Anne, did not seem to listen to him, so he spoke louder and more forcefully. Eventually Rae-Anne responded, leading Darby, a single parent, to yell increasingly frequently. While his actions may have worked at first, Rae-Anne eventually became good at screening out her father's screams. Darby entered therapy saying, "Nothing works with her!" He had, unfortunately, chosen a strategy that

According to one Native American story, our life is like a house with four rooms: physical, spiritual, social, and intellectual. I think about these rooms as varying in size. For instance, some may be larger and more lived in than others. Some may be nicely decorated, while others are full of cobwebs. For a satisfying life, however, we should enter each room at least briefly every day. How I live in my rooms, though, may be different from how you live in yours.

Do you visit your "rooms" regularly? How? How big is each room? Does this work for you? What could you do to bring your rooms into a healthier balance?

was occasionally reinforced just often enough to keep Darby using it, but infrequently enough to keep him frustrated.

Melba (from chapter 13) was frustrated and overwhelmed by the pain in her life. She eventually discovered that cutting herself seemed to relieve the pain, and she told her therapist Dena, "It's the only thing that helps!" It may have helped, but it only worked in the short term. After that, she was overwhelmed by guilt, and her problems were still there. The self-inflicted injuries removed the pain without doing anything to heal the problems that caused it. In fact, the cutting tended to move her further and further from healing (cf. Waters & Lawrence, 1993). With each cutting episode, she increasingly felt guilty and ashamed and avoided the things that were healing for her. In turn, avoiding the things that worked for her increased her negative feelings, suicidal thoughts, and cutting episodes.

Sometimes, people attempt to slavishly follow cultural ideals to solve problems. Euro-American adolescent girls, for example, may diet and develop eating disorders. Some Native Americans, facing the cultural mandate to avoid expressing anger, may instead resort to alcohol to handle their feelings (LaFramboise, 2000; Tafoya, 1990). More is not necessarily better, even when the goal is a good one.

Looking for Causes and Solutions

Think about a problem that you have had in your life. How do you think it began? Does thinking about its origins give you clues about how to resolve this problem? If you have already resolved the problem, how was your solution related to your analysis of its cause?

It may be clear when someone is out of balance, and it may be clear what he or she needs to do to get back into balance, but it can sometimes be unclear (and even irrelevant) how the person *got* out of balance. Garry, an isolated gay man in a committed, but distant relationship, entered therapy both dysthymic and depressed. Did he become isolated and depressed because his childhood was neglectful and somewhat abusive? Was he born this way, as his mother had claimed? Were the communication patterns and boundaries in his family overly rigid and maladaptive?

As other writers have argued (Minuchin, 1974; O'Hanlon, 1999), it does not matter how Garry became withdrawn. The therapist's goal is to identify how he can move back into balance. What *maintains* the problem behavior? Sometimes it takes a small step like engaging in pleasurable behaviors again. At other times, it may require identifying cognitive or physical obstacles that prevent a person from moving into balance and seeing ways to overcome these obstacles. Garry, for example, assumed he was "bad" because even his own mother had been abusive and neglectful. He saw his affectional orientation as just one more piece of evidence of his worthlessness. As he challenged these beliefs in therapy, he became more comfortable with himself and in his interactions with others, and as a result, his depression lifted.

This approach is much more reality focused and action-oriented than therapies that focus on the past. Nonetheless, how the client thinks about the past, present, and future plays a central role in the change process. How people think about themselves and their problems can make a significant difference in how they cope with stressors and develop their ability to grow. It makes a difference whether Melba (in chapter 13) sees herself as broken after being raped or as having survived a difficult time.

We are not our past, and our future was not predetermined for us. We do not need a time machine to change the past so we can go forward. We can change without knowing how we ended up in the problem situation. The present and future can be changed one step at a time by acknowledging what happened (or what is), yet continuing anyway. Although the cards dealt us may not be what we would choose, we can make them into a winning hand.

Watch people who are struggling with solving a problem. How do they attempt to solve it? What kinds of actions or attitudes seem helpful? Which ones do not?

THE WAY BACK TO BALANCE

Because of the idiosyncratic nature of balance points, discovering them is sometimes difficult. It may be clear that Garry's current approach is ineffective and that his balance point might be different from Mia's (his therapist), but a healthy approach may not be immediately apparent. It's easy to look at a 4-year-old who is given age-inappropriate expectations and little opportunity to play and then identify ways to bring his life into balance: Just give him more opportunities for play. But it's more difficult to pinpoint how Martha, a single African American professional, is out of balance. Is she spending too much time at work, too little time with peers, or too little time with her church?

Understanding Cultural and Developmental Norms

There are several ways to begin differentiating among these hypotheses. Relative to other African American women her age, Martha was more isolated from her home community and was working harder. At 37, she had never been in a serious dating relationship and had no children. Her friends from high school had between three and five teenage children, and she often felt out of place whenever she was with them, as she did with the White professionals and their partners at her job.

Martha would have been as unhappy living the lives of her high school friends as her own. However, cultural and developmental norms can begin to highlight problem areas. Being unmarried and without children, Martha was often isolated from other African American women. She was working

60 to 70 hours each week and taking little time for her friends or her church.

Slavishly following or completely avoiding cultural and developmental norms is not useful. But, seeking out paths that fit a client's personal values within the broader cultural framework definitely is useful. There may be one valuing system that guides the culture and keeps its members in balance, but there will be many paths through it.

Making It Work

Another strategy is to examine *when* a person experiences less of the problem or when they experience more of the hoped-for solution than usual (Berg, 1994; O'Hanlon, 1999). This can be assessed in the following manner, as Leone did with Martha:

> LEONE: *I know that most of the time things feel bleak and over-whelming. (Martha grimaces and nods.) When is it a little bit better? (Paraphrase, open question)*
> MARTHA: *(Pause) It often feels overwhelming, but I do sometimes feel better at my sister's, just playing with her kids . . .*
> LEONE: *I'm curious. Tell me about one of these good times. (Self-disclosure, directive)*

Exceptions to the normal patterns are clues to what works (Berg, 1994; O'Hanlon, 1999). With just Martha's single response, however, it remained unclear why things were better when she was at her sister's. Was she feeling less judged or less lonely with good adult company? Was she really enjoying the time with her nieces? As Leone recognized, this is a first step in making this assessment. Therapist and client can begin looking for patterns when Martha spends time at her sister's house. In collaboratively identifying a hypothesis, such as when Martha is less lonely at her sister's, and allowing her to explore its validity, Leone is supporting Martha's autonomy and her sense of competency.

Two important aspects of Leone's assessment strategy are worth noting. First, he made sure that Martha and he were on the same page (by paraphrasing her description of her mood over the last months). In that way he made sure that she felt understood. She was also less likely to dismiss his interventions as being based on a premature and inadequate understanding. Second, from that supportive base, he was able to use an open question as an indirect and mild challenge of her belief that her life was *always* terrible. Closed questions like, "Is it ever better?" suggest that things may never be better. But when phrased as an open question, such as "When are things a little bit better?" exceptions to the problem can become clear.

Open-question words such as "when," "where," and "how" are especially useful with this type of assessment. Closed-question words such as "do," "is," and "are" are not. Closed questions tend to elicit short responses, but open questions tend to encourage talking. Consequently, people are often able to report smaller amounts of change when answering open questions. Closed questions, however, encourage people to make dichotomous distinctions between successes and failures. With closed questions, reporting even partial successes is more difficult.

Using Psychosocial Histories

Another way to assess when a person experiences less of a problem is to compose psychosocial histories between periods of low and higher functioning. Mervyn (from chapter 2), for example, was able to identify the period before his son's death as a relatively happy time. Although he could not bring his son back to life, he could explore some of the ways in which his current life was now different and less effective (see table 15.1). Specifically, he now had fewer friends and poorer relationships with his wife and extended family. He was less involved with his church and community, and he worked very long hours. While he was not convinced that he needed or wanted to have his life like it had been before, the comparison between these two psychosocial histories gave him new ideas about how to make his life work better.

The psychosocial histories also suggested how Mervyn's philosophy of life had changed. He acknowledged that he tended to use Job, his father, and employer as models and, as a result, had a work-focused and joyless life. However, as a young adult he had been able to see options in his future and work toward his goals. He recognized the hopeful and committed aspects of his earlier life, and he acknowledged how much he missed them, how much he felt defeated, and how much he missed the action of his youth.

Finding Success

Some clients will attempt to deny that things have ever been good. At such times, listening for successes can be very useful (Meichenbaum, 2000b). When giving a timeline or psychosocial history, many people will highlight the problems, but the fact is that they will have been successful in some ways in the past. Melba (chapter 13) spontaneously talked about the problems in her life. However, she had graduated at the top of her high school class, had consistently succeeded in many parts of her life, and had strong, supportive relationships with many people, especially with her family (see

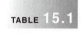

TABLE 15.1 COMPARISONS BETWEEN MERVYN'S PSYCHOSOCIAL HISTORIES FOR THE HAPPIEST PERIOD OF HIS LIFE AND THE PRESENT

Happiest Period (1981–1986)	The Present
Individual resources Responsible, dedicated, and determined. He reports having enjoyed gardening and camping.	Responsible, dedicated, and determined, but does not know how to focus his energy. He likes playing with his dog, but he generally falls asleep immediately after finishing the work he brought home for the evening.
Social resources, such as friends and family Had one good friend and several friendly relationships at work, church, and in his neighborhood.	Has a superficial friendship with a neighbor. He reports being afraid that he might "overwhelm" his friend were he to really share his concerns.
Had never been close to his father or siblings, but had been close to his wife, mother, and son. His mother died shortly before this period. He resents his siblings because they did not share more of the caretaking for his mother. His son drowned in 1986.	Has distant and conflictual family relationships for the most part. He continues in a caretaking role for his father, but he dreads the time they spend together.
Work Had a responsible well-paying job with a good pension. When things were stressful, he tended to work more.	Describes himself as a "workaholic," but does not enjoy the amount of time he spends on the job. He worries about losing his position if he were to suggest changes at work. He worries about not having a livable pension.
Models and mentors Admired President Kennedy's commitment to his country and community. He saw JFK as someone who could do anything and could energize the people around him. Mervyn liked his mother, whom he saw as decisive, efficient, and capable.	Sees himself as being like Job—stoic under significant adversity. He admires his employer whom he describes as capable and competent. He viewed his father's approach to relationships negatively and accepts this.
Community resources Had positive attitudes toward David's school, their church, and the Boy Scout troop.	Has regular yearly physicals with his doctor and almost monthly visits for minor stress-related ailments.
Community contributions Was a Boy Scout leader and an usher in his church until his son's death.	Has none currently.

table 15.2). She saw the glass as being half empty rather than half full, but the facts pointed out that it truly was more nearly full than empty.

DENA: *Wow! You know, I'm impressed. Given all that's happened in your life, how'd you make it back into college and do so well? (Self-disclosure, open question)*

TABLE 15.2	A POSITIVE TIMELINE FOR MELBA
1970	Melba was born.
1971	Melba's sister Maeve was born. They have been inseparable since early childhood.
1972	She and her mother have been especially close and supportive of one another since Melba was hospitalized for a bout of pneumonia.
1975	Although she had been nervous about going to school, Melba did very well in school and developed friends with whom she continues to be close.
1977	Her second-grade teacher was very supportive. She actively mentored Melba and recommended her for the gifted program.
1979	Melba skipped fourth grade and did well in fifth grade after a period of nervousness.
1981	She worked in her church's summer program and was relied upon to take an active role in caring for the youngest children.
1982	Although her best friend moved away, the two remained in contact. Her social group widened, and she developed several close friends.
1984	She became an active participant in a community service group in her high school and spent time working in the inner city.
1987	She became salutatorian of her class and won several awards for her community service. She received several scholarships that paid for a portion of her college education. She was accepted at several universities, including her first choice.
1989	She dropped out of school after posttraumatic symptoms interfered with her ability to concentrate on her major courses. She married her high school sweetheart, who was generally supportive, even though he had difficulty understanding her depression and flashbacks. He does not know what to do when she is suicidal.
1992	Her daughter (also Maeve) is born. Their relationship is close and supportive.
1995	Her son Jake is born. They have a very good relationship, although she describes him as a "pill."
1998	She returns to school and changes her major to nursing, with great trepidation about the effect this will have on her family and about whether she will be able to go to school successfully. She earns a 3.3 GPA in her first semester.
1999	Her advisor is actively supportive of her schooling and work, but strongly encourages her to enter therapy. She does, unsuccessfully. She receives the first of several departmental and university-wide awards and scholarships.
2000	She is elected president of the Nursing Club. She receives the top award among nursing students from her department. Her advisor encourages her to consider getting a master's degree in nursing. She enters therapy again with a new, more supportive therapist.

MELBA: *I don't know . . . (Pause) I think I'm just dogged sometimes and won't let things get in the way of what I want. (Pause) And my mom always supported me and believed in me, even though most of the time I thought she was crazy for doing so.*

Dena is not being naïve or glossing over Melba's life when she is impressed by Melba's successes in the face of adversity. She acknowledges the bad ("Given all that's happened in your life . . . ") without overlooking the good, which Melba consistently does. In so doing, Dena's open question reframes Melba's life story from someone who has repeatedly failed to someone who has succeeded against the odds.

When recognized, positive life events can moderate stress-related depression (Dixon & Reid, 2000). In addition to reframing Melba's life story, Dena also began to identify situations and traits that might later serve as resources. Melba's doggedness is a real strength that the two were able to use as a touchstone throughout the rest of therapy: Melba was not a quitter, but rather someone who continued, no matter what. This characterization of her as a "dogged" person was helpful in reframing Melba's thinking about her cutting herself, which were attempts to relieve the pain rather than attempts to commit suicide. She wanted to keep going, but could not identify other ways to do this. She was not weak and hopeless, but courageous and persistent in continuing, despite the odds against her.

Lambert (Asay & Lambert, 1999; Lambert, 1992) identified four factors accounting for the variability in therapeutic outcomes. In decreasing degree of importance, these are

- Extratherapeutic factors such as client resources and the quality of the support system (40%)
- Therapeutic alliances (30%)
- Hope and expectancies (15%)
- Model-specific techniques (15%)

Note how Dena's interventions addressed the first three of these. In asking "How'd you make it back into college and do so well?" she encouraged Melba to identify personal resources (her doggedness) as well as systemic supports (her mom). She built their therapeutic alliance by hearing Melba's successes as well as her stressors. She fostered hope when she recognized successes and implied that they would continue into the future. These aspects of her intervention are as helpful as the more specifically clinical interventions of identifying the pattern and the exceptions to her behavior.

Doing Something Different

Kohler (1917/1925) described the *umweg* task, a task that parallels the kind of difficulties that many people face on a daily basis. He put a goal (food) on one side of a U-shaped wire mesh fence, with the two arms of the U extending down behind the animal. Many animals, rather than going around the barrier, attempted to go through the fence or dig under it to reach the food. It took a measure of cognitive flexibility to recognize the problem and look for other approaches to it. The chicken's difficulty in solving this problem may seem ridiculous, but Darby and Rae-Anne approached their problem in a similar way. Each found a simplistic and rigid solution to a complicated problem and gave up searching for approaches that might be more successful and satisfying.

Skinner (1948) described pigeons' process of solving an insoluble problem as initially unfocused and random. As their behavior was accidentally reinforced, specific and unusual "superstitious" behaviors developed. Darby's and Melba's behaviors resemble this. They committed to partly effective solutions that they believed would work long-term. Because there was some reinforcement for their solutions, they continued them, although simpler and more effective solutions were possible.

Both Darby and Rae-Anne would be better off had they tried something different. What is Rae-Anne doing well? Why aren't their problems worse than they are (cf. O'Hanlon, 1999)? When does Rae-Anne listen to Darby? Darby reported that they fight about chores and homework, but that they often have long talks about her friends and boyfriends. When asked to think about what was different, Darby reported that he often "told" his daughter what to do with her homework and housework, but that he listened more when Rae-Anne talked about her frustrations with her friends. Although he didn't think he could just listen to Rae-Anne in either problem situation, Darby did think he could use a more collaborative tone of voice — one that was more like the tone he used when they talked about her friends. This small change got them back on track and to a place where they could work together.

Similarly, Melba described several things that were helpful (see table 15.3). When she felt heard and validated, she was usually able to handle her feelings more successfully and could more easily recognize the impulse to cut early enough in the cycle that she could deal with it effectively. If she waited, however, the difficulty would increase. She was more likely to run into problems when, from her point of view, her needs conflicted with someone else's (cf. Levenkron, 1998). However, she was less likely to run into problems when she was able to identify a win-win solution, but was more likely to cut when exposed to explicit stimuli related to her history of abuse. This was especially true when she did not anticipate the cutting impulses. When she recognized them early and dealt with them immediately, she had fewer problems.

For people who have a difficult time identifying exceptions in the pattern ("It always happens") tracking behaviors and their antecedents and consequences can be helpful. This is true even in the beginning of therapy when few, if any, successes are spontaneously described. Identifying the patterns characterizing the problematic behavior can lead to successes.

TABLE 15.3 SITUATIONS THAT MELBA IDENTIFIED AS HAVING HANDLED WELL (−) OR LESS WELL (+)

Antecedent	Behavior	Consequences
+ Husband was concerned about how they have split household chores.	Melba assertively described her concerns while listening to him.	Initially nervous, but they had a "productive" conversation. Had a sense of accomplishment about the conversation.
− "Day from hell" with many minor stressors.	Pretended that nothing was bothering her.	Increasingly anxious and cut.
− Learned that two employees will be laid off at work.	Wondered who these employees were. Aware of impulses to cut and tried to distract herself.	Cut. Initially relieved, then guilty and ashamed.
+ Supervisor was in a bad mood, gave Melba "too much work," and criticized her.	Talked to a friend at work who helped her understand the pressures her supervisor was under. She journaled briefly.	Calmed down. Recognized this was a "high-risk" situation for her and was proud that she handled it well.
− Read a novel a friend had given her that included a graphic description of a violent sexual act.	Got flustered and did not know what to do.	Was increasingly anxious until she cut.
+ Went to a family reunion where she knew she would encounter the man who raped her.	Spent afternoon with a cousin who knew about the abuse and challenged her thoughts that she was "bad" or that the abuse was her fault.	Felt somewhat anxious, but also supported by her cousin's presence. Felt empowered that she made it through this high-risk situation intact.

WHEN BALANCING GETS DIFFICULT

Some people have such chronic feelings of hopelessness that they have difficulty identifying even short periods of relative calm and happiness. This is especially true for people who grew up in very chaotic or abusive families. They may never have had a period of healthy functioning that could be used either as a touchstone through hard times or as a guide toward change. Sometimes, the solutions they identify are approaches that will create even greater problems (as Melba's cutting did). Furthermore, their vision of the future may be, at best, a *poor* guide. For example, Garry's ideal for the future includes few specifics and, thus, identifies few steps toward his ultimate goals. For this type of client, it may be useful to create small successes.

Using the Tricks of the Trade

Most therapists have a bag of tricks they use when clients feel especially hopeless about their future. Some refer their clients for antidepressant medication therapies. Others give simple homework assignments that everyone can do that will be successful regardless of the outcome, such as teaching them some interesting concept or fact. Still others teach relaxation and breathing techniques ("Breathe in and hold two, three, and breathe all the way out") when stress and anxiety are significant problems. When depression is a greater problem, other tricks include encouraging clients to identify a list of things they enjoy and then ask that they engage in at least one of them each day. These interventions are generally successful enough to decrease clients' feelings of hopelessness and increase their perceptions of self-efficacy ("I *can* do something to make things different!). When they have experienced even small successes, clients are much more likely to feel successful with the larger systemic issues they face in their lives.

One caveat about these assignments: Giving people something positive *to do* is generally more effective than telling them what *not* to do (Walter & Peller, 1993). An example is telling a client *not* to think about pink elephants dancing in tutus! Suggesting things that people should avoid often paradoxically increases their focus on the problematic behavior and simultaneously increases the difficulty of avoiding it (Wegner, 1994). Olive, for example, had spent the last several years trying to stop smoking. Now, much of her time centers on smoking. She continually thinks about when she could smoke, where she could smoke, and even how she could stop smoking. Her therapist Caitlyn suggested that they try a different focus for a change. Rather than focus on smoking at this point in therapy, Caitlyn suggested that they deal with Olive's pervasive depression. They initially used some of the simple interventions just discussed. Olive's smoking and, just as importantly, her obsessive thoughts about smoking, decreased almost immediately. Paradoxically, Olive's focus on not smoking when she felt hopeless about stopping *increased* her desire to smoke. But a different focus reduced her desire to smoke.

Attacking the Fear

What keeps people doing things that are ineffective, that keep them stuck, that alienate them from the people around them? Ambivalence and fear are often the reasons. When depressed, stressed, or afraid, people begin thinking rigidly and dichotomously and even about extreme options. Darby, for example, thought that he should stay on top of Rae-Anne's behavior or his daughter would *really* get out of control. Melba thought that she could cut herself and either get a brief respite from her emotional pain or be completely overwhelmed by it. She could not imagine other possibilities. Even when Melba's therapist helped her identify other options, she still had difficulty with change. She could see things that might be helpful, but she was immobilized by the fear that they might really become worse. As a result, she had difficulty doing anything.

What role has fear played in your life? Does it motivate you to try new things or prevent you from changing? What allows you to change despite the fear?

O'Hanlon (1999) tells a story of Tibetan monks facing a similar dilemma. Buddhist students lined up for an enlightenment ceremony offered only once every one hundred years (only once in a person's life). Their teachers told them that, although successfully completing the ceremony had significant benefits (enlightenment), it also had significant costs—they would have to enter and cross a room filled with 1000 demons and successfully exit on the other side through the only door that could be opened. But the *presence* of demons wasn't bad enough. Each demon was capable of taking the form of one's worst fears. People who were afraid of heights would see themselves on a narrow ledge on a high mountaintop. Those afraid of spiders would see the room full of hairy eight-legged creatures and would feel spiders crawling on them.

The students had to cross the room on their own and many became trapped and overwhelmed by their fears. But others didn't. Like them, clients have choices: they can become trapped by their fears, or they can remember that their demons are self-created illusions; they can become stuck, or they can remind themselves that when they keep moving they will make it to a better place.

Clients in therapy have an advantage over the students seeking enlightenment. While the students needed to face their fears completely on their own, clients can ask for help from their families, their friends, and of course, their therapists. They are not in their *situation,* nor are they in the *solutions,* by themselves. We, as their therapists, should remind them that their fears are not real, that they can and should move forward, and that they can ask for help whenever they need it. We can help them remember the places where they have been courageous in the past and can help them transfer those skills into the present. Here is yet another advantage of using timelines in therapy:

> DENA: *Melba, it sounds like it feels scary and impossible to think about doing the things that we have talked about here. Because you have been equally courageous on other people's behalf, I wonder if you can do the same thing for yourself. (Reflection of feeling, reframe, implied directive in the form of a self-disclosure)*

WHEN DOING THE SAME OLD THING WON'T WORK

People often fear that things will get worse rather than better if they make a change. When doing the same old thing takes all the energy they have, it is difficult to imagine doing anything different. Instead, like Melba, many people just keep trying the same old thing. When that doesn't work, they just do it harder, faster, or louder.

If a rat is placed in a box where it must press a bar for food, its behavior will include random exploratory behaviors. When it finally begins to press the bar for food, the rat's behavior will become more focused until it first satiates then sleeps. If the bar suddenly breaks or starts working sporadically, the rat will press the bar for extended periods of time, even when another solution to the problem is available. This illustrates Kohler's (1917/1925) chickens stuck in the *umweg* task.

Sometimes doing one thing differently can be the only way to improve one's lot in life (O'Hanlon, 1999). Still, it takes hope to make things different. It takes courage to recognize life's problems and to believe that things will go well. Creech's (1994) narrator summarizes it like this:

> [B]ravery is looking Pandora's box full in the eye as best you can, and then turning to the other box, the one with the smoothbeautiful fold inside. (p. 277)

Neither looking at the beautiful nor seeing the painful alone represents real courage.

Luckily, people are different from rats and dogs in being able to step back from a situation and brainstorm solutions, even when they don't always recognize this as a possibility. Thom had been depressed to a greater or lesser degree for years. He had been working in therapy for a while, at first very ambivalently, and would often "keep his head in the sand" rather than do anything that could really make a difference. One morning, after he had been feeling better for a while, he woke up depressed again. He normally would have gone back to bed and complained about the terrible hand he had been dealt in life, but on that morning he got out of bed and went running. He surprised himself by doing something different and was excited that running seemed to help. Things in his life started to improve.

When people get off-track, doing the same old thing simply moves them farther and farther away and more and more out of balance (Watzlawick et al., 1974). When Thom stayed in bed, skipped work, and avoided friends because he felt bad, his actions seemed to him to make sense, and he couldn't imagine the energy it would take to face the world again. However, when he stayed in bed, he stopped doing the things that made him feel connected to the people around him, the things that made him feel competent with something to offer. Along with its natural physiological benefits and antidepressant qualities, running also got him out of bed and doing the things he enjoyed, which moved him back toward his natural balance point (Tkachuk & Martin, 1999).

Who has served as a model or mentor in your life? How has he or she been helpful? How has he or she *not* been helpful? If your mentor is a real person in your life, what did he or she do that was supportive? Talk to friends and family about the people who have served as mentors for them. What worked?

MODELS AND MENTORS

Sometimes, it is difficult for many people to see what might work or to see those times when they were already successful ("We always fight!"). In those situations, it is helpful to find others who are already successful and to model their behavior. When Mervyn was asked who his models were, he identified Job. His choice of models was somewhat problematic because he chose someone who faced endless and overwhelming obstacles. There were, however, some real lessons Mervyn could learn from Job. First, Mervyn remembered that it was Job's faith in God that got him through the hard times. Second, he remembered that Job eventually did overcome his problems successfully.

But Job was a difficult model for another reason. Mervyn had a difficult time seeing exactly what Job did to get through the hard times. Generally, it is better to carefully observe live models rather than fictional models (Watson & Tharp, 1997). While these can be friends, relatives, or successful political figures or sports personalities, people who are warm and perceived to share important similarities are preferable (Kazdin, 1984). Furthermore, people who struggled to learn a task and were successful at it make better models than people who always found tasks easy. Job's stoicism made him a useful model, but turning to President Kennedy helped Mervyn to think about ways of overcoming, rather than only tolerating, adversity.

This is one reason why small self-disclosures are useful in therapy. In describing our own struggles with a similar problem we both increase our similarity to our clients as well as provide a better model of how to cope:

> FELICIA: *My daughter and I have the same sort of problem. It's okay when either one of us is tired, but when we both are—Watch out! We've learned to agree to go to our rooms to read and talk later.*

Therapy often provides a warm person after whom clients can model their own behavior.

Although clients may ask their model what he or she would do to solve a similar problem, observations are often more useful than listening to their beliefs about what they do (Watson & Tharp, 1997). Most people have a difficult time describing what they do anyway, especially highly practiced behaviors.

Self-reports are often a poor source of data and are strongly influenced by the form of the questions (Schwarz, 1999). The information gained may be vague at best and may even be misleading. If we choose to ask questions, specific questions are better than more general ones. It is better to ask, "How do you handle coming home from work hungry?" than "How do you stay thin?"

Try describing how you ride a bicycle without getting on one! What steps do you imagine?

When people are stressed, depressed, anxious, or tired they will tend to think dichotomously and fail to identify available solutions. The behavior of their models and mentors may be a ready source of possible solutions. Some solutions may be usefully transferred to a second person, but others may be inappropriate. Sheryl, for example, really admired one of the older teachers at her school. She thought Ernest was very creative and developed good classroom projects for his students. While Sheryl was sensitive to Ernest's suggestion that she wasn't "tough enough" on her students and would often let them get out of control, she wanted to use a different disciplinary strategy with her own students. Ernest was skeptical about her approach, but was supportive as Sheryl made changes in her teaching practices. In fact, her new approach to teaching was more successful for her than her attempts at Ernest's approach, which was quite successful for him. Watching his style of approaching students was very useful for her because it helped her recognize that multiple styles of disciplining children can work.

Of course, another way that a model or mentor can be helpful is as a touchstone. When clients are struggling with a difficult experience, we can ask them to recall the feelings they have with someone who truly accepts them and believes in them (Ivey et al., 1997). When they are able to recall that experience and accept its validity, they often feel more capable of coping with life's stressors. In this way also, their self-concept will be more balanced, as strengths, adaptive coping mechanisms, and their own perception of weaknesses and failures are integrated into their experience.

DIFFERENT BALANCE POINTS FOR DIFFERENT PEOPLE

No single balance point exists that works every time for everyone. If this were the case, we would have Recommended Daily Allowances for each "room" in our house, just as we have for vitamins. Each individual has significantly different needs for intimacy, autonomy, stimulation, and productivity, and these needs are often influenced by cultural factors. Returning to the house metaphor, one person's rooms may be different sizes than another's. Each person needs to enter their rooms in ways that work specifically with *them*.

As we begin helping our clients redecorate their rooms, we need to be aware of our values and recognize how these may be different from our clients'. This problem is seen in Mia's work with Garry. Their work was influenced by differences in race, class, gender, affectional orientation, and family communication styles (see table 15.4). When he entered therapy, Garry knew that he was having problems. His real self was significantly different from his ideal. He had no friends or even friendly interactions with people other than his partner and was spending significant time in fan-

TABLE 15.4   REAL AND IDEAL PSYCHOSOCIAL HISTORIES OF GARRY AND HIS THERAPIST MIA

Garry's Real	Garry's Ideal	Mia's Ideal
Problem		
Current symptoms Moderately depressed with occasional suicidal ideation.	No depression, although does not expect to be wildly happy.	"I'd like to be able to approach every day, even the bad ones, with a measure of acceptance and joy."
Beliefs about symptoms "It's just the way I am. Some people are depressed. I am one of them."		"While some people are more likely to become depressed, it's the stressors and the way we think about them that make us depressed."
Personal history of psychological disorders Probably has been dysthymic most of his life, at least from early adolescence. He was seriously suicidal at several points during his adolescence and even made several attempts at suicide.		Was very anxious in graduate school. She handled this with some help from her friends. Later, she resolved milder episodes in therapy.
Family history of psychological disorders Has mother whose side of the family adopts a generally somber approach to life. His mother is probably dysthymic.		Mild anxiety and depression tends to run in the family. Her family tends to take an active, problem solving approach to these.
Current Context		
Recent events No recent stressors were identified, although his job and friendships are unsatisfying.	Would like to be able to rebound, even in the face of moderate stressors.	Leads a moderately and chronically stressful life.
Physical condition Is out of shape and thinks he would be more accepted if he looked better. He is concerned about getting HIV, although he is in a committed relationship.	Would like to be more attractive—like Cary Grant—but sees this as unlikely.	Would like to lose 15 pounds, although generally in good health and likes her body.
Drug and alcohol use Moderate alcohol intake.	Not seen as a problem.	Tends to drink somewhat heavily at times.
Intellectual and cognitive functioning Is of average intelligence, with above-average persistence. He tends to think concretely and dichotomously.	Would like to be able to be a person who handles problems more flexibly.	Is a very bright, creative, and flexible problem solver.
Coping style Daydreams for many hours a day and reads and watches movies. He is often unassertive interpersonally.	Would like to daydream less frequently and be more assertive in solving his problems.	Drinks more frequently than she would like to, but otherwise generally takes a positive and problem-focused coping strategy to match her internal locus of control.

(continued)

TABLE 15.4 *(continued)*

Garry's Real	Garry's Ideal	Mia's Real and Ideal
Self-concept Has difficulty identifying things about himself that he likes. He tends to see himself as a person who has made a number of bad mistakes, and he expects to continue to make bad mistakes and to be criticized.	Wants to like himself better, more like he perceives Mia doing, and would like to see himself as someone who has made some big mistakes but has rebounded from them. He hopes for a better future. He wants to turn his life around and be able to talk to the people around him without worrying whether or not he will be ridiculed or rejected.	Generally pleased with the person she has become and thinks she is on the right path in life. She sees herself as someone who has done the best she could under the conditions, and she views herself as a "lucky" person. She expects that this will continue in her future.
Sociocultural background Rarely feels part of his community and attributes this feeling to being gay in a homophobic society. He is "out" with few people other than his partner.	Would like to be out and accepted in his community, although he can barely imagine this.	Would like to feel more accepted in her adopted community and neighborhood, but generally feels comfortable in them. She is proud of her racial background, although she wishes other African American professionals were in her community.
Religion and spirituality Has been estranged from his church since early adolescence and believes that the church condemns him.	Not interested in attending church, but interested in feeling forgiven.	Drives 35 miles to the nearest African Methodist Episcopal (AME) Church and gets significant satisfaction from her religion.
Resources and Barriers *Individual resources* Is an imaginative daydreamer and is comfortable being alone. He is serious, realistic, and persistent.	Would like to be more self-confident in new situations and be a flexible and creative problem solver.	Bright, hopeful, and playful. She readily engages with other people.
Social resources, such as friends and family Has no friendships and has few friendly relationships.	Would like cordial relationships at work and in the community.	Has several intimate friends and friendly relationships with her colleagues and with people in her community.
Has a formal, but cordial, relationship with his parents. All but one brother is distant and uninvolved in his life because of the conflictual nature of the relationship. His family does not accept his partner.	Wants cordial and friendly relationships with his parents and his brother.	Enjoys friendly and supportive relationships with her family. She would like them to be geographically closer than they are and wants to see them more often.
Is in a distant but committed relationship and has no children.	Wishes his relationship with his partner were more intimate, but is afraid of taking any steps to make it more satisfying.	Is married and has two children. She enjoys spending time with her husband and children.
Work Often feels incompetent at a very challenging job and feels that his coworkers make fun of him.	Would like to do his job competently and have cordial relationships with his coworkers.	Hopes to become a truly excellent therapist and to continue to enjoy her profession in the future as much as she does now. She belongs to a very supportive peer supervision group.

(continued)

TABLE 15.4 *(continued)*

Garry's Real	Garry's Ideal	Mia's Real and Ideal
Community resources Has none.	Thinks that becoming a member of a gay support group might be a good idea, despite the fact that it terrifies him.	Has a positive relationship with her daughter's babysitter and has a positive attitude toward her son's school, but wants a more supportive relationship with her neighbors.
Community contributions Has none.	None desired.	Very active in her state's social work association and active in son's school and her church.
Mentors and models Idealizes Katharine Hepburn and Cary Grant.	Same.	Admires the approaches toward work and life taken by several friends. She was openly mentored by two professors in her training program.
Obstacles to change Tends to see his depression as biological in origin, but does not want to take medication. Sees himself as able to decrease his depression.		Wonders about Garry's commitment to change. She is not as hopeful about the change process as she typically is.
Therapeutic relationship Has a good relationship with therapist, but he tends to take a one-down stance in therapy. He expects Mia to tell him how to solve this problem.		Wants an egalitarian relationship and is frustrated by Garry's demands for greater directiveness.

tasy. His relationships with his family were often distant, stilted, and guilt-ridden. He did not enjoy his work and often felt incompetent at it. However, his ideal self was also different from Mia's. She was in a number of close and satisfying relationships and tended to get mildly depressed when she was isolated for too long. Garry wanted interactions that were more cordial, but he became restless and overwhelmed whenever he was around people for extended periods. Mia wanted to become an excellent therapist and saw this realm of her life as central to her self-esteem. Garry wanted to feel competent at his work, but saw it as "just a job" and wanted to keep it that way. The differences between their values and goals created significant potential for a value conflict in their work together.

Garry admittedly had an uninvolved and unsatisfying life. Mia preferred a more highly stimulating lifestyle and was closer to meeting her goals. Even if Mia had been able to disregard her own values completely, looking only at Garry's absolute levels of involvement in satisfying activities might cause Mia to misidentify some areas as problematic. For example,

Garry did not value his spirituality and community involvement, and he was satisfied with the quality and quantity of his hobbies and relaxation activities. From his point of view, these were only minor problems at best. Mia was very active in her church and community. She saw his hobbies as "escapist" and wondered whether they might exacerbate his problems rather than reduce them. Nonetheless, she recognized that he did not want to address these goals in therapy. Value conflicts often occur when (1) there are significant discrepancies between the therapist's and the client's valuing systems and when (2) absolute rather than relative involvement in particular areas is considered. This is an especially important consideration when cultural differences are large.

It would be easy to believe that as Garry progressed in therapy, his values and goals would look more like those of Mia (cf. T. A. Kelly & Strupp, 1992). However, this is a "therocentric" view of life in which therapeutic values and goals are seen as ideal and other values and goals are seen as good *only* when they approximate our own (as though all therapists had the same values and goals!). This type of thinking leads to the potential for the kinds of value clashes and potential abuses described in chapter 6. Many clients idealize their therapist and emulate their therapist's behavior, values and goals, which can have the effect of greater self-confidence, autonomy, and interpersonal sensitivity over the course of therapy (T. A. Kelly & Strupp, 1992). However, clients should eventually begin to make decisions for themselves based on their own values, and therapy should strengthen their own voice rather than teach them to copy another's.

We should encourage people to make progress toward their own goals for several reasons. Progress toward their own goals is likely to be more rapid and successful than progress toward others' goals (Prochaska, 1999; Walter & Peller, 1992). However, when we suggest that our clients should approach our goals (or when they believe they should), they are likely to experience anxiety and depression to the degree that their new goals differ from their core values (Higgins, 1987). They may be left believing, "I *should* be more empathic, successful, wise . . . "

Are we more Rogerian, believing that clients can make healthy decisions for themselves? Or do we believe, like Freudians, that clients are in some ways incompetent, self-centered, selfish, and unable to make healthy decisions for themselves on their own? If the latter is true, we will have more difficulty empowering our clients to make decisions for themselves.

> Think about whether and why you might want to empower your clients. What would you look for in yourself that could help others? What steps might you take to move them toward making decisions for themselves?

Setting Mutually Agreed-Upon Goals

Some clients enter therapy willingly and are able to identify the direction they want to go. Others, however, enter therapy less so. They may not initially identify therapeutic goals and, when they do, their goals may be discrepant from those of their therapists and referral agent. In the following example, Angelo and Minnie begin their discussion with goals that appear different. Angelo is able to negotiate mutual goals, such as improving the quality of his parenting and changing her pattern of drinking.

ANGELO: *What is your goal in coming here? (Open question.)*
MINNIE: *The judge and social worker have decided that I need to come here.*
ANGELO: *So, this was their idea. What makes them think you need to come here? (Paraphrase, open question.)*
MINNIE: *They recently took my two kids away from me because they said I was neglecting them. The kids are in a foster home and the court has taken custody. The school social worker made the report. The judge says that if I want to get my kids back, I have to come and see you.*
ANGELO: *Oh, I'm sorry about your kids, you must miss them very much. (Self-disclosure, interpretation.)*
MINNIE: *Yes, a lot. They are the world to me. All I have are my children and I don't know what to do with myself.*
ANGELO: *So, they are saying you need to parent differently? Is this your goal too? (Clarification)*
MINNIE: *Yes, I haven't been too good with the kids sometimes. They just get to be too much and I get myself in trouble with my drinking.* (Walter & Peller, 1992, p. 248. Names added for clarity, therapeutic leads added for consistency)

Especially with involuntary clients like Minnie, setting treatment goals can be difficult. Some therapists respond to this problem by labeling their clients as "resistant" and refusing to work with them. Others continue to work with them, but align with their clients and refuse to set goals. Angelo's decision provides a third, more useful path. He recognized that the judge and social worker had made the referral, yet was also respectful of Minnie's viewpoint and then listened carefully to her. He recognized that her goals might be somewhat different than the court's or his own. Rather than making a decision for her, Angelo highlighted her choice, "Is this your goal too?," then he put the alternatives on the table and allowed her to choose them. This was her choice, even if it was one that she would rather not make. Highlighting her choice also implied that any action, even the choice of failing to act, was *hers*.

Three things (1) respectful attitude, (2) reflective listening, and (3) empowering actions are essential aspects of the contextual viewpoint. We may not always share essential values with the people with whom we work, but it is extremely important to remember to stop and listen to their viewpoint. Had Angelo told Minnie that she had to do things the court's way, he would have lost her. By listening to her, by helping her feel respected and heard, he was able to create an alliance with her. By hearing her strengths (being a loving parent and missing her children very much), he was able to help her set positive goals rather than a negative one, such as resisting the court's wishes. Note that her goals are very similar to the court's.

CONCLUSIONS

When dogs are given an insoluble task, they eventually give up on attempting *both* insoluble and solvable tasks (Alloy & Seligman, 1979; Seligman, 1968). Seligman (1975) suggests that this research is a good model for human depression. Like Seligman's dogs, we may become "stuck" in one style of approaching a problem and give up on this and other tasks when our problem solving is unsuccessful.

Finding a way out of a problem is often difficult. This chapter identifies a variety of ways to help people get back on track or back "in balance." The entire book provides assessment strategies that help us identify places where we may have focused less on or areas in which we may have put too much focus. As Garry's psychosocial history illustrates, when identifying treatment goals, it is important to recognize both group and individual values and to examine how these can be valid *and* different from the therapist's own. Timelines and psychosocial histories can be used to highlight successes, as well as to identify periods when life has been more satisfying. Comparing psychosocial histories for the two periods—times of greater success and times of less success—can identify clues for therapeutic shifts.

Sometimes, it is not clear what can be done to identify a balance point. In this case, we can encourage problem-solving strategies that are already successful. When we are stressed we tend to think dichotomously and rigidly, but successful problem solving comes from brainstorming a wide range of potential solutions and choosing from among them:

- We can look at periods of success and repeat them.
- We can try something different from what we have done in the past.
- We can focus on things other than the problem.
- We can remember places where we have been successful in the past.
- We can recognize the role that fear plays in preventing change.

Finally, having a respectful attitude toward clients, being a reflective listener to their viewpoints, and facilitating the client's exploration of empowering actions are essential elements for success in a contextual therapeutic approach.

HIGHLIGHTING THEMES

LISTEN FOR CONTEXT
RESPECT INDIVIDUAL AND CULTURAL DIFFERENCES
DENIGRATED AND PATHOLOGIZED DIFFERENCES AMONG CULTURES
VALUES AND THEIR EFFECTS ON ASSESSMENTS
CARICATURES OF CULTURAL VALUES

RECOGNIZE AND ADDRESS POWER DIFFERENTIALS
OPPRESSION AND UNEARNED PRIVILEGE
SOCIAL JUSTICE
GIVE UP POWER AND EXPERTISE TO BE EFFECTIVE
ACCEPT AND USE POWER WHEN IT IS HELPFUL

THINK SYSTEMATICALLY
PROVIDE SERVICES RELEVANT TO CLIENTS' LIVES AND WORLDVIEWS
HELP CLIENTS RECOGNIZE AVAILABLE SUPPORTS
HELP CLIENTS REGAIN BALANCE

RECONSIDER THE GOALS OF THERAPY
CLIENTS' FEARS OF CHANGE
SYMPTOM REDUCTION VERSUS GOOD OUTCOMES
RISKS OF CULTURALLY AWARE THERAPY
USE SAFETY NETS

MAKE THE JOURNEY TOWARD CULTURAL COMPETENCY

This book has emphasized a holistic approach to seeing people in the larger racial, sociological, historical, and personal contexts that influence them. The assessment and intervention processes were broken into smaller pieces for ease of teaching and learning. This final chapter highlights themes and brings together concepts that were explicitly and implicitly discussed throughout the book.

LISTEN FOR CONTEXT

Other people's behavior, especially when it is very different from what we (as therapists) would choose to do in the same situation, can sometimes seem "crazy." It looks the most crazy when the context has been overlooked, which is something that Western observers, in particular, tend to do (Morris & Peng, 1994). In general, however, people's behavior makes sense to themselves, though they may not be able to explain their motivations.

Examining a client's context has several advantages. First, it helps explain the person's symptoms. For example, baseless anxiety may turn out to be justified worry. Second, as we recognize the situations that influence a person, we are more able to empathize with them and their behavior, and our assessment becomes more useful. Third, as we respond more empathically, the therapeutic relationship often becomes stronger.

Respect Individual and Cultural Differences

"The sparrow is sorry for the peacock at the burden of his tail," said Rabindranath Tagore. Like the sparrow, we often equate different with bad, unless we see it as "exotic," which is a condescending response. *A multicultural framework assumes that multiple valuing stances can be equally valid.* Choosing to be independent and autonomous in one's life decisions is not necessarily better or worse than maintaining closer, more dependent relationships with family and friends. In working with clients the question can be asked, "Does it work for the person and system in this given situation?"

Broadly speaking, culture is one cause of differences among people. Even within a culture, members can have disparate values, goals, and concerns. So, respecting the differences involves recognizing that members of a single group can be very different from one another. Roseanne Barr (brash and over-the-top comedienne), Hillary Clinton (smart, savvy, and assertive senator and former first lady), and Laura Bush (refined and supportive first lady and librarian) are each Euro-American women, yet each has different values, goals, and experiences! Each has taken center stage, but Clinton and Bush work within the system, while Barr attacks it. Clinton drafts laws to make change, while Bush advocates for changes within the school system. Clinton appears to be her husband's professional equal, while Bush has taken a quieter and more supportive role.

Although this book covers a number of differences, the similarities among people can be much greater than the differences. When listening to others, become aware of the similarities as well as the differences. A Euro-American man and a Korean American woman may feel significant loss (among other feelings) when their last child leaves home, but the extent of the loss and the range of other emotions can be vastly different.

Denigrated and Pathologized Differences Among Cultures

A behavior that is denigrated and pathologized in one culture may be respected and valued in another. One's worldview and values influence what is seen as normal and right. Gonzalez-Ramos and her colleagues (1998), for example, suggest that Anglos are more likely to describe respectfulness and compliance—behaviors that are culturally normative and desirable for Puerto Rican children—as "shy," "inhibited," or "withdrawn." Wearing a veil may be no more oppressive for Arab Americans than wearing a miniskirt and high heels is for Western women (Erickson & Al-Timimi, 2001). These may even be symbols of ethnic pride within the two cultures. Rather than being oppressive, arranged marriages also have advantages. Listen to your clients' values from *their* point of view rather than only your own. Recognize their strengths.

Values and Their Effects on Assessments

Know your values and how they can affect your assessments in therapy. Clients generally take a position on whether problems were caused by themselves or by someone or something else. They may also draw conclusions about their ability to change the "problem." In the same situation, some may recognize their responsibility and may exert control, and others may not. Clients' and therapists' perspectives on the world can be a way of connecting with and understanding others, or they can be excuses for blaming.

Given that our own personal values necessarily influence our assessments (Erickson & Al-Timimi, 2001; Gonzalez-Ramos et al., 1998), how should we handle clients who have a different set of values, goals, and experiences than our own? Fontaine and Hammond (1994) suggest becoming aware of both sets of values and alternate perspectives. This can highlight potential traps that may be faced in therapy. As we become aware of other viewpoints, we can also identify multiple effective strategies for handling concerns. Learning to recognize alternate perspectives *and* their strengths and limitations, can help us respond more empathically to clients.

Caricatures of Cultural Values

Challenge caricatured expressions of cultural values. Many people do more of their typical coping strategy when they hit a bump in the road (O'Hanlon, 1999). An example of this is, "If telling your children doesn't work, yell at them." More is not necessarily better. Many Euro-Americans see direct expressions of anger as "cathartic and therapeutic," despite research to the contrary (Tavris, 1989). They often have difficulty seeing the difference between healthy levels (and types) of catharsis and unhealthy ones. Some Native Americans see anger as "toxic" and as a break in group harmony, and they have difficulty expressing even moderate amounts of anger (Tafoya, 1990).

Both of these approaches are distortions of cultural messages about anger. Although yelling, screaming, and throwing things are rarely advantageous, talking about feelings and voicing concerns, especially with someone who is trusted and supportive, can be very helpful (Tavris, 1989). Similarly, Tafoya (1990) attributes the high rates of alcoholism in Native American groups to avoiding "toxic" anger, rather than using healthy culturally appropriate outlets.

RECOGNIZE AND ADDRESS POWER DIFFERENTIALS

Most therapeutic approaches do not consider the role of power and its effects on clients and the therapeutic process. This model directly considers power differentials between therapists and clients, as well as between clients and their families and community. When clients have less power and freedom than their age and abilities would predict, they are at risk. Power differentials in therapy can either follow cultural help-seeking patterns or slow therapeutic growth.

Oppression and Unearned Privilege

Acknowledge and challenge oppression and unearned privilege. Oppression and privilege have very real consequences for a person's psychological and physical health (cf. Elligan & Utsey, 1999; Guyll et al., 2001; Harris & Kuba, 1997; Horne, 1999; Landrine & Klonoff, 1996; Tull et al., 1999). Clients at more complex ego statuses may be aware of this impact (Helms & Cook, 1999). Clients who are aware of oppression, yet unable to have it acknowledged by their therapists, may feel misunderstood and may question the helpfulness of their therapist, or even of therapy itself, like Mr. C. in chapter 7 (Holmes, 1992, as cited in Yi, 1998). Other clients may be less aware of oppression and privilege, yet feel validated and make positive psychological and social changes when they enter an environment that supports their exploration of prejudice, discrimination, and oppression. Of course, increased anxiety and anger sometimes are positive outcomes of recognizing oppression.

This can be difficult work, however, when therapists do not keep pace with their clients. Effective work by the therapist involves acting with or slightly ahead of the client. When therapists focus too heavily or exclusively on the roles of prejudice and oppression, clients may feel disbelieved, bullied, or unheard. When therapists do not address issues of culture and oppression, clients may feel blamed or misunderstood and have difficulty disclosing in therapy (C. E. Thompson et al., 1994).

Social Justice

Work for social justice. Recognizing oppression and privilege is not enough. We must also *work* for social justice (D. W. Sue et al., 1999). Rather than staying in the safety of our therapy rooms, we must enter our community and address factors that allow and give privilege to misogyny, racism, heterosexism, ageism, classism, and all the other *isms* that are part of the fabric of different societies. By challenging oppression and unearned privilege, a therapeutically helpful community can be created. Failing to act in this regard suggests that the status quo is acceptable.

While we should work for justice, it is often a therapeutic process as well as a therapeutic outcome when our clients also work for social justice (Watts et al., 2002). Working for social justice can be empowering and can give healthy expression to anger. It can also reflect an awareness of oppressive influences, as well as an increasingly internal locus of control and appropriate assertiveness.

Give Up Power and Expertise to Be Effective

Rather than assuming that there is one and only one way to do therapy, we may need to recognize multiple paths and give up power and expertise to be effective. We need to listen to our clients and follow their lead. We need to become comfortable enough with ourselves to admit that we may not be right, at least not right for every individual client. Some clients just need to have their power reaffirmed. Examples include:

- Immigrants who surrendered power in their new country.
- An adult male with an unstable position in his family.
- A woman who lost faith in herself after being beaten and verbally abused.
- A gay teen who struggled to find his place in a homophobic community.

Listen carefully to your clients' *explicit* and *implicit* messages about their problems, their perceptions of the problems, the causes of their problems, and their ability to change them. Assume that your clients' direction in therapy makes sense. Not all clients are able to describe their concerns. Common reasons include:

- They cannot put words to their feelings.
- They are used to placating those in power.
- They have a history of oppression that silences them (Atkinson et al., 1992; Fischer & Good, 1997; Gim et al., 1991; Propst et al., 1992; C. E. Thompson et al., 1994).

Therapists do not have to be "guilty" to silence clients; as many clients bring their experiences with oppressive forces into the therapy room. Therapists must directly behave differently ("Not all dominant group members behave in an oppressive fashion"), and they must help clients brainstorm effective ways of responding to culturally related factors.

Clients and therapists may address cultural concerns without talking about them directly. Sonja, formerly a computer programmer in Bosnia, was only able to get a menial job in the United States because (1) her degrees were not accepted locally, (2) she did not have a driver's license, and (3) her English was poor. She began having a variety of panic symptoms and flashbacks secondary to her experiences during the war. She entered the clinic as an emergency walk-in and agreed to complete the intake materials before her second appointment and to keep a structured diary about when and where she was having symptoms.

Sonja forgot her paperwork and diary at her next appointment and at subsequent ones. However, she did an extensive Internet search on PTSD and panic disorder and was able to speak knowledgeably about treatment options and to contribute toward identifying treatment goals. She moved in a different direction than her therapist, but an equally valid one. Although Marc, her Euro-American therapist, initially wondered about identifying her behavior as resistance, he decided to follow her lead. In doing so, he honored her goals as well as her competencies, something that she desperately needed since coming to this country.

Accept and Use Power When It Is Helpful

Accepting and using power can be helpful. Talk with a client about your rationale for setting up a particular type of service and come to an agreement about the nature of the therapeutic process (Erickson & Al-Timimi, 2001). Many groups expect experts to be healers and will relate to them as such they become uncomfortable when a different type of role is set up. A culturally aware therapist may need to move comfortably into the expert role when this expectation can facilitate change and share power when it will be helpful.

THINK SYSTEMATICALLY

Systematic thinking is integral to this approach. Considering clients in a familial, community, cultural, developmental, and temporal framework can change not only how clients are perceived, but also make services more acceptable and effective. Furthermore, systematic thinking can lead clients and therapists to identify internal and external resources that will enable clients to become successful.

Provide Services Relevant to Clients' Lives and Worldviews

Services must be relevant to clients' lives and worldviews. The Americans with Disabilities Act (United States Congress, 1990) mandates that public buildings and services be accessible to people with disabilities. Physical accessibility is mandated by the ADA, but good counseling services should also be "culturally accessible."

Cultural accessibility can be met in several ways. Services should be provided in a culturally relevant location, such as an African American neighborhood or a GLBT community center. Symbols suggesting openness to local cultures should be present, like having a diverse staff, flyers, intake materials written in languages common to the locale, and culturally relevant artwork. Services should be offered in native languages when possible and through an interpreter when not. Office hours should be appropriate for the population. Evenings and weekends should be available for people working full-time, especially people working minimum wage jobs, who often have less flexible work hours than some white collar workers. As discussed in chapter 7, a diverse staff can decrease the probability of cultural mismatches, and therapist assignments should consider the racial identities of clients *and* staff (Atkinson et al., 1986; Atkinson & Wampold, 1993; Bennett & Bigfoot-Sipes, 1991; Liddle, 1996; C. E. Thompson et al., 1994).

Services must also be culturally relevant. This was a primary impetus to the development of wraparound and family-based services for highly distressed children, teens, and their families (Slattery & Knapp, 2003). Traditional mental health services had failed to offer the range of services necessary to stabilize these families. Among these were family therapy, parenting groups, wraparound services, respite, short-term foster care, and advocacy in the school and in medical systems. Similarly, Tafoya (1990) suggests involving traditional healers and healing ceremonies when working with Native Americans. Culturally different clients often prefer more relationship building at the beginning of therapy than do many task-oriented Euro-Americans (S. Sue et al., 1994). Given the taboos that Asian, Arab, and Native Americans, for example, often have about disclosing to strangers, expecting clients to rapidly disclose difficult information in a culturally inappropriate manner may lead to premature terminations (see table 8.3, p. 173; Erickson & Al-Timimi, 2001; D. W. Sue & Sue, 1999; Tafoya, 1990; Zhang, 2003g).

Help Clients Recognize Available Supports

A primary goal of effective contextual therapy is to help clients recognize available supports. The research on support systems suggests that people who are well-supported do better than those who are insufficiently supported or have individually inappropriate or culturally inappropriate supports (Aquino et al., 1996; S. L. Brown, 1991; T. Elliott et al., 1992; T. Elliott & Shewchuk, 1995; Kurdek, 1988; Zemore & Shepel, 1989). When the support system is insufficient or ineffective, we can help clients find ways to gather support. This may involve putting additional programs into place. In other cases, it may involve recognizing and accessing services or people within the client's system who are already available and supportive. Examples include grandparents, neighbors, principals, and the like. In still other instances, it may require fine-tuning these resources, such as

- Helping a grandparent to be supportive in a positive, rather than a critical manner.
- Asking neighbors to listen rather than give advice.
- Giving a principal a list of priorities for handling a child who is out of control.

Supports can take any form. We can ignore a problem, see it as overwhelming and impossible to resolve, solve the problem for them, guide their use of our solutions, or encourage them to discover their own solutions. When possible, we should choose interventions that help clients discover their own power. We should listen to their values, help them discover their own solutions, and recognize their ability to succeed in achieving their goals. Being empowering with a child may involve giving choices ("Do you want the red or green crayon?"). With an adult, empowering may involve recognizing and nurturing their skills of empathy, insight, technical ability, or problem solving. Also, it will generally involve using metaphors and stories appropriate for the culture.

How one empowers, of course, is influenced by the client's values, skills, and level of crisis. Furthermore, being empowering to one individual (a child) may be disempowering to another in that person's system (a parent). It is important to consider the needs of the entire system and the treatment goals that go into the planning of interventions. We do not have to choose whom we empower; we can empower an entire system.

Help Clients Regain Balance

Change may involve recognizing and regaining balance. People often change their behavior when they are in crisis. Whether the change causes or follows the crisis is unclear, however. Nonetheless, when depressed, eating and sleeping habits change. People withdraw from others, stop going to church, and avoid the things they used to enjoy. Learning more about how the client's world has changed between more satisfying and less satisfying periods is generally helpful in developing a plan for treatment. A timeline or psychosocial history can be very useful in this process.

Although general heuristics exist about what a healthy life should look like, there are also significant individual and cultural differences. Rediscovering balance must be within the client's individual and cultural valuing system, with the balance for a Native American client often different than that for a Euro-American client.

RECONSIDER THE GOALS OF THERAPY

In several ways, contextualized therapy deviates from the goals of other therapies. Clients are recognized as unique individuals who may require individualized interventions based not only upon their race, but also their racial identity, gender, age, religion, class, temporal history, their readiness for change, and their strengths and weaknesses. This can make each new client a challenge. Wise therapists will anticipate these challenges and prepare for them.

In addition, resistance to change may be positive, while removing symptoms may not be. Therapists and clients should carefully consider the meaning of symptoms and their potential adaptiveness.

Clients' Fears of Change

Acknowledge the client's fears about change and about working within the system. Many people who have worked in a variety of systems and with a variety of providers will enter therapy expecting that they will be treated disrespectfully and will not be understood (and then only from the dominant culture's framework). They already know what services will be provided, which typically are services that *providers* think are important and that these services will be provided in an enabling or disempowering manner. Therapists and caseworkers must challenge inaccurate and nonproductive expectations directly.

Furthermore, therapy—especially with someone who appears different or who holds significantly different values—is a significant risk. Clients may be misunderstood or blamed. Things may get worse before they get better. The problem may be unfixable. Fixing one problem may cause significant additional problems. Leaving an abusive spouse may separate children from a beloved parent, cause a drop in the standard of living, and encourage family and church members to shun them for their decision. Accepting the risk to change when there are often many reasons not to shows considerable courage (Waters & Lawrence, 1993).

Symptom Reduction Versus Good Outcomes

Symptom reduction is not necessarily a good outcome to therapy. Some symptoms are adaptive responses to trauma or injustice, such as anxiety and anger in response to sexual harassment. Identifying oppression and discrimination as such may increase anxiety and anger, depending upon the person's level of racial identity. Rather than being unhealthy, recognizing oppression can be adaptive, especially when one can also identify a useful response to it. Rather than working to decrease symptoms, normalizing symptoms and identifying healthy outlets can make good sense.

Conversely, not being angry, depressed, or anxious *can* be a *bad* outcome. This is most easily seen with the avoidant-dissociative aspects of post-traumatic stress disorder, but it can also be seen in Helms' description of Conformity and Dissonance ego statuses (Helms & Cook, 1999). Development and growth are often initially associated with an increase rather than a decrease in symptoms.

Risks of Culturally Aware Therapy

Culturally aware therapy is risky. Becoming aware of previously unrecognized and unearned privilege, oppressive acts, and one's own involvement in maintaining oppression can be threatening. Culturally aware therapy means remaining open to the fact that there is always more to learn about the relationships among race, class, gender, age, and other cultural variables. It means admitting that one's own valuing system and decisions in life are not necessarily the only "right" ones, and it requires one to remain open to other viewpoints. It means being comfortable enough to say, "I don't know," then to learn more about a group or cultural practice. Each of these actions requires us to walk slightly outside our comfort zone, which is something many people find challenging.

It is a significant psychological risk to really listen to someone else ("What if I can't do it this time?"). Recognize this risk and, rather than pretend that it's not there, use it to encourage personal growth as a person and as a therapist. Frame this process in a positive manner. It is challenging to admit that the psychology field's knowledge base (and our own) is incomplete, but it is also exciting to listen with a fresh ear to each new client and to be part of an effort to extend this knowledge base. We should listen carefully when someone reminds us that we have more to learn (and that they believe we *can* learn) and accept it as a compliment. At least they feel safe enough to challenge us. Our ability to listen nondefensively can be part of this education, as well as being part of the therapy. How empowering it can be to have someone really listen to you when you've challenged them!

Use Safety Nets

As in any therapy experience, some things will be easy, and others will be more difficult. Use safety nets, develop strengths, and identify ways to strengthen relative weaknesses. Important safety nets include the field's ethical guidelines, our theory of change, and the treatment plans we develop with our clients (Slattery & Knapp, 2003). Journaling and talking to supervisors and peer consultants can help us navigate difficult areas.

Our ethical guidelines are useful in identifying many of therapy's trouble spots. However, many humane responses have traditionally been taboo in psychotherapy, although they may be normative in some cultures. This is yet another problem with using models first designed for upper-class Euro-Americans from urban areas. D. W. Sue (2000) argued that our identification of these behaviors as taboo came from a deficit rather than a strength-based model and suggested that we expand the counseling repertoire to include advice giving, self-disclosures, accepting gifts—which in many cultures are both culturally normative and an extension of self—bartering, and some kinds of dual relationships.

Taboos develop for a reason. Dietary taboos in the Jewish faith arose because some foods had been risky and were associated with disease. Many taboo behaviors in counseling have a higher risk of problems, but are not inevitably risky. In fact, consulting psychology, a field with similar methods and goals, has explicitly rejected the deficit model associated with psychotherapy's ethical guidelines in favor of strength-based strategies (V. Littlefield, personal communication, August 6, 2000). Rather than presuming that one approach is *never* or is *always* correct, we should be like consulting psychologists and stop to consider *what actually works.*

We should consider both the short-term and long-term advantages and disadvantages, especially when we consider coloring outside the lines. How might this be useful now? How might it be difficult? What long-term benefits are predictable? What long-term costs can be anticipated?

Although ethical guidelines are often treated in a dichotomous fashion (i.e., right or wrong), it may be more useful to think about *how* to handle a problem, rather than only identifying a single solution. Although our ethical guidelines can identify places where we may run into a problem, our treatment plans and theoretical orientation can help us choose among potential solutions. For example, Slattery and Knapp (2003) suggested that providers in wraparound systems (i.e., work with seriously at-risk children that "wraps around" the child's and family's multiple needs and goals) recognize the ethical concerns raised by their work, but use theory (culturally aware, systemically aware, and empowering) and treatment plans to choose among interventions that may meet a family's needs.

MAKE THE JOURNEY TOWARD CULTURAL COMPETENCE

Cultural competency is a journey. Wachtel (2002) argues that our focus on prejudice and discrimination alone becomes problematic when it obscures the very real problem of indifference, which, "in the face of severe human suffering is not a minor offense" (Wachtel, 1999, p. 39, as quoted in Wachtel, 2002). No single book can teach everything that one needs to know about race, culture, class, age, gender, affectional orientation, ability, and all their intersections. There are just too many groups and permutations among groups for any one person to be an expert on all of them. But, educating oneself about culture and context can open the therapist's eyes to different options and valuing stances. It will also challenge the indifference that can be a real barrier to empathy (Wachtel, 2002). Continue to read widely, travel to diverse parts of the country and world, and listen to different worldviews. Expect to make mistakes, but learn from them.

Learn from people, including clients, throughout life and career. At the end of my internship year, while saying goodbye, a family asked, "What did you learn?" I was a bit taken aback and thought, "Weren't they the ones who were supposed to be learning?" While therapy is not designed to help the therapist and should not be steered toward meeting our needs, I now know that I am learning at least as much as my clients. (Thank you.) Learning to see and understand people, their context, values, and goals, as well as how we can best adapt our work to individual clients is and will be a lifelong journey.

References

Abramson, L., Metalsky, G., & Alloy, L. (1989). Hopelessness depression: A theory-based subtype of depression. *Psychological Review, 96,* 358–372.

Adams, E. M., & Betz, N. E. (1993). Gender differences in counselors' attitudes toward and attributions about incest. *Journal of Counseling Psychology, 40,* 210–216.

Affleck, G., Tennen, H., Croog, S., & Levine, S. (1987). Causal attribution, perceived benefits, and morbidity after a heart attack: An 8-year study. *Journal of Consulting and Clinical Psychology, 55,* 29–35.

Affleck, G., Tennen, H., & Rowe, J. (1991). *Infants in crisis: How parents cope with newborn intensive care and its aftermath.* New York, NY: Springer-Verlag.

Albee, G. W. (2000). The Boulder Model's fatal flaw. *American Psychologist, 55,* 247–248.

Alexander, J. F., Waldron, H. B., Barton, C., & Mas, C. H. (1989). The minimizing of blaming attributions and behaviors in delinquent families. *Journal of Consulting and Clinical Psychology, 57,* 19–24.

Al-Issa, I. (1982). *Culture and psychopathology.* Baltimore, MD: University Park Press.

Alloy, L. & Seligman, M. (1979). On the cognitive component of learned helplessness. In G. Bower (Ed.), *The psychology of learning and motivation* (Vol. 13). San Diego, CA: Academic Press.

Amer, M. M. (2002). Mental health considerations and coping behaviors among Arab Americans. In J. Ghannam, *Culturally-sensitive mental health treatment for Arab Americans.* Paper presented at the annual meeting of the American Psychological Association, Chicago, IL.

American Counseling Association. (1995). *ACA code of ethics and standards of practice.* Retrieved January 13, 2002, from http://www.counseling.org/resources/codeofethics.htm

American Law Institute, Model Penal Code and Commentaries (Official draft and revised comments) § 4.01 (1985).

American Psychiatric Association. (2000). *Diagnostic and statistical manual of mental disorders* (4th ed., text revision). Washington, DC: Author.

American Psychological Association. (2002). Ethical principles of psychologists and code of conduct. *American Psychologist, 57,* 1060–1073.

Angelou, M. (1981). *The heart of a woman.* New York, NY: Random House.

Anonymous. (2000, March). Boundaries in therapy: The limits of care. *Pennsylvania Psychologist Update, 1,* 3.

APA Task Force on Promotion and Dissemination of Psychological Procedures. (1995). Training in and dissemination of empirically validated psychological treatments: Report and recommendation. *The Clinical Psychologist, 48,* 3–23.

Aquino, J. A., Russell, D. W., Cutrona, C. E., & Altmaier, E. M. (1996). Employment status, social support, and life satisfaction among the elderly. *Journal of Counseling Psychology, 43,* 480–489.

Aronson, J., Blanton, H., & Cooper, J. (1995). From dissonance to disidentification: Selectivity in the self-affirmation process. *Journal of Personality and Social Psychology, 68,* 986–996.

Arroyo, C. G., & Zigler, E. (1995). Racial identity, academic achievement, and the psychological well-being of economically disadvantaged adolescents. *Journal of Personality and Social Psychology, 69,* 903–914.

Asay, T. P., & Lambert, M. J. (1999). The empirical case for common factors in therapy: Quantitative findings. In M. A. Hubble, B. L. Duncan, & S. D. Miller (Eds.), *The heart and soul of change: What works in therapy* (pp. 33–55). Washington, D. C.: American Psychological Association.

Atkinson, D. R., Brown, M. T., Parham, T. A., Matthews, L. G., Landrum-Brown, J., & Kim, A. U. (1996). African American client skin tone and clinical judgments of African American and European American psychologists. *Professional Psychology: Research and Practice, 27,* 500–505.

Atkinson, D. R., Casas, A., & Abreu, J. (1992). Mexican-American acculturation, counselor ethnicity and cultural sensitivity, and perceived counselor competence. *Journal of Counseling Psychology, 39,* 515–520.

Atkinson, D. R., Furlong, M. J., & Poston, W. C. (1986). Afro-American preferences for counselor characteristics. *Journal of Counseling Psychology, 33,* 326–330.

Atkinson, D. R., Maruyama, M., & Matsui, S. (1978). The effects of counselor race and counseling approach on Asian Americans' perceptions of counselor credibility and utility. *Journal of Counseling Psychology, 25,* 76–83.

Atkinson, D. R., Morten, G., & Sue, D. W. (1998). *Counseling American minorities* (5th ed.). Boston, MA: McGraw-Hill.

Atkinson, D. R., & Wampold, B. E. (1993). Mexican Americans' initial preferences for counselors: Simple choice can be misleading: Comment on Lopez, Lopez, and Fong (1991). *Journal of Counseling Psychology, 40,* 245–248.

Bachelor, A., & Horvath, A. (1999). The therapeutic relationship. In M. A. Hubble, B. L. Duncan, & S. D. Miller (Eds.), *The heart and soul of change: What works in therapy* (pp. 133–178). Washington, D. C.: American Psychological Association.

Bailey, W., Nowicki, S., Jr, & Cole, S. P. (1998). The ability to decode nonverbal information in African American, African and Afro-Caribbean, and European American adults. *Journal of Black Psychology, 24,* 418–431.

Banaji, M. R., Hardin, C. D., & Rothman, A. J. (1993). Implicit stereotyping in person judgment. *Journal of Personality and Social Psychology, 65,* 272–281.

Bandura, A. (1982). The self and mechanisms of agency. In J. Suls (Ed.), *Psychological perspectives on the self* (Vol. 1, pp. 3–39). Hillsdale, NJ: Erlbaum.

Bandura, A. (1997). *Self-efficacy: The exercise of control.* New York, NY: W.H. Freeman and Company.

Baumrind, D. (1991). Effective parenting during the early adolescent transition. In P. E. Cowan & E. M. Hetherington (Eds.), *Advances in family research* (Vol. 2, pp. 111–163). Hillsdale, NJ: Erlbaum.

Bean, T., Jones Bean, D., Slattery, J. M., & Becker, R. (2000, April). *Family and agency teamwork throughout the system: Walking the walk.* Workshop presented at the annual PA CASSP conference, State College, PA.

Beattie, M. C., & Longabough, R. (1999). General and alcohol-specific social support following treatment. *Addictive Behaviors, 24,* 593–606.

Beck, A. T. (1991). Cognitive therapy: A 30-year retrospective. *American Psychologist, 46,* 368–375.

Becker, D., & Lamb, S. (1994). Sex bias in the diagnosis of borderline personality disorder and posttraumatic stress disorder. *Professional Psychology: Research and Practice, 25,* 55–61.

Becker, D. F., Weine, S. M., Vojvoda, D., & McGlashan, T. H. (1999). Case series: PTSD symptoms in adolescent survivors of "ethnic cleansing": Results from a 1-year follow-up study. *Journal of the American Academy of Child and Adolescent Psychiatry, 38,* 775–781.

Beckman, H. B., & Frankel, R. M. (1984). The effect of physician behavior on the collection of data. *Annals of Internal Medicine, 101,* 692–696.

Belar, C. D., & Deardorff, W. W. (1995). *Clinical health psychology in medical settings: A practitioner's guidebook.* Washington, D. C.: American Psychological Association.

Belenky, M. F., Clinchy, B., Goldberger, N., & Tarule, J. M. (1986). *Women's ways of knowing: The development of self, voice, and mind.* New York, NY: Basic Books.

Bennett, S. K., & Bigfoot-Sipes, D. S. (1991). American Indian and White college student preferences for counselor characteristics. *Journal of Counseling Psychology, 38,* 440–445.

Berg, I. K. (1994). *Family-based services: A solution-focused approach.* New York, NY: Norton.

Bergin, A. E. (1991). Values and religious issues in psychotherapy and mental health. *American Psychologist, 46,* 394–403.

Bergin, A. E., & Garfield, S. L. (1994). Overview, trends, and future issues. In A. E. Bergin & S. L. Garfield (Eds.), *Handbook of psychotherapy and behavior change* (4th ed., pp. 821–830). New York, NY: John Wiley & Sons.

Berman, J. (1979). Counseling skills used by Black and White male and female counselors. *Journal of Counseling Psychology, 26,* 81–84.

Bianchi, F. T., Zea, M. C., Belgrave, F. Z., & Echeverry, J. J. (2002). Racial identity and self-esteem among Black Brazilian men: Race matters in Brazil too! *Cultural Diversity and Ethnic Minority Psychology, 8,* 157–169.

Bloom, S. L. (1998). By the crowd they have been broken, by the crowd they shall be healed: The social transformation of trauma. In R. G. Tedeschi, C. L. Park & L. G. Calhoun (Eds.), *Posttraumatic growth: Positive changes in the aftermath of crisis* (pp. 179–213). Mahwah, NJ: Lawrence Erlbaum.

Bogart, C. J. (1999). A feminist approach to teaching theory use to counseling psychology graduate students. *Teaching of Psychology, 26,* 46–47.

Boninger, D. S., Gleicher, F., & Strathman, A. (1994). Counterfactual thinking: From what might have been to what may be. *Journal of Personality and Social Psychology, 67,* 297–307.

Boraine, A. (1996, July). Alternatives and adjuncts to criminal prosecutions. Speech presented at *Justice in cataclysm: Criminal tribunals in the wake of mass violence,* Brussels, Belgium. Retrieved March 4, 2002, from http://www.polity.org.za/html/govdocs/speeches/1996/sp0720.html

Bourgeois, L., Sabourin, S., & Wright, J. (1990). Predictive validity of therapeutic alliance in group marital therapy. *Journal of Consulting and Clinical Psychology, 58,* 608–613.

Bower, J. E., Kemeny, M. E., Taylor, S. E., & Fahey, J. L. (1998). Cognitive processing, discovery of meaning, CD4 decline, and AIDS-related mortality among bereaved HIV-seropositive men. *Journal of Consulting and Clinical Psychology, 66,* 979–986.

Bowers, K. S., & Farvolden, P. (1996). Revisiting a century-old Freudian slip—From suggestion disavowed to the truth repressed. *Psychological Bulletin, 119,* 355–380.

Boyd-Franklin, N. (1990). Five key factors in the treatment of Black families. In G. W. Saba, B. M. Karrer, & K. V. Hardy (Eds.), *Minorities and family therapy* (pp. 53–69). New York, NY: Haworth.

Bradley, B. P., Gossop, M., Brewin, C. R., Phillips, G., & Green, L. (1992). Attributions and relapse in opiate addicts. *Journal of Consulting and Clinical Psychology, 60,* 470–472.

Branscombe, N. R., Schmitt, M. T., & Harvey, R. D. (1999). Perceiving pervasive discrimination among African Americans: Implications for group identification and well-being. *Journal of Personality and Social Psychology, 77,* 135–149.

Brewin, C. R., Andrews, N., & Valentine, J. D. (2000). Meta-analysis of risk factors for posttraumatic stress disorder in trauma-exposed adults. *Journal of Consulting and Clinical Psychology, 68,* 748–766.

Brokenleg, M. (1996, March). *Culture and helping.* Workshop presented at University of Pittsburgh Medical Center, Warrendale, PA.

Brown, J. D. (1986). Evaluations of self and others: Self-enhancement biases in social judgments. *Social Cognition, 4,* 353–376.

Brown, L. M. (1998). *Raising their voices: The politics of girls' anger.* Cambridge, MA: Harvard University Press.

Brown, S. L. (1991). *Counseling victims of violence.* Alexandria, VA: American Association for Counseling and Development.

Buber, M. (1970). *I and Thou* (W. A. Kaufmann, Trans.). New York, NY: Scribner.

Campbell, P. R. (1996). *Population projections for states by age, sex, race, and Hispanic origin: 1995 to 2025.* U.S. Bureau of the Census, Population Division, PPL-47. Retrieved on December 8, 2002, from http://www.census.gov/population/www/projections/ppl47.html

Carkhuff, R. (1969). *Helping and human relations* (Vols. 1 & 2). New York, NY: Holt, Rinehart & Winston.

Carlton-LaNey, I. (1999). African American social work pioneers' response to need. *Social Work, 44,* 311–321.

Carroll, J. (1996). *An American requiem: God, my father, and the war that came between us.* Boston, MA: Houghton Mifflin.

Carroll, L. (1865/1960). *The annotated Alice: Alice's adventures in wonderland and Through the looking glass.* New York, NY: Bramhall House.

Carver, C. S., Pozo, C., Harris, S., Noriega, V., Scheier, M. F., Robinson, D. S., Ketcham, A. S., Moffat, F. L., & Clark, K. C. (1993). How coping mediates the effect of optimism on distress: A study of women with early stage breast cancer. *Journal of Personality and Social Psychology, 65,* 375–390.

Catlin, G., & Epstein, S. (1992). Unforgettable experiences: The relation of life events to basic beliefs about self and world. *Social Cognition, 10,* 189–209.

Ceballo, R. (1999). Negotiating the life narrative: A dialogue with an African American social worker. *Psychology of Women Quarterly, 23,* 309–321.

Chadwick, W. (1990). *Women, art, and society.* London: Thames and Hudson.

Chan, C. S. (1997). Don't ask, don't tell, don't know: The formation of a homosexual identity and sexual expression among Asian American lesbians. In B. Greene (Ed.), *Ethnic and cultural diversity among lesbians and gay men: Vol. 3. Psychological perspective on lesbian and gay issues* (pp. 240–248). Thousand Oaks, CA: Sage.

Cheng, N. (1986). *Life and death in Shanghai.* New York, NY: Penguin.

Cheryan, S., & Bodenhausen, G. V. (2000). When positive stereotypes threaten intellectual performance: The psychological hazards of "model minority" status. *Psychological Science, 11,* 399–402.

Chin, D., & Kroesen, K. W. (1999). Disclosure of HIV infection among Asian/Pacific Islander American women: Cultural stigma and support. *Cultural Diversity and Ethnic Minority Psychology, 5,* 222–235.

Chodorow, N. J. (1999). *The power of feelings: Personal meaning in psychoanalysis, gender and culture.* New Haven, CT: Yale University Press.

Clark, M. D. (1998). Strength-based practice: The ABC's of working with adolescents who don't want to work with you. *Federal Probation, 62,* 46–53.

Cochran, S. D. (2001). Emerging issues in research on lesbians' and gay men's mental health: Does sexual orientation really matter? *American Psychologist, 56,* 931–941.

Cohen, D. (1998). Culture, social organization, and patterns of violence. *Journal of Personality and Social Psychology, 75,* 408–419.

Cohen, D., Nisbett, R. E., Bowdle, B. F., & Schwarz, N. (1996). Insult, aggression, and the southern culture of honor: An "experimental ethnography." *Journal of Personality and Social Psychology, 70,* 945–960.

Cohen, L. H., Towbes, L. C., & Flocco, R. (1988). Effects of induced mood on self-reported life events and perceived and received social support. *Journal of Personality and Social Psychology, 55,* 669–674.

Cohen, S., & Wills, T. (1985). Stress, social support, and the buffering hypothesis. *Psychological Bulletin, 98,* 310–357.

Columbia World of Quotations. (1996). Columbia University Press. Retrieved on January 24, 2003, from http://www.bartleby.com/66/66/65066.html

Cook, S. W. (1985). Experimenting on social issues: The case of school desegregation. *American Psychologist, 40,* 452–460.

Cotterell, N. (1999, June). Applying cognitive therapy: Seven steps to anger management. *Cognitive Therapy Today.* Retrieved March 4, 2002, from http://www.beckinstitute.org/june99/therapy.html

Courtois, C. (1988). *Healing the incest wound.* New York, NY: Norton.

Cowen, E. L. (1991). In pursuit of wellness. *American Psychologist, 46,* 404–408.

Creech, S. (1994). *Walk two moons.* New York, NY: HarperCollins.

Crocker, J., Cornwell, B., & Major, B. (1993). The stigma of overweight: Affective consequences of attributional ambiguity. *Journal of Personality and Social Psychology, 64,* 60–70.

Crocker, J., Thompson, L.L., McGraw, K. M., & Ingerman, C. (1987). Downward comparison, prejudice, and evaluations of others: Effects of self-esteem and threat. *Journal of Pesonality and Social Psychology, 52,* 907–916.

Croteau, J. M., & Hedstrom, S. M. (1993). Integrating commonality and difference: The key to career counseling with lesbian women and gay men. *Career Development Quarterly, 41,* 201–209.

Curry, L. A., Snyder, C. R., Cook, D. L., Ruby, B. C. & Rehm, M. (1997). Role of hope in academic and sport achievement. *Journal of Personality and Social Psychology, 73,* 1257–1267.

Cutrona, C. E. (1989). Ratings of social support by adolescents and adult informants: Degree of correspondence and prediction of depressive symptoms. *Journal of Personality and Social Psychology, 57,* 723–730.

Dasgupta, N., & Greenwald, A. G. (2001). On the malleability of automatic attitudes: Combating automatic prejudice with images of admired and disliked individuals. *Journal of Personality and Social Psychology, 81,* 800–814.

Davison, A. J., & Higgins, N. C. (1993). Observer bias in perceptions of responsibility. *American Psychologist, 48,* 584.

de Shazer, S. (1988). *Clues: Investigating solutions in brief therapy.* New York, NY: Professional Books.

Delahanty, D. L., Herberman, H. B., Craig, K. J., Hayward, M. C., Fullerton, C. S., Ursano, R. J., & Baum, A. (1997). Acute and chronic distress and posttraumatic stress disorder as a function of responsibility for serious motor vehicle accidents. *Journal of Consulting and Clinical Psychology, 65,* 560–567.

DeMaio, T. J. (1984). Social desirability and survey measurement: A review. In C. F. Turner & E. Martin (Eds.), *Surveying subjective phenomena* (Vol. 2, pp. 257–281). New York, NY: Russell Sage Foundation.

DeParle, J. (1999, May 15). Project to rescue needy stumbles against persistence of poverty. *The New York Times.* Retrieved February 11, 2002, from http://query.nytimes .com/search/abstract?res=FA0710F73D5A0C768DDDAC0894D1494D81

DeSouza, E. (2000, March). Multicultural and gender issues in teaching, counseling and therapy. In J. Sigal (Chair), *Multicultural and gender issues in teaching, counseling and therapy.* Symposium presented at the annual meetings of the Eastern Psychological Association, Baltimore, MD.

Diller, J. V. (1999). *Cultural diversity: A primer for the human services.* Belmont, CA: Brooks/Cole.

Dixon, W. A., & Reid, J. K. (2000). Positive life events as a moderator of stress-related depressive symptoms. *Journal of Counseling & Devlopment, 78,* 343–347.

Dorfman, L. T. & Moffet, M. M. (1987). Retirement satisfaction in married and widowed rural women. *The Gerontologist, 27,* 215–221.

Dovidio, J. F., & Gaertner, S. L. (1999). Reducing prejudice: Combating intergroup biases. *Current Directions in Psychological Science, 8,* 101–105.

Duncan, B. L. (1976). Differential social perception and attribution of intergroup violence: Testing the lower limits of stereotyping of Blacks. *Journal of Personality and Social Psychology, 34,* 590–598.

Eagly, A. (2000, August). *Prejudice: A social role analysis.* Presented at the annual meetings of the American Psychological Association, Washington, D.C.

Elligan, D., & Utsey, S. (1999). Utility of an African-centered support group for African American men confronting societal racism and oppression. *Cultural Diversity and Ethnic Minority Psychology, 5,* 156–165.

Elliot, J. (1999). *An unexpected light: Travels in Afghanistan.* New York, NY: Picador.

Elliott, D. M., & Guy, J. D. (1993). Mental health professionals versus non-mental-health professionals: Childhood trauma and adult functioning. *Professional Psychology: Research and Practice, 24,* 83–90.

Elliott, T., Herrick, S., Witty, T., Godshall, F. & Spruell, M. (1992). Social support and depression following spinal cord injury. *Rehabilitation Psychology, 37,* 37–48.

Elliott, T., & Shewchuk, R. (1995). Social support and leisure activities following severe physical disability: Testing the mediating effects of depression. *Basic and Applied Social Psychology, 16,* 471–487.

Elliott, T. R., Shewchuk , R. M., & Richards, J. S. (1999). Caregiver social problem-solving abilities and family member adjustment to recent-onset physical disability. *Rehabilitation Psychology, 44,* 104–123.

Emery, R. E., Fincham, R. E., & Cummings, E. M. (1992). Parenting in context: Systemic thinking about parental conflict and its influence on children. *Journal of Consulting and Clinical Psychology, 60,* 909–912.

Emmons, R. A., & Colby, P. M. (1995). Emotional conflict and well-being: Relation to perceived availability, daily utilization, and observer reports of social support. *Journal of Personality and Social Psychology, 68,* 947–959.

Enns, C. Z. (1992). Toward integrating feminist psychotherapy and feminist philosophy. *Professional Psychology: Research and Practice, 23,* 453–466.

Epp, L. (1998). The courage to be an existential counselor: An interview of Clemmont Vontress. *Journal of Mental Health Counseling, 20,* 1–12.

Epstein, M. H. (1999). The development and validation of a scale to assess the emotional and behavioral strengths of children and adolescents. *Remedial and Special Education, 20,* 258–262.

Epstein, R. M., Quill, T. E., & McWhinney, I. R. (1999). Somatization reconsidered: Incorporating the patient's experience of illness. *Archives of Internal Medicine, 159,* 215–222.

Epstein, S. (1973). The self-concept revisited: Or a theory of a theory. *American Psychologist, 28,* 404–416.

Erdoes, R., & Ortiz, A. (Eds.). (1984). *American Indian myths and legends.* New York, NY: Pantheon.

Erickson, C. D., & Al-Timimi, N. R. (2001). Providing mental health services to Arab Americans: Recommendations and considerations. *Cultural Diversity and Ethnic Minority Psychology, 7,* 308–327.

Esterling, B. A., Antoni, M. H., Fletcher, M. A., Margulies, S., & Schneiderman, N. (1994). Emotional disclosure through writing or speaking modulates latent Epstein-Barr virus antibody titers. *Journal of Consulting and Clinical Psychology, 62,* 130–140.

Fang, L. (1995). *The ch'i-lin purse: A collection of ancient Chinese stories.* New York, NY: Farrar Straus Giroux.

Fauber, R. L., & Long, N. (1991). Children in context: The role of the family in child psychotherapy. *Journal of Consulting and Clinical Psychology, 59,* 813–820.

Festinger, L. (1957). *A theory of cognitive dissonance.* Stanford, CA: Stanford University Press.

Fischer, A. R., & Good, G. E. (1997). Men and psychotherapy: An investigation of alexithymia, intimacy, and masculine gender roles. *Psychotherapy: Theory, Research, Practice, Training, 34,* 160–170.

Fischer, A. R., Tokar, D. M., & Serna, G. S. (1998). Validity and construct contamination of the Racial Identity Attitude Scale—Long Form. *Journal of Counseling Psychology, 45,* 212–224.

Fiske, S. T. (1993). Controlling other people: The impact of power on stereotyping. *American Psychologist, 48,* 621–628.

Folkman, S. (2001). Coping and health. In J. S. Halonen & S. F. Davis (Eds.). *The many faces of psychological research in the 21st century* (chap. 1). Retrieved December 16, 2001, from http://teachpsych.lemoyne.edu/teachpsych/faces/script/Ch01.htm

Follette, V. M., Alexander, P. C, & Follette, W. C. (1991). Individual predictors of outcome in group treatment for incest survivors. *Journal of Consulting and Clinical Psychology, 59,* 150–155.

Fontaine, J. H., & Hammond, N. L. (1994). Twenty counseling maxims. *Journal of Counseling and Development, 73,* 223–226.

Fontes, L. A., & Piercy, F. P. (2000). Engaging students in qualitative research through experiential class activities. *Teaching of Psychology, 27,* 174–179.

Ford, M. R., & Widiger, T. A. (1989). Sex bias in the diagnosis of histrionic and antisocial personality disorders. *Journal of Consulting and Clinical Psychology, 57,* 301–305.

Frances, A. J., First, M. B., Widiger, T. A., Miele, G. M., Tilly, S. M., Davis, W. W., & Pincus, H. A. (1991). An A to Z guide to DSM-IV conundrums. *Journal of Abnormal Psychology, 100,* 407–412.

Francisco, P. W. (1999). *Telling: A memoir of rape and recovery.* New York, NY: HarperCollins.

Frank, J. D. (1961). *Persuasion and healing: A comparative study of psychotherapy.* Baltimore, MD: Johns Hopkins.

Frankl, V. (1959). *Man's search for meaning: An introduction to logotherapy.* Boston, MA, Beacon Press.

Frazier, P. A. (1990). Victim attributions and post-rape trauma. *Journal of Personality and Social Psychology, 59,* 298–304.

Freedman, S. R., & Enright, R. D. (1996). Forgiveness as an intervention goal with incest survivors. *Journal of Consulting and Clinical Psychology, 64,* 983–992.

Fukuyama, M. (1990). Taking a universal approach to multicultural counseling. *Counselor Education and Supervision, 30,* 6–17.

Fygetakis, L. M. (1997). Greek American lesbians: Identity odysseys of honorable good girls. In B. Greene (Ed.), *Ethnic and cultural diversity among lesbians and gay men:* Vol. 3. *Psychological perspective on lesbian and gay issues* (pp. 152–190). Thousand Oaks, CA: Sage.

Garbarino, J. (2000). The soul of fatherhood. *Marriage and Family Review, 29,* 11–21.

Gauvain, M., & Huard, R. D. (1999). Family interaction, parenting style, and the development of planning: A longitudinal analysis using archival data. *Journal of Family Psychology, 13,* 75–92.

Gelso, C. J. (2000, August). Toward a positive psychotherapy: Focus on human strength. In W. B. Walsh (Chair), *Fostering human strength–A counseling psychology perspective.* Symposium at the annual meeting of the American Psychological Association, Washington, D. C.

Gilbert, D. T., & Malone, P.S. (1995). The correspondence bias. *Psychological Bulletin, 117,* 21–38.

Gil, E. (1999). *The healing power of play : Working with abused children.* New York, NY: Guilford.

Gilligan, C. (1982). *In a different voice: Psychological theory and women's development.* Cambridge, MA: Harvard University Press.

Gilligan, C. (1991). Women's psychological development: Implications for psychotherapy. In C. Gilligan, A. G. Rogers, & D. L. Tolman (Eds.), *Women, girls, & psychotherapy: Reframing resistance* (pp. 5–31). New York, NY: Harrington Park Press.

Gilligan, C., & Brown, L. M. (1992). *Meeting at the crossroads: Women's psychology and girls' development.* Cambridge, MA: Harvard University Press.

Gim, R.H., Atkinson, D. R., & Kim, S. J. (1991). Asian-American acculturation, counselor ethnicity and cultural sensitivity, and ratings of counselors. *Journal of Counseling Psychology, 38,* 57–62.

Giner-Sorolla, R., & Chaiken, S. (1994). The causes of hostile media judgments. *Journal of Experimental Social Psychology, 30,* 165–180.

Giordano, J., & McGoldrick, M. (1996). Italian families. In M. McGoldrick, J. Giordano, & J. K. Pearce (Eds.), *Ethnicity and family therapy* (2nd ed., pp. 567–582). New York, NY: Guilford Press.

Glinder, J. G., & Compas, B. E. (1999). Self-blame attributions in women with newly diagnosed breast cancer: A prospective study of psychological adjustment. *Health Psychology, 18,* 475–481.

Goldfried, M. R. (2001). Integrating gay, lesbian and bisexual issues into mainstream psychology, *American Psychologist, 56,* 977–988.

Gollwitzer, P. M. (1999). Implementation intentions: Strong effects of simple plans. *American Psychologist, 54,* 493–503.

Gonzalez-Ramos, G., Zayas, L. H., & Cohen, E. V. (1998). Child-rearing values of low-income, urban Puerto Rican mothers of preschool children. *Professional Psychology: Research and Practice, 29,* 377–382.

Goode, K. T., Haley, W. E., Roth, D. L., & Ford, G. R. (1998). Predicting longitudinal changes in caregiver physical and mental health: A stress process model. *Health Psychology, 17,* 190–198.

Gray-Little, B., & Hafdahl, A. R. (2000). Factors influencing racial comparisons of self-esteem: A quantitative review. *Psychological Bulletin, 126,* 26–54.

Greenberg, G. (1997). Right answers, wrong reason: Revisiting the deletion of homosexuality from the DSM. *Review of General Psychology, 1*, 256–270.

Greenberg, J., Pyszczynski, T., & Solomon, S. (1982). The self-serving attributional bias: Beyond self-presentation. *Journal of Experimental Social Psychology, 29*, 229–251.

Greenberg, L. S. (1995). The use of observational coding in family therapy research: Comment on Alexander et al. *Journal of Family Psychology, 9*, 366–37.

Greene, B. A. (1985). Considerations in the treatment of Black patients by White therapists. *Psychotherapy, 22*, 389–393.

Greene, B. (1997). Ethnic minority lesbians and gay men: Mental health and treatment issues. In B. Greene (Ed.), *Ethnic and cultural diversity among lesbians and gay men: Vol. 3. Psychological perspective on lesbian and gay issues* (pp. 216–239). Thousand Oaks, CA: Sage.

Greene, B. (2000). Beyond heterosexism and across the cultural divide. In B. Greene & G. L. Croom (Eds.), *Education, research, and practice in lesbian, gay, bisexual, and transgendered psychology: A resource manual* (pp. 1–45). Thousand Oaks, CA: Sage.

Greenwald, A., McGhee, D., & Schwartz, J. (1998). Measuring individual differences in implicit cognition: The Implicit Association Test. *Journal of Personality and Social Psychology, 74*, 1464–1480.

Greif, G. L. (1990). Twenty-five basic joining techniques in family therapy. *Journal of Psychoactive Drugs, 22*, 89–90.

Greif, G. L., Hrabowski, F.A., & Maton, K. I. (1998). African American fathers of high-achieving sons: Using outstanding members of an at-risk population to guide intervention. *Families in Society, 79*, 45–52.

Guyll, M., Matthews, K. A., & Bromberger, J. T. (2001). Discrimination and unfair treatment: Relationship to cardiovascular reactivity among African American and European American women. *Health Psychology, 20*, 315–325.

Gurung, R. A. R., & Mehta, V. (2001). Relating ethnic identity, acculturation, and attitudes toward treating minority clients. *Cultural Diversity and Ethnic Minority Psychology, 7*, 139–151.

Guthrie, R. V. (1997). *Even the rat was white* (2nd ed.). Boston, MA: Allyn & Bacon.

Haaga, D. A., & Stewart, B. L. (1992). Self-efficacy for recovery from a lapse after smoking cessation. *Journal of Consulting and Clinical Psychology, 60*, 24–28.

Hagerty, B. M., & Williams, R. A. (1999). The effects of sense of belonging, social support, conflict, and loneliness on depression. *Nursing Research, 48*, 215–219.

Hagerty, B. M., Williams, R. A., Coyne, J. C., & Early, M. R. (1996). Sense of belonging and indicators of social and psychological functioning. *Archives of Psychiatric Nursing, 10*, 235–244.

Hahn, W. K. (1998). Gifts in psychotherapy: An intersubjective approach to patient gifts. *Psychotherapy, 35*, 78–86.

Haley, J. (1993). *Uncommon therapy: The psychiatric techniques of Milton H. Erickson, M.D.* New York, NY: W. W. Norton.

Haley, W. E., Roth, D. L., Coleton, M. I., Ford, G. R., West, C. A. C., Collins, R. P., & Isobe, T. L. (1996). Appraisal, coping, and social support as mediators of well-being in black and white family caregivers of patients with Alzheimer's Disease. *Journal of Consulting and Clinical Psychology, 64*, 121–129.

Hall, G. C. N. (1997). Misunderstandings of multiculturalism: Shouting fire in crowded theaters. *American Psychologist, 52,* 654–655.

Halonen, J. S., & Santrock, J. W. (1997). *Human adjustment* (2nd ed.). Madison, WI: Brown & Benchmark.

Han, S-P, & Shavitt, S. (1994). Persuasion and culture: Advertising appeals in individualistic and collectivistic societies. *Journal of Experimental Social Psychology, 30,* 326–350.

Hanna, F. J., & Ritchie, M. H. (1995). Seeking the active ingredients of psychotherapeutic change: Within and outside the context of therapy. *Professional Psychology: Research and Practice, 26,* 176–183.

Harackiewicz, J. M., Sansone, C., Blair, L. W., Epstein, J. A., & Maderlink, G. (1987). Attributional processes in behavior change and maintenance: Smoking cessation and continued abstinence. *Journal of Consulting and Clinical Psychology, 55,* 372–378.

Hardin, S. I., Subich, L. M., & Holvey, J. M. (1988). Expectancies for counseling in relation to premature termination. *Journal of Counseling Psychology, 35,* 37–40.

Hardy, K. V. (1990). The theoretical myth of sameness: A critical issue in family therapy training and treatment. In G. W. Saba, B. M. Karrer, & K. V. Hardy (Eds.), *Minorities and family therapy* (pp. 17–33). New York, NY: Haworth.

Hardy, K. V. (2001, September/October). Soul work. *Psychotherapy networker,* 36–39, 53.

Harris, D. J., & Kuba, S. A. (1997). Ethnocultural identity and eating disorders in women of color. *Professional Psychology: Research and Practice, 28,* 341–347.

Hays, P. A. (1995). Multicultural applications of cognitive-behavior therapy. *Professional Psychology: Research and Practice, 26,* 309–315.

Hegi, U. (1997). *Tearing the silence: On being German in America.* New York, NY: Simon & Schuster.

Heider, F. (1946). Attitudes and cognitive organization. *Journal of Psychology, 21,* 107–112.

Helgeson, V. S., & Cohen, S. (1996). Social support and adjustment to cancer: Reconciling descriptive, correlational, and intervention research. *Health Psychology, 15,* 135–148.

Helms, J. E. (1984). Toward a theoretical explanation of the effects of race on counseling: A Black and White model. *The Counseling Psychologist, 12,* 153–165.

Helms, J. E. (1994). How multiculturalism obscures racial factors in the therapy process: Comment on Ridley et al. (1994), Sodowsky et al. (1994), Ottavi et al. (1994), and Thompson et al. (1994). *Journal of Counseling Psychology, 41,* 162–165.

Helms, J. E. (1999). A new racial world order. In J. E. Helms & D. A. Cook. *Using race and culture in counseling and psychotherapy: Theory and process* (pp. 36–37). Boston, MA: Allyn & Bacon.

Helms, J. E. (2000, August). Racial identity interaction model: Current status, future directions. In G. Roysicar-Sodowsky & E. Delgado-Romero (Chairs), *Millennium multicultural counseling psychologists.* Symposium at the annual meetings of the American Psychological Association, Washington, D. C.

Helms, J. E., & Cook, D. A. (1999). *Using race and culture in counseling and psychotherapy: Theory and process.* Boston, MA: Allyn & Bacon.

Helms, J. E., & Richardson, T. Q. (1997). How "multiculturalism" obscures race and culture as differential aspects of counseling competency. In D.B. Pope-Davis & H. L. K. Coleman (Eds.), *Multicultural counseling competencies: Assessment, education, training and supervision* (pp. 60–79). Thousand Oaks, CA: Sage.

Higgins, E. T. (1987). Self-discrepancy: A theory relating self and affect. *Psychological Review, 94,* 319–340.

Hinawer, H., & Wetzel, N. A. (1996). German families. In M. McGoldrick, J. Giordano, & J. K. Pearce (Eds.), *Ethnicity and family therapy* (2nd ed., pp. 496–516). New York, NY: Guilford Press.

Hindman, J. (1989). *Just before dawn.* Ontario, OR: AlexAndria Associates.

Hines, P., M., & Boyd-Franklin, N. (1996). African American families. In M. McGoldrick, J. Giordano, & J. K. Pearce (Eds.), *Ethnicity and family therapy* (2nd ed., pp. 66–84). New York, NY: Guilford Press.

Hofstede, G. (1980). *Culture's consequences: International differences in work-related values.* Beverly Hills, CA: Sage.

Holmes, T. H., & Rahe, R. H. (1967). The Social Readjustment Rating Scale. *Journal of Psychosomatic Research, 11,* 214–218.

Horenczyk, G., & Nisan, M. (1996). The actualization balance of ethnic identity. *Journal of Personality and Social Psychology, 70,* 836–843.

Horne, S. (1999). Domestic violence in Russia. *American Psychologist, 54,* 55–61.

Howard, G. S. (1992). Behold our creation! What counseling psychology has become and might yet become. *Journal of Counseling Psychology, 39,* 419–442.

Howard, K. I., Lueger, R. J., Maling, M. S., & Martinovich, Z. (1993). A phase model of psychotherapy outcome: Causal mediation of change. *Journal of Consulting and Clinical Psychology, 61,* 678–685.

Hoyt, D., Kaiser, M., Peters, G., & Babchuck, N. (1980). Life satisfaction and activity theory: A multidimensional approach. *Journal of Gerontology, 35,* 935–941.

Hoyt, S. (1999). Beyond prejudiced thoughts: Conceptual links between classism and discrimation (Doctoral dissertation, Miami University, 1998). *Dissertation Abstracts International, 59,* AAT 9841251.

Hubble, M. A., Duncan, B. L., & Miller, S. D. (1999a). Introduction. In M. A. Hubble, B. L. Duncan, & S. D. Miller (Eds.), *The heart and soul of change: What works in therapy* (pp. 1–19). Washington, D. C.: American Psychological Association.

Hubble, M. A., Duncan, B. L., & Miller, S. D. (Eds.). (1999b). *The heart and soul of change: What works in therapy.* Washington, D. C.: American Psychological Association.

Humphreys, H., & Rapoport, J. (1993). From the community mental health movement to the war on drugs: A study in the definition of social problems. *American Psychologist, 48,* 892–901.

Hyde, J. S., Fennema, E., & Lamon, S. J. (1990). Gender differences in mathematics performance: A meta-analysis. *Psychological Bulletin, 107,* 139–155.

Hyde, J. S., & Plant, E. A. (1995). Magnitude of psychological gender differences: Another side to the story. *American Psychologist, 50,* 159–161.

Ibrahim, F. A. (1985). Effective cross-cultural counseling and psychotherapy: A framework. *The Counseling Psychologist, 13,* 625–638.

Ingram, R. E., & Kendall, P. C. (1986). Cognitive clinical psychology: Implications of an information processing perspective. In R. E. Ingram (Ed.), *Information processing approaches to clinical psychology* (pp. 3–21). San Diego, CA: Academic Press.

Ituarte, P. H. G., Kamarck, T. W., Thompson, H. S., & Bacanu, S. (1999). Psychosocial mediators of racial differences in nighttime blood pressure dipping among normotensive adults. *Health Psychology, 18,* 393–402.

Ivey, A. E., & Ivey, M. B. (2003). *Intentional interviewing and counseling: Facilitating client development in a multicultural society* (5th ed.). Pacific Grove, CA: Brooks/Cole.

Ivey, A. E., Ivey, M. B., & Simek-Morgan, L. (1997). *Counseling and psychotherapy: A multicultural perspective* (4th ed.). Boston, MA: Allyn & Bacon.

Jackson, J. (1999, August). *What ought Psychology to do?* Paper presented at the meetings of the American Psychological Association, Boston, MA.

Jackson, J. (2000). What ought Psychology to do? *American Psychologist, 55,* 328–330.

Janoff-Bulman, R. (1979). Characterological versus behavioral self-blame: Inquiries into depression and rape. *Journal of Personality and Social Psychology, 37,* 1798–1809.

Janoff-Bulman, R. (1992). *Shattered assumptions: Towards a new psychology of trauma.* New York, NY: Free Press.

Jarrett, R. L. (1999). Successful parenting in high-risk neighborhoods. *Future of Children, 9,* 45–50. Retrieved February 11, 2002, from http://www.futureofchildren.org/information2826/information_show.htm?doc_id=71897

Jones, E. E. (1979). The rocky road from acts to disposition. *American Psychologist, 34,* 107–117.

Josephs, R. A., Larrick, R. P., Steele, C. M., & Nisbett, R. E. (1992). Protecting the self from the negative consequences of risky decisions. *Journal of Personality and Social Psychology, 62,* 26–37.

Kadlek, D. (1997, May 5). The new world of giving. *Time, 149,* 62–64.

Karrer, B. M. (1990). The sound of two hands clapping: Cultural interactions of the minority family and the therapist. In G. W. Saba, B. M. Karrer, & K. V. Hardy (Eds.), *Minorities and family therapy* (pp. 209–237). New York, NY: Haworth.

Katz, J. (1985). The sociopolitical nature of counseling. *The Counseling Psychologist, 13,* 615–624.

Kazdin, A. E. (1984). Covert modeling. In P. C. Kendall (Ed.), *Advances in cognitive-behavioral research and therapy* (Vol. 3, pp. 103–129). New York, NY: Academic Press.

Kelly, E. W., Jr. (1995). Counselor values: A national survey. *Journal of Counseling and Development, 73,* 648–653.

Kelly, T. A., & Strupp, H. H. (1992). Patient and therapist values in psychotherapy: Perceived changes, assimilation, similarity, and outcome. *Journal of Consulting and Clinical Psychology, 60,* 34–40.

Keltner, D. (1995). Signs of appeasement: Evidence for the distinct displays of embarrassment, amusement, and shame. *Journal of Personality and Social Psychology, 68,* 441–454.

Kennedy, F. R. (1976). *Color me Flo: My hard life and good times.* Englewood Cliffs, NJ: Prentice-Hall.

Kenrick, D. T., Neuberg, S. L., & Caldini, R. B. (1999). *Social psychology: Unraveling the mystery.* Boston, MA: Allyn & Bacon.

Kerwin, C., Ponterotto, J. G., Jackson, B. L., & Harris, A. (1993). Racial identity in biracial children: A qualitative investigation. *Journal of Counseling Psychology, 40,* 221–231.

Kettl, P. A. (1999, October). *Our violent society: The scope of the problem.* Paper presented at Violence in youth: Home, school and community perspectives, Clarion, PA.

King, M-C., & Wilson, A. C. (1975). Evolution at two levels in humans and chimpanzees. *Science, 188,* 107–116.

Kingsolver, B. (2002). Going to Japan. In B. Kingsolver (Ed.), *Small wonder* (pp. 176–179). New York, NY: HarperCollins.

Kinzie, J. D., Sack, W., Angell, R., Clarke, G., & Ben, R. (1989). A three-year follow-up of Cambodian young people traumatized as children. *Journal of the American Academy of Child and Adolescent Psychiatry, 28,* 501–504.

Kirsch, I., & Lynn, S. J. (1999). Automaticity in clinical psychology. *American Psychologist, 54,* 504–515.

Kluznik, J. C., Speed, N., Van Valkenberg, C., & Magraw, R. (1986). Forty-year follow-up of United States prisoners of war. *American Journal of Psychiatry, 143,* 1443–1446.

Knight, B. G., & McCallum, T. J. (1998). Adapting psychotherapeutic practice for older clients: Implications of the contextual, cohort-based, maturity, specific-challenge model. *Professional Psychology: Research and Practice, 29,* 15–22.

Kohlberg, L. (1966). A cognitive-developmental analysis of children's sex role concepts and attitudes. In E. E. Maccoby (Ed.), *The development of sex differences.* Palo Alto, CA: Stanford University.

Kohlberg, L. (1981). *The philosophy of moral development: Moral stages and the idea of justice.* San Francisco, CA: Harper & Row.

Kohler, W. (1917/1925). *The mentality of apes.* London: Routledge & Kegan Paul.

Koltko-Rivera, M. E. (1999, August). *World views and multicultural counseling: Two teaching activities.* Paper presented at the annual meeting of the American Psychological Association, Boston, MA.

Kopta, S. M., Howard, K. I., Lowry, J. L., & Beutler, L. E. (1994). Patterns of symptomatic recovery in psychotherapy. *Journal of Consulting and Clinical Psychology, 62,* 1009–1016.

Krech, S. (1999). *The ecological Indian: Myth and history.* New York, NY: W. W. Norton.

Kurdek, L. A. (1988). Perceived social support in gays and lesbians in cohabitating relationships. *Journal of Personality and Social Psychology, 54,* 504–509.

Kurosawa, A. (Director), & Minoura, J. (Producer). (1950). *Rashomon* [Motion picture]. Japan: Daiei.

LaFramboise, T. D. (2000, August). Implications of research with Native American adolescents: For current and future practice. In G. Roysicar-Sodowsky & E. Delgado-Romero (Chairs), *Millennium multicultural counseling psychologists.* Symposium at the annual meetings of the American Psychological Association, Washington, D. C.

Lahr, J. (1997, January 27). Speaking across the divide. *The New Yorker, 72,* pp. 35–42.

Laing, R. D. (1967). *The politics of experience.* New York, NY: Pantheon.

Lambert, M. J. (1992). Implications of outcome research for psychotherapy integration. In J. C. Norcross & M. R. Goldfried (Eds.), *Handbook of psychotherapy integration* (pp. 94–129). New York, NY: Basic Books.

Landrine, H., & Klonoff, E. A. (1996). The Schedule of Racist Events: A measure of racial discrimination and a study of its negative physical and mental health consequences. *Journal of Black Psychology, 22,* 144–168.

Latané, B., & Darley, J. M. (1968). Group inhibition of bystander intervention in emergencies. *Journal of Personality and Social Psychology, 10,* 215–221.

Lazarus, A. (1993). Tailoring the therapeutic relationship, or being an authentic chamaeleon. *Psychotherapy, 30,* 404–407.

Lee, E. (1990). Assessment and treatment of Chinese-American immigrant families. In G. W. Saba, B. M. Karrer, & K. V. Hardy (Eds.), *Minorities and family therapy* (pp. 99–122). New York, NY: Haworth.

LeGuin, U. K. (1994). Dancing to Ganam. In U. K. LeGuin (Ed.), *A fisherman of the inland sea* (pp. 115–157). New York, NY: HarperPrism.

Lepore, S. J., Evans, G. W., & Schneider, M. L. (1991). Dynamic role of social support in the link between chronic stress and psychological distress. *Journal of Personality and Social Psychology, 61,* 899–909.

Levenkron, S. (1998). *Cutting: Understanding and overcoming self-mutilation.* New York, NY: Norton.

Levinson, D. (2000). Helping to create a new kind of family. *Newsweek* (May 29), 9.

Liddle, B. J. (1996). Therapist sexual orientation, gender, and counseling practices as they relate to ratings on helpfulness by gay and lesbian clients. *Journal of Counseling Psychology, 43,* 394–401.

Liu, W. M. (2002). The social class-related experiences of men: Integrating theory and practice. *Professional Psychology: Research and Practice, 33,* 355–360.

Locke, D. (1990). A not so provincial view of multicultural counseling. *Counselor Education and Supervision, 30,* 18–25.

Lorde, A. (1984a). Age, race, class, and sex: Women redefining difference. In A. Lorde, *Sister outsider: Essays and speeches* (pp. 114–123). Freedom, CA: Crossing Press.

Lorde, A. (1984b). The transformation of silence into language and action. In A. Lorde, *Sister outsider: Essays and speeches* (pp. 40–44). Freedom, CA: Crossing Press.

Lorde, A. (1984c). The uses of anger: Women responding to racism. In A. Lorde, *Sister outsider: Essays and speeches* (pp. 124–133). Freedom, CA: Crossing Press.

Lussier, Y., Sabourin, S., & Wright, J. (1993). On causality, responsibility, and blame in marriage: Validity of the entailment model. *Journal of Family Psychology, 7,* 322–332.

Madanes, C. (1999, July/August). Rebels with a cause: Honoring the subversive power of psychotherapy. *Family Therapy Networker, 57,* 44–49.

Mah, A. Y. (1997). *Falling leaves: The true story of an unwanted Chinese daughter.* New York, NY: John Wiley & Sons.

Marlatt, A. (1996). Models of relapse and relapse prevention: A commentary. *Experimental and Clinical Psychopharmacology, 4,* 55–60.

Martin, J. K., & Hall, G. C. N. (1992). Thinking Black, thinking internal, thinking feminist. *Journal of Counseling Psychology, 39,* 509–514.

Martz, J. M., Verette, J., Arriaga, X. B., Slovik, L. F., Cox, C. L., & Rusbult, C. E. (1998). Positive illusion in close relationships. *Personal Relationships, 5,* 159–181.

Marvel, K. M., Epstein, R. M., Flowers, K., & Beckman, H. B. (1999). Soliciting the patient's agenda: Have we improved? *JAMA, 281,* 283–287.

Mason, H. R. C., Marks, G., Simoni, J., Ruiz, M. S., & Richardson, J. L. (1995). Culturally sanctioned secrets? Latino men's nondisclosure of HIV infection to family, friends, and lovers. *Health Psychology, 14,* 6–12.

May, R. (1967). *Psychology and the human dilemma.* New York, NY: Van Nostrand Reinhold.

Mayer, E., Kosmin, B. A., & Keysar, A. (2001). *American Religious Identification Survey. Retrieved* on December 8, 2002, from http://www.gc.cuny.edu/studies/key_findings.htm

May, R. (1989). Black and impotent: The life of Mercedes. In D. Wedding & R. J. Corsini (Eds.), *Case studies in psychotherapy* (pp. 165–176). Itasca, IL: Peacock.

McBride, J. (1996). *The color of water: A Black man's tribute to his White mother.* New York, NY: Riverhead.

McClure, F. H. (1999). Comments on "Keeping and crossing professional and racialized boundaries." *Psychology of Women Quarterly, 23,* 305–308.

McConnell, A. R., & Leibold, J. M. (2001). Relations between the Implicit Association Test, explicit racial attitudes, and discriminatory behavior. *Journal of Experimental Social Psychology, 37,* 435–442.

McCullough, M. E., Worthington, E. L., & Rachal, K. C. (1997). Interpersonal forgiving in close relationships. *Journal of Personality and Social Psychology, 73,* 321–336.

McGill, D. W., & Pearce, J. K. (1996). American families with English ancestors from the colonial era: Anglo Americans. In M. McGoldrick, J. Giordano, & J. K. Pearce (Eds.), *Ethnicity and family therapy* (2nd ed., pp. 451–466). New York, NY: Guilford Press.

McGoldrick, M., Gerson, R., & Shellenberger, S. (1999). *Genograms: Assessment and intervention* (2nd ed.). New York, NY: Norton.

McGoldrick, M., Giordano, J., & Pearce, J. K. (1996). *Ethnicity and family therapy* (2nd ed.). New York, NY: Guilford Press.

McGuire, J., Nieri, D., Abbott, D., Sheridan, K., & Fisher, R. (1995). Do Tarasoff principles apply in AIDS-related psychotherapy? Ethical decision making and the role of therapist homophobia and perceived client dangerousness. *Professional Psychology: Research and Practice, 26,* 608–611.

McIntosh, P. (1989). White privilege: Unpacking the invisible knapsack. *Peace and Freedom,* July/August, pp. 10–12.

McLean, R. (1998). *Zen fables for today: Stories inspired by the zen masters.* New York, NY: Avon.

Meichenbaum, D. (2000a). *Core tasks of psychotherapy: What "expert" therapists do.* Invited address presented at the Evolution of Psychotherapy Conference, Anaheim, CA.

Meichenbaum, D. (2000b). *Treatment of Post Traumatic Stress Disorder in Adults.* Workshop presented at the Evolution of Psychotherapy Conference, Anaheim, CA.

Melidonis, G. G., & Bry, B. H. (1995). Effects of therapist exceptions questions on blaming and positive statements in families with adolescent behavior problems. *Journal of Family Psychology, 9,* 451–457.

Michener, A. (1998). *Becoming Anna: The autobiography of a sixteen-year-old.* Chicago, IL: University of Chicago Press.

Mikkelson, B., & Mikkelson, D. P. (2001). Urban legends reference pages. Retrieved March 15, 2002, from http://www.snopes2.com/humor/jokes/landmine.htm

Mikulincer, M. (1998). Attachment working models and the sense of trust: An exploration of interaction goals and affect recognition. *Journal of Personality and Social Psychology, 74,* 1209–1224.

Milloy, C. (1999, May 2). A look at tragedy in black, white. *Washington Post,* p. C01.

Minuchin, S. (1974). *Families and family therapy.* Cambridge, MA: Harvard Univesity Press.

Minuchin, S., & Nichols, M. P. (1993). *Family healing: Strategies for hope and healing.* New York, NY: Free Press.

Moncur, M. (n.d.) *Michael Moncur's (cynical) quotations.* Rerieved on May 19, 2003, from http://www.quotationspage.com

Montalvo, B., & Gutierrez, M. J. (1990). Nine assumptions for work with ethnic minority families. In G. W. Saba, B. M. Karrer, & K. V. Hardy (Eds.), *Minorities and family therapy* (pp. 35–52). New York, NY: Haworth.

Morris, M. W., & Peng, K. (1994). Culture and cause: American and Chinese attributions for social and physical events. *Journal of Personality and Social Psychology, 67,* 949–971.

Moskowitz, J. T., Folkman, S., Collette, L., & Vittinghoff, E. (1996). Coping and AIDS-related caregiving and bereavement. *Annals of Behavioral Medicine, 18,* 49–57.

Motter, T. A., Slattery, J. M., & Bean, T. (1999, April). *Assessment of in-home family therapy outcomes with high-risk families.* Paper presented at the annual meetings of the Eastern Psychological Association, Providence, RI.

Mueller, P., & Major, B. (1989). Self-blame, self-efficacy, and adjustment to abortion. *Journal of Personality and Social Psychology, 57,* 1059–1068.

Mueser, K. T., Goodman, L. B., Trumbetta, S. L., Rosenberg, S. D., Osher, F. C., Vidaver, R., Auciello, P., & Foy, D. W. (1998). Trauma and posttraumatic stress disorder in severe mental illness. *Journal of Consulting and Clinical Psychology, 66,* 493–499.

Nash, M. R., Hulsey, T. C., Sexton, M. C., Harralson, T. L., & Lambert, W. (1993). Long-term sequelae of childhood sexual abuse: Perceived family environment, psychopathology, and dissociation. *Journal of Consulting and Clinical Psychology, 61,* 276–283.

Nash, M. R., Neimeyer, R. A., Hulsey, T. L., & Lambert, W. (1998). Psychopathology associated with sexual abuse: The importance of complementary designs and common ground. *Journal of Consulting and Clinical Psychology, 66,* 568–571.

National Association of Social Workers. (1999). *National Association of Social Workers code of ethics.* Retrieved January 13, 2002, from http://www.socialworkers.org/pubs/code/code.htm

Nickerson, K. J., Helms, J. E., & Terrell, F. (1994). Cultural mistrust, opinions about mental illness, and Black students' attitudes toward seeking psychological help from White counselors. *Journal of Counseling Psychology, 41,* 378–385.

Noel, J. G., Wann, D. L., & Branscombe, N. R. (1995). Peripheral ingroup membership status and public negativity toward outgroups. *Journal of Personality and Social Psychology, 68,* 127–137.

Nolen-Hoeksema, S., & Davis, C. G. (1999). "Thanks for sharing that": Ruminators and their social support networks. *Journal of Personality and Social Psychology, 77,* 801–814.

Nolen-Hoeksema, S., Girgus, J. S., & Seligman, M. E. P. (1992). Predictors and consequences of childhood depressive symptoms: A 5-year longitudinal study. *Journal of Abnormal Psychology, 101,* 405–422.

Nolen-Hoeksema, S., & Morrow, J. (1991). A prospective study of depression and post-traumatic stress symptoms after a natural disaster: The 1989 Loma Prieta Earthquake. *Journal of Personality and Social Psychology, 61,* 519–527.

Norcross, J. (2000). *Empirically supported therapy relationships—Task force of APA's Psychotherapy Division.* Symposium presented at the annual meeting of the American Psychological Association, Washington, D.C.

Ogbu, J. U. (1986). The consequences of the American caste system. In U. Neisser (Ed.), *The school acheivement of minority children* (pp. 19–56). Hillsdale, NJ: Lawrence Erlbaum.

O'Hanlon, B. (1999). *Do one thing different and other uncommonly sensible solutions to life's persistent problems.* New York, NY: William Morrow.

O'Hanlon, W. H., & Weiner-Davis, M. (1989). *In search of solutions: A new direction in psychotherapy.* New York, NY: Norton.

Ohio Public Images. (nd). *Public Images Network: Think "People first."* Retrieved January 7, 2002, from http://www.publicimagesnetwork.org/first.html

Omoto, A. M., & Snyder, M. (1995). Sustained helping without obligation: Motivation, longevity of service, and perceived attitude change among AIDS volunteers. *Journal of Personality and Social Psychology, 68,* 671–686.

Osborne, J. W. (1997). Race and academic disidentification. *Journal of Educational Psychology, 89,* 728–735.

Ottavi, T. M., Pope-Davis, D. B., & Dings, J. G. (1994). Relationship between white racial identity attitudes and self-reported multicultural counseling competencies. *Journal of Counseling Psychology, 41,* 149–154.

Oyserman, D., Coon, H. M., & Kemmelmeier, M. (2002). Rethinking individualism and collectivism: Evaluation of theoretical assumptions and meta-analyses. *Psychological Bulletin, 128,* 3–72.

Oz, S. (1995). A modified balance-sheet procedure for decision making in therapy: Cost-cost comparisons. *Professional Psychology: Research and Practice, 26,* 78–81.

Painter, N. I. (1996). *Sojourner Truth: A life, a symbol.* New York, NY: W.W. Norton.

Painter, N. (1999, April 21). *Sojourner Truth visits Abraham Lincoln.* Lecture given at Clarion University. Clarion, PA.

Palmer, S. E., Brown, R. A., Rae-Grant, N. I., & Loughlin, M. J. (1999). Responding to children's disclosure of familial abuse: What survivors tell us. *Child Welfare, 78,* 259–282.

Paniagua, F. A. (1998). *Assessing and treating culturally diverse clients: A practical guide* (2nd ed.). Thousand Oaks, CA: Sage.

Parham, T. A., & Helms, J. E. (1985). The relationship of racial identity attitudes to self-actualization and affective states of Black students. *Journal of Counseling Psychology, 32,* 431–440.

Park, C. L. (1998). Implications of posttraumatic growth for individuals. In R. G. Tedeschi, C. L. Park & L. G. Calhoun (Eds.), *Posttraumatic growth: Positive changes in the aftermath of crisis* (pp. 153–177). Mahwah, NJ: Lawrence Erlbaum.

Park, C. L. (1999, August). *Religion and the making of meaning in stressful times.* Paper presented at the annual meeting of the American Psychological Association, Boston, MA.

Park, C. L., & Folkman, S. (1997). Meaning in the context of stress and coping. *Review of General Psychology, 1,* 115–144.

Parrott, L. (1997). *Counseling and psychotherapy.* New York, NY: McGraw-Hill.

Pedro-Carroll, J. (2001). The promotion of wellness in children and families: Challenges and opportunities. *American Psychologist, 56,* 993–1004.

Peng, K., & Nisbett, R. E. (1999). Culture, dialectics, and reasoning about contradiction. *American Psychologist, 54,* 741–754.

Pennebaker, J. W., & Beall, S. (1986). Confronting a traumatic event: Toward an understanding of inhibition and disease. *Journal of Abnormal Psychology, 95,* 274–281.

Pennebaker, J. W., Colder, M., & Sharp, L. K. (1990). Accelerating the coping process. *Journal of Personality and Social Psychology, 58,* 528–537.

Pennebaker, J. W., Hughes, C., & O'Heeron, R. C. (1987). The psychophysiology of confession: Linking inhibitory and psychosomatic processes. *Journal of Personality and Social Psychology, 52,* 781–793.

Pennebaker, J. W., Kiecolt-Glaser, J. K., & Glaser, R. (1988). Disclosure of traumas and immune function: Health implications for psychotherapy. *Journal of Consulting and Clinical Psychology, 56,* 239–245.

Perlow, R., & Latham, L. L. (1993). Relationship of client abuse with locus of control and gender: A longitudinal study in mental retardation facilities. *Journal of Applied Psychology, 78,* 831–834.

Perozynski, L. M., & Kramer, L. (1999). Parental beliefs about managing sibling conflict. *Developmental Psychology, 35,* 489–499.

Petrie, K. J., Booth, R. J., Pennebaker, J. W., Davison, K. P., & Thomas, M. G. (1995). Disclosure of trauma and immune response to a Hepatitis B vaccination program. *Journal of Consulting and Clinical Psychology, 63,* 787–792.

Peyser, M. (1998). Battling backlash. *Newsweek,* August 17, 50–52.

Pfendler, B. A., Slattery, J. M., Hollis, M. L., & Bean, T. (1996, August). *In-home family therapy: Apparent gender differences in outcome.* Paper presented at the annual meetings of the American Psychological Association, Toronto.

Piaget, J. (1960). *The child's conception of the world.* Totowa, NJ: Littlefield.

Pickett, T. (2002). Unexplored oppression: A theory of classism. In W. M. Liu (Chair), *Perpetuating oppression and prejudice: Classism theory, White trashism, and ableism.* Symposium presented at the annual meeting of the American Psychological Association, Chicago, IL.

Pinel, E. C. (1999). Stigma consciousness: The psychological legacy of social stereotypes. *Journal of Personality and Social Psychology, 76,* 114–128.

Poindexter-Cameron, J. M., & Robinson, T. L. (1997). Relationships among racial identity attitudes, womanist identity attitudes, and self-esteem in African American college women. *Journal of College Student Development, 38,* 288–296.

Pollack, W. S., & Levant, R. F. (Eds.). (1998). *New psychotherapy for men.* New York, NY: John Wiley & Sons.

Polster, E. (2000). Shaping and re-shaping the self. Workshop presented at the Evolution of Psychotherapy Conference, Anaheim, CA.

Ponterotto, J. G. (1987). Counseling Mexican Americans: A multimodal approach. *Journal of Counseling & Development, 65,* 308–312.

Pope, M. (1995). The "salad bowl" is big enough for us all: An argument for the inclusion of lesbians and gay men in any definition of multiculturalism. *Journal of Counseling and Development, 73,* 301–304.

Powell, D. S., Batsche, C. J., Ferro, J., Fox, L., & Dunlap, G. (1997). A strength-based approach in support of multi-risk families: Principles and issues. *Topics in Early Childhood Special Education, 17,* 1–26.

Prochaska, J. O. (1999). How do people change, and how can we change to help more people? In M. A. Hubble, B. L. Duncan, & S. D. Miller (Eds.), *The heart and soul of change: What works in therapy* (pp. 227–255). Washington, D. C.: American Psychological Association.

Prochaska, J. O., & DiClemente, C. C. (1982). Transtheoretical therapy: Toward a more integrative model of change. *Psychotherapy: Theory, Research and Practice, 19,* 276–288.

Propst, L. R., Ostrom, R., Watkins, P., Dean, T., & Mashburn, D. (1992). Comparative efficacy of religious and nonreligious cognitive-behavior therapy for the treatment of clinical depression in religious individuals. *Journal of Consulting and Clinical Psychology, 60,* 94–103.

Pryor, J. B., LaVite, C., & Stoller, L. (1993). A social psychological analysis of sexual harassment: The person/situation interaction. *Journal of Vocational Behavior, 42,* 68–83.

Pyant, C. T., & Yanico, B. J. (1991). Relationship of racial identity and gender-role attitudes to Black women's psychological well-being. *Journal of Counseling Psychology, 38,* 315–322.

Quindlen, A. (2000). The problem of the color line. *Newsweek,* March 13, 76.

Rabasca, L. (2000, January). No goal out of reach. *Monitor on Psychology, 31,* 20–22.

Raine, N. V. (1998). *After silence: Rape and my journey back.* New York, NY: Crown.

Ramírez, E., Maldonado, A., & Martos, R. (1992). Attributions modulate immunization against learned helplessness in humans. *Journal of Personality and Social Psychology, 62,* 139–146.

Razack, S. H. (1998). *Looking white people in the eye: Gender, race, and culture in courtrooms and classrooms.* Toronto: University of Toronto.

Reed, G. M., Taylor, S. E., & Kemeny, M. E. (1993). Perceived control and psychological adjustment in gay men with AIDS. *Journal of Applied Social Psychology, 23,* 791–824.

Reiter, E. (1999, July). Sacagawea, we hardly knew you. *COINage,* p. 6.

Renjilian, D. A., Perri, M. G., Nezu, A. M., McKelvey, W. F., Shermer, R. L., & Anton, S. D. (2001). Individual versus group therapy for obesity: Effects of matching participants to their treatment preferences. *Journal of Consulting and Clinical Psychology, 69,* 717–721.

Richie, B. S., Fassinger, R. E., Linn, S. G., Johnson, J., Prosser, J., & Robinson, S. (1997). Persistence, connection, and passion: A qualitative study of the career development of highly achieving African American-Black and White women. *Journal of Counseling Psychology, 44,* 133–148.

Richter, C. (1957). On the phenomenon of sudden death in animals and men. *Psychosomatic Medicine, 19,* 191–198.

Ridley, C. R. (1984). Clinical treatment of the nondisclosing client: A therapeutic paradox. *American Psychologist, 39,* 1234–1244.

Ridley, C. R., Mendoza, D. W., Kanitz, B. E., Angermeier, L., & Zenk, R. (1994). Cultural sensitivity in multicultural counseling: A perceptual schema model. *Journal of Counseling Psychology, 41*, 125–136.

Rind, B., Tromovitch, P., & Bauserman, R. (1998). A meta-analytic examination of assumed properties of child sexual abuse using college samples. *Psychological Bulletin, 124*, 22–53.

Roberts, C. (1998). First-class mechanic. In C. Roberts (Ed.), *We are our mothers' daughters* (pp. 77–86). New York, NY: William Morrow and Company.

Robinson, N. S. (1995). Evaluating the nature of perceived support and its relation to perceived self-worth in adolescents. *Journal of Research in Adolescence, 5*, 253–280.

Robinson, T., & Ward, J. V. (1991). "A belief is far greater than anyone's disbelief": Cultivating resistance among African American female adolescents. In C. Gilligan, A. G. Rogers, & D. L. Tolman (Eds.), *Women, girls, & psychotherapy: Reframing resistance* (pp. 87–103). New York, NY: Harrington Park Press.

Roche, T. (2002). The Yates odyssey. *Time*, January 28, 42–50.

Rockland, L. H. (1992). *Supportive therapy for borderline patients: A psychodynamic approach.* New York, NY: Guilford.

Rodin, J. (1986). Aging and health: Effects of the sense of control. *Science, 233*, 1271–1276.

Rodriguez, N., Ryan, S. W., Vande Kemp, H., & Foy, D. W. (1997). Posttraumatic stress disorder in adult female survivors of child sexual abuse: A comparison study. *Journal of Consulting and Clinical Psychology, 65*, 53–59.

Rogers, C. R. (1957). The necessary and sufficient conditions of therapeutic personality change. *Journal of Consulting Psychology, 21*, 95–103.

Rogers, C. R. (1983). *Freedom to learn for the '80s.* Columbus, OH: Merrill.

Rosenbaum, M. E. (1986). The repulsion hypothesis: On the nondevelopment of relationships. *Journal of Personality and Social Psychology, 61*, 1156–1166.

Rosenhan, D. L. (1973). On being sane in insane places. *Science, 179*, 250–258.

Rothbaum, B., Foa, E., Riggs, D., Murdock, T., & Walsh, W. (1992). A prospective examination of post-traumatic stress disorder in rape victims. *Journal of Traumatic Stress, 5*, 455–475.

Rotheram-Borus, M. J. (1990). Adolescents' reference-group choices, self-esteem, and adjustment. *Journal of Personality and Social Psychology, 59*, 1075–1081.

Rowley, S. J., Sellers, R. M., Chavous, T. M., & Smith, M. A. (1998). The relationship between racial identity and self-esteem in African American college and high school students. *Journal of Personality and Social Psychology, 74*, 715–724.

Ruggiero, K. M., & Taylor, D. M. (1995). Coping with discrimination: How disadvantaged group members perceive the discrimination that confronts them. *Journal of Personality and Social Psychology, 68*, 826–838.

Saba, G. W., & Rodgers, D. V. (1990). Discrimination in urban family practice: Lessons from minority poor families. In G. W. Saba, B. M. Karrer, & K. V. Hardy (Eds.), *Minorities and family therapy* (pp. 177–207). New York, NY: Haworth.

Safran, J. D., & Wallner, L. K. (1991). The relative predictive validity of two therapeutic alliance measures in cognitive therapy. *Psychological Assessment, 3*, 188–195.

Sandler, K. (1993). *A question of color* [Film]. (Available from California Newsreel, 149 Ninth St., San Francisco, CA 94103)

Sartre, J. P. (1946/1965). *Anti-Semite and Jew.* New York, NY: Schocken Books.

Schiller, L., & Bennett, A. (1994). *The quiet room: A journey out of the torment of madness.* New York, NY: Warner Books.

Schlenker, B. R., Britt, T. W., Pennington, J., Murphy, R., & Doherty, K. (1994). The triangle model of responsibility. *Psychological Review, 101,* 632–652.

Schlink, B. (1998). *The reader.* (C. B. Janeway, trans.). New York, NY: Vintage. (Original work published 1995).

Schwarz, N. (1999). Self-reports: How the questions shape the answers. *American Psychologist, 54,* 93–105.

Sedikides, C., & Campbell, W. K. (1998). The self-serving bias in relational context. *Journal of Personality and Social Psychology, 74,* 378–386.

Seligman, M. E. P. (1968). Chronic fear produced by unpredictable shock. *Journal of Comparative and Physiological Psychology, 66,* 402–411.

Seligman, M. E. P. (1975). *Helplessness: On depression, development and death.* San Francisco, CA: Freeman.

Seligman, M. E. P., Walker, E. F., & Rosenhan, D. L. (2001). *Abnormal psychology* (4th ed.). New York, NY: Norton.

Shapiro, J. P. (1989). Self-blame versus helplessness in sexually abused children: An attributional analysis with treatment recommendations. *Journal of Social and Clinical Psychology, 8,* 442–455.

Shapiro, J. P. (1995). Attribution-based treatment of self-blame and helplessness in sexually abused children. *Psychotherapy, 32,* 581–591.

Shaw, F. (1998). *Composing myself: A journey through postpartum depression.* South Royalton, VT: Steerforth.

Shaw, L. L., Batson, C. D., & Todd, R. M. (1994). Empathy avoidance: Forestalling feeling for another in order to escape the motivational consequences. *Journal of Personality and Social Psychology, 67,* 879–887.

Sherif, M., Harvey, O. J., White, B. J., Hood, W. R., & Sherif, C. W. (1961/1988) *The Robbers Cave experiment: Intergroup conflict and cooperation.* Middletown, CT: Wesleyan University Press.

Shimrat, I. (1997). *Call me crazy: Stories from the mad movement.* Vancouver: Press Gang.

Shostak, M. (1981). *Nisa: The life and words of a !Kung woman.* New York, NY: Vintage Books.

Siegel, J. M., Yancey, A. K., & McCarthy, W. J. (2000). Overweight and depressive symptoms among African-American women. *Preventive Medicine: An International Journal Devoted to Practice and Theory. 31,* 232–240.

Silver, E., Cirincione, C., & Steadman, H. J. (1994). Demythologizing inaccurate perceptions of the insanity defense. *Law and Human Behavior, 18,* 63–70.

Simoneau, T. L., Miklowitz, D. J., & Saleem, R. (1998). Expressed emotion and interactional patterns in the families of bipolar patients. *Journal of Abnormal Psychology, 107,* 497–507.

Simoni, J. M., Mason, H. R. C., Marks, G., Ruiz, M. S., Reed, D., & Richardson, J. L. (1995). Women's self-disclosure of HIV infection: Rates, reasons, and reactions. *Journal of Consulting and Clinical Psychology, 63,* 474–478.

Simpson, J. B. (1988). *Simpson's contemporary quotations.* Boston, MA: Houghton Mifflin.

Skinner, B. F. (1948). 'Superstition' in the pigeon. *Journal of Experimental Psychology, 38,* 168–172.

Slattery, J. M. (2000a). Boundaries in therapy: A confused definition of care. *Pennsylvania Psychologist Update,* October 1, 3.

Slattery, J. M. (2000b, November 9). Changing the sign and keeping the sermon was cowardice. *Clarion News,* 5.

Slattery, J. M., Ferringer, S., & Grigsby, J. (1997, September). *Bridging the gap: Acknowledging and empowering our GLB population.* Presented at "Invisible and excluded? Issues impacting the gay, lesbian and bisexual community," Clarion, PA.

Slattery, J. M., & Knapp, S. (2003). In-home family therapy and wraparound services for working with seriously at-risk children and adolescents. In L. VandeCreek & T.L. Jackson (Eds.), *Innovations in clinical practice: focus on children and adolescents* (pp. 135–149). Sarasota, FL: Professional Resource Press.

Smaby, B., Slattery, J. M., Creany, A., & Motter, T. (2000). *Gender balance in the workplace at Clarion University.* Clarion, PA: Clarion University, Presidential Commission on the Status of Women.

Sodowsky, G. R., Taffe, R. C., Gutkin, T. B., & Wise, S. L. (1994). Development of the Multicultural Counseling Inventory: A self-report measure of multicultural competencies. *Journal of Counseling Psychology, 41,* 137–148.

Solzhenitsyn, A. I. (1963). *One day in the life of Ivan Denisovich* (M. Hayward and R. Hingley, trans.). New York, NY: Praeger. (Original work published 1962).

Stangor, C., Carr, C., & Kiang, L. (1998). Activating stereotypes undermines task performance expectations. *Journal of Personality and Social Psychology, 75,* 1191–1197.

Steele, C. M. (1997). A threat in the air: How stereotypes shape intellectual identity and performance. *American Psychologist, 52,* 613–629.

Steele, C. M. (1998). Stereotyping and its threat are real. *American Psychologist, 53,* 680–681.

Steele, C. M., & Aronson, J. (1995). Stereotype threat and the intellectual test performance of African Americans. *Journal of Personality and Social Psychology, 69,* 797–811.

Steele, C. M., Spencer, S. J., & Lynch, M. (1993). Self-image resilience and dissonance: The role of affirmational resources. *Journal of Personality and Social Psychology, 64,* 885–896.

Steingarten, J. (1997). *The man who ate everything.* New York, NY: Vintage.

Steinpreis, R. E., Ritzke, D., & Anders, K. A. (1999). The impact of gender on the review of the curricula vitae of job applicants and tenure candidates: A national empirical study. *Sex Roles, 41,* 509–528.

Stevenson, H. C., & Renard, G. (1993). Trusting ole wise owls: Therapeutic use of cultural strengths in African-American families. *Professional Psychology: Research and Practice, 24,* 433–442.

Stevenson, R. (Director), & Walsh, B. (Producer). (1964). *Mary Poppins* [Motion picture]. United States: Walt Disney Company.

Stice, E., Presnell, K., & Spangler, D. (2002). Risk factors for binge eating onset in adolescent girls: A 2-year prospective investigation. *Health Psychology, 21,* 131–138.

Stoddard, S., Jans, L., Ripple, J., & Kraus, L. (1998). *Chartbook on Work and Disability in the United States, 1998.* Washington, D.C.: U.S. National Institute on Disability and Rehabilitation Research. Retrieved on December 8, 2002, from http://www.infouse.com/disabilitydata/workdisability_1_1.html

Sue, D., Sue, D. W., & Sue, S. (2000). *Understanding abnormal behavior* (6th ed.). Boston, MA: Houghton Mifflin.

Sue, D. W. (2000, August). Discussant. In W. B. Walsh (Chair), *Fostering human strength: A counseling psychology perspective.* Symposium at the annual meeting of the American Psychological Association, Washington, D. C.

Sue, D. W., Bingham, R. P., Porché-Burke, L., & Vasquez, M. (1999). The diversification of Psychology: A multicultural revolution. *American Psychologist, 54,* 1061–1069.

Sue, D. W., & Sue, D. (1999). *Counseling the culturally different: Theory and practice* (3rd ed.) New York, NY: John Wiley & Sons.

Sue, S. (1999). Science, ethnicity, and bias: Where have we gone wrong? *American Psychologist, 54,* 1070–1077.

Sue, S., Zane, N., & Young, K. (1994). Research on psychotherapy with culturally diverse populations. In A. E. Bergin & S. L. Garfield. *Handbook of psychotherapy and behavior change* (4th ed.), (pp. 783–817). New York, NY: John Wiley & Sons.

Szasz, T. S. (1963). *Law, liberty and psychiatry: An inquiry into the social uses of mental health practices.* New York, NY: Macmillan.

Tafoya, T. (1990). Circles and cedar: Native Americans and family therapy. In G. W. Saba, B. M. Karrer, & K. V. Hardy (Eds.), *Minorities and family therapy* (pp. 71–98). New York, NY: Haworth.

Tallman, K., & Bohart, A. C. (1999). The client as a common factor: Clients as self-healers. In M. A. Hubble, B. L. Duncan, & S. D. Miller (Eds.), *The heart and soul of change: What works in therapy* (pp. 91–131). Washington, D. C.: American Psychological Association.

Tatum, B. (2000, August). Black women in college: Identity in context. In R. L. Hall (Chair), *Identity and Black women.* Symposium at the annual meeting of the American Psychological Association, Washington, D. C.

Tavris, C. (1989). *Anger: The misunderstood emotion* (rev. ed.). New York, NY: Touchstone.

Tennant, C. C., Goulston, K. J., & Dent, O.F. (1986). The psychological effects of being a prisoner of war: Forty years after release. *American Journal of Psychiatry, 143,* 618–621.

Tennen, H., & Affleck, G. (1990). Blaming others for threatening events. *Psychological Bulletin, 108,* 209–232.

Terrell, F., & Terrell, S. L. (1981). An inventory to measure cultural mistrust among blacks. *Western Journal of Black Studies, 5,* 180–184.

Terrell, F., & Terrell, S. L. (1984). Race of counselor, client sex, cultural mistrust level, and premature termination from counseling among black clients. *Journal of Counseling Psychology, 31,* 371–375.

Thompson, C. E., & Jenal, S. T. (1994). Interracial and intraracial quasi-counseling interactions when counselors avoid discussing race. *Journal of Counseling Psychology, 41,* 484–491.

Thompson, C. E., Worthington, R., & Atkinson, D. R. (1994). Counselor content orientation, counselor race, and black women's cultural mistrust and self-disclosures. *Journal of Counseling Psychology, 41,* 155–161.

Thompson, C. P., Anderson, L. P., & Bakeman, R. A. (2000). Effects of racial socialization and racial identity on acculturative stress in African American college students. *Cultural Diversity and Ethnic Minority Psychology, 6,* 196–210.

Thompson, S. C., & Spacapan, S. (1991). Perceptions of control in vulnerable populations. *Journal of Social Issues, 47,* 1–21.

Thompson, T. (1999). An illness no one understands: Tourette's syndrome. *Washington Post,* January 19, p. Z12.

Tkachuk, G. A., & Martin, G. L. (1999). Exercise therapy for patients with psychiatric disorders: Research and clinical implications. *Professional Psychology: Research and Practice, 30,* 275–282.

Tolman, D. L. (1991). Adolescent girls, women and sexuality: Discerning dilemmas of desire. In C. Gilligan, A. G. Rogers, & D. L. Tolman (Eds.), *Women, girls, & psychotherapy: Reframing resistance* (pp. 55–69). New York, NY: Harrington Park Press.

Trierweiler, S. J., Neighbors, H. W., Munday, C., Thompson, E. E., Binion, V. J., & Gomez, J. P. (2000). Clinician attributions associated with the diagnosis of schizophrenia in African American and non-African American patients. *Journal of Consulting and Clinical Psychology, 68,* 171–175.

Tsai, J. L., Ying, Y-W., & Lee, P. A. (2001). Cultural predictors of self-esteem: A study of Chinese American female and male young adults. *Cultural Diversity and Ethnic Minority Psychology, 7,* 284–297.

Twenge, J. M., & Crocker, J. (2002). Race and self-esteem: Meta-analyses comparing Whites, Blacks, Hispanics, Asians, and American Indians and comment on Gray-Little and Hafdahl (2000). *Psychological Bulletin, 128,* 371–408.

Tull, E. S., Wickramasuriya, T., Taylor, J., Smith-Burns, V., Margot, B., Champagnie, G., Daye, K., Donaldson, K., Solomon, N., Walker, S., Fraser, H., & Jordan, O. (1999). Relationship of internalized racism to abdominal obesity and blood pressure in Black women: Implications for the Insulin Resistance Syndrome in African Americans. *Diabetes, 48,* SA323.

United States Congress. (1990). *Americans with Disabilities Act of 1990.* Retrieved June 12, 2002, from http://www.usdoj.gov/crt/ada/statute.html

Van den Bos, K., Wilke, H. A. M., & Lind, E. A. (1998). When do we need procedural fairness? The role of trust in authority. *Journal of Personality and Social Psychology, 75,* 1449–1458.

Vontress, C. E., Johnson, J. A., & Epp, L. R. (1999). *Cross-cultural counseling: A casebook.* Alexandria, VA: American Counseling Association.

Wachtel, P. L. (2002). Psychoanalysis and the disenfranchised: From therapy to justice. *Psychoanalytic Psychology, 19,* 199–215.

Walter, J. L., & Peller, J. E. (1992). *Becoming solution-focused in brief therapy.* New York, NY: Brunner/Mazel.

Walters, K. L., & Simoni, J. M. (1993). Lesbian and gay male group identity attitudes and self-esteem: Implications for counseling. *Journal of Counseling Psychology, 40,* 94–99.

Wang, Y.W. (1999, August). Asian cultural values and indigenous coping styles. In C. J. Yeh (Chair), *Indigenous coping styles across cultures: Implications for counseling and training.* Paper presented presented at the annual meeting of the American Psychological Association, Boston, MA.

Waters, D. B., & Lawrence, E. C. (1993). *Competence, courage, and change: An approach to family therapy.* New York, NY: Norton.

Watkins, C. E., & Terrell, F. (1988). Mistrust level and its effects on counseling expectations in Black client-White counselor relationships: An analogue study. *Journal of Counseling Psychology, 35,* 194–197.

Watkins, C. E., Terrell, F., Miller, F. S., & Terrell, S. L. (1989). Cultural mistrust and its effects on expectational variables in Black client-White counselor relationships. *Journal of Counseling Psychology, 36,* 447–450.

Watson, D. L., & Tharp, R. G. (1997). *Self-directed behavior: Self-modification for personal growth* (7th ed.). Pacific Grove, CA: Brooks/Cole.

Watts, R. J., Abdul-Adil, J. K., & Pratt, T. (2002). Enhancing critical consciousness in young African American men: A psychoeducational approach. *Psychology of Men and Masculinity, 3,* 41–50.

Watzlawick, P., Weakland, J. H., & Fisch, R. (1974). *Change: Principles of problem formation and problem resolution.* New York, NY: Norton.

Wegner, D. M. (1994). Ironic processes of mental control. *Psychological Review, 101,* 34–52.

Weine, S., Kulenovic, A. D., Pavkovic, I., & Gibbons, R. (1998). Testimony psychotherapy in Bosnian refugees: A pilot study. *American Journal of Psychiatry, 155,* 1720–1726.

Weine, S. M., Vojvoda, D., Becker, D. F., McGlashan, T. H., Hodzic, E., Laub, D., Hyman, L., Sawyer, M., & Lazrove. S. (1998). PTSD symptoms in Bosnian refugees one year after resettlement in the United States. *American Journal of Psychiatry, 155,* 562–564.

Weisberg, M. B., & Clavel, A. L. (1999). Why is chronic pain so difficult to treat? Psychological conditions from simple to complex care. *Postgraduate Medicine, 106.* Retrieved February 11, 2002, from http://www.postgradmed.com/issues/1999/11_99/weisberg.htm

Wentzel, K. R. (1997). Student motivation in middle school: The role of perceived pedagogical caring. *Journal of Educational Psychology, 89,* 411–419.

Whaley, A.L. (1998). Issues of validity in empirical tests of stereotype threat theory. *American Psychologist, 53,* 679–680.

Whitaker, C., & Bumberry, W. (1987). Dancing with the family: A symbolic experiential approach. New York, NY: Brunner/Mazel.

Widom, C. S. (1999). Posttraumatic stress disorder in abused and neglected children grown up. *American Journal of Psychiatry, 156,* 1223–1229.

Wiesel, E. (1982). *One generation after.* New York, NY: Schocken Books.

Williams, G. C., Rodin, G. C., Ryan, R. M., Grolnick, W. S., & Deci, E. L. (1998). Autonomous regulation and long-term medication adherence in adult outpatients. *Health Psychology, 17,* 269–276.

Williams, G. H. (1995). *Life on the color line.* New York, NY: Plume.

Wood, P. S., & Mallinckrodt, B. (1990). Culturally sensitive assertiveness training for ethnic minority clients. *Professional Psychology: Research and Practice, 21,* 5–11.

Worthington, E. L. (1988). Understanding the values of religious clients: A model and its application to counseling. *Journal of Counseling Psychology, 35,* 166–174.

Worthington, E. L., Kurusu, T. A., McCollough, M. E., & Sandage, S. J. (1996). Empirical research on religion and psychotherapeutic processes and outcomes: A 10-year review and research prospectus. *Psychological Bulletin, 119,* 448–487.

Wright, G., & Millar, S. (1999, April 22). A clique within a clique, obsessed with guns, death and Hitler. *The Guardian.* Retrieved February 11, 2002, from http://www.guardian.co.uk/Archive/Article/0,4273,3856954,00.html

Wright, J. W. (Ed.). (1998). *1999 The New York Times Almanac.* New York, NY: Penguin Reference.

Wright, M. A. (1998). *I'm chocolate, you're vanilla: Raising healthy black and biracial children in a race-conscious world.* San Francisco, CA: Jossey-Bass.

Yalom, I. D. (1989). "The wrong one died." In I. D. Yalom. *Love's executioner and other tales of psychotherapy.* New York, NY: Harper Perennial.

Yau, T. Y., Sue, D., & Hayden, D. (1992). Counseling style preference of international students. *Journal of Counseling Psychology, 39,* 100–104.

Yi, K. (1995). Psychoanalytic psychotherapy with Asian clients: Transference and therapeutic considerations. *Psychotherapy, 32,* 308–316.

Yi, K. Y. (1998). Transference and race: An intersubjective conceptualization. *Psychoanalytic Psychology, 15,* 245–261.

Zaharlick, A. (2000). Southeast Asian-American women. In M. Julia (Ed.), *Constructing gender: Multicultural perspectives in working with women* (pp. 177–204). Belmont, CA: Brooks/Cole.

Zane, N. W., Sue, S., Hu, L-T., & Kwon, J-H. (1991). Asian-American assertion: A social learning analysis of cultural differences. *Journal of Counseling Psychology, 38,* 63–70.

Zayas, L. H., & Solari, F. (1994). Early childhood socialization in Hispanic families: Context, culture, and practice implications. *Professional Psychology: Research and Practice, 25,* 200–206.

Zemore, R., & Shepel, L. F. (1989). Effects of breast cancer and mastectomy on emotional support and adjustment. *Social Science and Medicine, 28,* 19–27.

Zhang, W. (1994). American counseling in the mind of a Chinese counselor. *Journal of Multicultural Counseling and Development, 22,* 79–85.

Zhang, W. (1999). Did you really hear what I said? In A. E. Ivey & M. B. Ivey. *Intentional interviewing and counseling: Facilitating client development in a multicultural society* (4th ed., pp. 118–119). Pacific Grove, CA: Brooks/Cole.

Zhang, W. (2003a). Can I trust what I see? In A. E. Ivey & M. B. Ivey. *Intentional interviewing and counseling: Facilitating client development in a multicultural society* (5th ed., pp. 112–113). Pacific Grove, CA: Brooks/Cole.

Zhang, W. (2003b). Can we be "nonjudgmental" about crime? In A. E. Ivey & M. B. Ivey. *Intentional interviewing and counseling: Facilitating client development in a multicultural society* (5th ed., pp. 190–191). Pacific Grove, CA: Brooks/Cole.

Zhang, W. (2003c). Confrontation in the real world. In A. E. Ivey & M. B. Ivey. *Intentional interviewing and counseling: Facilitating client development in a multicultural society* (5th ed., pp. 230–231). Pacific Grove, CA: Brooks/Cole.

Zhang, W. (2003d). Does he have any feelings? In A. E. Ivey & M. B. Ivey. *Intentional interviewing and counseling: Facilitating client development in a multicultural society* (5th ed., pp. 150–151). Pacific Grove, CA: Brooks/Cole.

Zhang, W. (2003e). Use with care: Culturally incorrect attending can be rude. In A. E. Ivey & M. B. Ivey. *Intentional interviewing and counseling: Facilitating client development in a multicultural society* (5th ed., p. 47). Pacific Grove, CA: Brooks/Cole.

Zhang, W. (2003f). What do you mean by "family"? In A. E. Ivey & M. B. Ivey. *Intentional interviewing and counseling: Facilitating client development in a multicultural society* (5th ed., pp. 84–85). Pacific Grove, CA: Brooks/Cole.

Zhang, W. (2003g). When is self-disclosure appropriate? In A. E. Ivey & M. B. Ivey. *Intentional interviewing and counseling: Facilitating client development in a multicultural society* (5th ed., pp. 320–321). Pacific Grove, CA: Brooks/Cole.

Zimmerman, S. L. (1991). Comment: Transgenerational patterns of suicide attempt. *Journal of Consulting and Clinical Psychology, 59,* 867–868.

Zuckerman, M. (1979). Attribution of success and failure revisited, or: The motivational bias is alive and well in attribution theory. *Journal of Personality, 47,* 245–287.

Author Index

Subject Index

Ability, group membership based on, 34, 35, 60–61

Abuse history. *See* Assault and abuse history

Acceptance of client's perspective, 141, 142t, 143–144, 159
  disclosure of information in, 200–201
  meaning making in, 253–254

Accessibility of services, cultural, 366

Accountability for behavior, 57–58
  justice and forgiveness in, 328, 329t
  responsibility and blame in, 282
    in invisible handicaps, 269–272
    in Tourette's syndrome, 268–269
  in strength-based approach, 282–283
  in unquestioning acceptance of client's perspective, 144

Action-oriented therapy, 47t, 96–97, 174
  empowering interventions in, 192, 226, 228–229

Aesthetic values, 47t, 209

Affectional orientation. *See* Sexual and affectional orientation

Affluence, guilt related to, 160–161, 164–165

African Americans
  attributions on behavior, 207
  developmental and cultural norms of, 49, 341–342
  expectations and goals for therapy, 96–97
  guilt related to affluence and assimilation, 160–161

individualism of, 315–316, 316f, 317

listening and disclosure patterns of, 172, 173t

in male support group, 248–250, 287

mistrust and resistance to therapy, 145–146

oppression of, 67, 69
  adaptive responses in, 248–250
  Rashelle example, 79, 80t–81t
  school performance in, 72–73, 82

preference for therapist characteristics, 157, 158, 174
  racial match in, 148, 155, 184–185

racial identity of, 147–151
  and self-esteem, 314, 317–318, 323

relationship-related values and beliefs of, 175t

responsibility and control locus of, 103

school performance of, 72–73, 82, 320

self-esteem of, 314, 315, 317–318, 320
  civil rights movement affecting, 323

social support of, 190t, 298, 299–300

strengths in family and community, 190t

Age
  and coping skills, 189
  group membership based on, 34, 35
  and self-esteem, 318, 320

and stressful issues in retirement, 182, 182t, 252, 253t

Alber, Josef, "Homage to the Square" painting by, 206, 282

Alcohol use. *See* Drug and alcohol use

Alliance, therapeutic, 177–179, 178t, 346

Alzheimer's disease, caregiver stress in, 291, 295

Ambiguous figure, interpretation of, 10–11, 11f

Ambivalence
  in change process, 349–350
  in disclosure of information, 199, 201

Amnesty, consequences of, 328, 329t

Anger, 172
  cultural differences in expression of, 363
  empowering interventions in, 227, 327
  positive use of, 326–328, 328f, 331

Anxiety, self-blame in, 286, 286t, 287

Arab Americans
  assertiveness-related values of, 52t
  listening and disclosure patterns of, 173t
  relationship-related values and beliefs of, 175t

Asian Americans
  assertiveness-related values of, 51, 52t, 218
  collectivism of, 98–99, 316–317
  diversity within group of, 38, 39
  listening and disclosure patterns of, 173t, 174, 175t–176t
  preference for style of therapy, 174, 228